BRADY

INTERMEDIATE Emergency Care

1985 Curriculum

Workbook

THIRD EDITION

Robert S. Porter

BRYAN E. BLEDSOE, DO, FACEP, EMT-P
Adjunct Associate Professor of Emergency Medicine
The George Washington University Medical Center
Washington, DC
and
Emergency Physician
Midlothian, Texas

ROBERT S. PORTER, MA, NREMT-P
Senior Advanced Life Support Educator
Madison County Emergency Medical Services
Canastota, New York
and
Flight Paramedic
AirOne, Onondaga County Sheriff's Department
Syracuse, New York

RICHARD A. CHERRY, MS, NREMT-P
Clinical Assistant Professor of Emergency Medicine
Technical Director for Medical Simulation
Upstate Medical University
Syracuse, New York

SCOTT R. SNYDER, BS, NREMT-P
Lecturer
Folsom, California
and
Adjunct Faculty Member, University of Maryland Department of Professional and Continuing Education
Baltimore, Maryland

PEARSON
Prentice Hall
Upper Saddle River, New Jersey 07458

AF886138

Publisher: Julie Levin Alexander
Publisher's Assistant: Regina Bruno
Executive Editor: Marlene McHugh Pratt
Senior Managing Editor for Development: Lois Berlowitz
Project Manager: Triple SSS Media Development
Editorial Assistant: Jonathan Cheung
Director of Marketing: Karen Allman
Executive Marketing Manager: Katrin Beacom
Marketing Specialist: Michael Sirinides
Managing Editor for Production: Patrick Walsh
Production Liaison: Faye Gemmellaro
Production Editor: Lynn Steines, Carlisle Publishing Services
Manufacturing Manager: Ilene Sanford
Manufacturing Buyer: Pat Brown
Senior Design Coordinator: Christopher Weigand
Cover Designer: Robert Aleman
Composition: Carlisle Publishing Services
Printing and Binding: Quebecor World Versailles
Cover Printer: Phoenix Color

NOTICE ON CARE PROCEDURES

This workbook reflects current EMS practices based on the 1985 U.S. Department of Transportation EMT-Intermediate National Standard Curriculum. It is the intent of the authors and publisher that this workbook be used as part of Formal Emergency Medical Technician-Intermediate education program taught by qualified instructors and supervised by a licensed physician. The procedures described in this workbook are based upon consultation with EMS and medical authorities. The authors and publisher have taken care to make certain that these procedures reflect currently accepted clinical practice; however, they cannot be considered absolute recommendations. The material in this workbook contains the most current information available at the time of publication. However, federal, state, and local guidelines concerning clinical practices, including, without limitation, those governing infection control and universal precautions, change rapidly. The reader should note, therefore, that the new regulations may require changes in some procedures. It is the responsibility of the reader to familiarize himself or herself with the policies and procedures set by federal, state, and local agencies as well as the Institution or agency where the reader is employed. The authors and the publisher of this workbook disclaim any liability, loss, or risk resulting directly or indirectly from the suggested procedures and theory, from any undetected errors, or from the reader's misunderstanding of the text. It is the reader's responsibility to stay informed of any new changes or recommendations made by any federal, state, and local agency as well as by his or her employing institution or agency.

NOTICE ON CPR AND ECC

The national standards for Cardiopulmonary Resuscitation (CPR) and Emergency Cardiovascular Care (ECC) are reviewed and revised on a regular basis and may change slightly after this workbook is printed. It is important that you know the most current procedures for CPR and ECC, both for the classroom and your patients. The most current information may be obtained from the appropriate credentialing agency.

Copyright © 2008 by Pearson Education, Inc., Upper Saddle River, New Jersey 07458. Pearson Prentice Hall. All rights reserved. Printed in the United States of America. This publication is protected by Copyright and permission should be obtained from the publisher prior to any prohibited reproduction, storage in a retrieval system, or transmission in any form or by any means, electronic, mechanical, photocopying, recording, or likewise. For information regarding permission(s), write to: Rights and Permissions Department.

Pearson Prentice Hall™ is a trademark of Pearson Education, Inc.
Pearson® is a registered trademark of Pearson plc
Prentice Hall® is a registered trademark of Pearson Education, Inc.

Pearson Education Ltd.
Pearson Education Australia Pty., Limited
Pearson Education Singapore, Pte. Ltd.
Pearson Education North Asia Ltd.
Pearson Education Canada, Ltd.
Pearson Educación de Mexico, S.A. de C.V.
Pearson Education—Japan
Pearson Education Malaysia, Pte. Ltd.
Pearson Education, Upper Saddle River, NJ

PEARSON
Prentice Hall

10 9 8 7 6 5
ISBN 10: 0-13-514783-2
ISBN 13: 978-0-13-514783-2

Dedication

This book is respectfully dedicated to the EMT professionals who toil each day in an environment that is unpredictable, often dangerous, and constantly changing. They risk their lives to aid the sick and the injured, driven only by their love of humanity and their devotion to this profession we call emergency medical services.

We remember the EMS, fire, and law enforcement personnel who have made the ultimate sacrifice for their communities and our nation. May they never be forgotten.

Contents

Self-Instructional Workbook

Intermediate Emergency Care: 1985 Curriculum

THIRD EDITION

INTRODUCTION

To the Self-Instructional Workbook

Intermediate Emergency Care: 1985 Curriculum

THIRD EDITION

Welcome to the self-instructional workbook for *Intermediate Emergency Care: 1985 Curriculum, Third Edition*. This workbook is designed to help guide you through an educational program for Intermediate-level training that follows the guidelines of the 1985 U.S. Department of Transportation EMT-Intermediate National Standard Curriculum. The workbook is designed to be used either in conjunction with your instructor or as a self-study guide you use on your own.

This workbook features many different ways to help you learn the material necessary to become an EMT-I, including those listed below.

Features

Review of Chapter Objectives

Each chapter of *Intermediate Emergency Care: 1985 Curriculum, Third Edition* begins with objectives that identify the important information and principles addressed in the chapter reading. To help you identify and learn this material, each workbook chapter reviews the important content elements addressed by these objectives as presented in the text.

Case Study Review

Each chapter of the textbook includes a case study, introducing and highlighting important principles presented in the chapter. The workbook reviews these case studies and points out much of the essential information and many of the applied principles they describe.

Content Self-Evaluation

Each chapter of the textbook presents an extensive narrative explanation of the principles of EMT-I practice. The workbook chapter contains between 10 and 50 multiple-choice questions to test your reading comprehension of the textbook material and to give you experience taking typical emergency medical service examinations.

Special Projects

The workbook contains several projects that are special learning experiences designed to help you remember the information and principles necessary to perform as an EMT-I. Special projects include crossword puzzles, personal benchmarking activities, and a variety of other exercises.

Emergency Drug Cards

This workbook contains alphabetized 3″ × 5″ cards that present the names/classes, descriptions, indications, contraindications, precautions, and routes and dosages of drugs you are most likely to encounter in prehospital care. Detach the cards and use them in flash card fashion. Practice until you can give the correct route, dosage, indications, and contraindications for each drug.

Acknowledgments

Reviewers

The reviewers listed below provided many excellent suggestions for improving this workbook. Their assistance is greatly appreciated.

Franco D. Piscitani, BSAS, NREMT-P
EMS Instructor
Columbus Division of Fire
Columbus, Ohio

Sean Kivlehan
EMS Instructor
St. Vincent's Hospital
New York, New York

How to Use

The Self-Instructional Workbook

Intermediate Emergency Care: 1985 Curriculum

THIRD EDITION

The self-instructional workbook accompanying *Intermediate Emergency Care: 1985 Curriculum, Third Edition* may be used as directed by your instructor or independently by you during your course of instruction. The recommendations listed below are intended to guide you in using the workbook independently.

- Examine your course schedule and identify the appropriate text chapter or other assigned reading.
- Read the assigned chapter in *Intermediate Emergency Care: 1985 Curriculum, Third Edition* carefully. Do this in a relaxed environment, free of distractions, and give yourself adequate time to read and digest the material. The information presented in the textbook is often technically complex and demanding, but it is very important that you comprehend it. Be sure that you read the chapter carefully enough to understand and remember what you have read.
- Carefully read the Review of Chapter Objectives at the beginning of each workbook chapter. This material includes both the objectives listed in the textbook and narrative descriptions of their content. If you do not understand or remember what is discussed from your reading, refer to the referenced pages and reread them carefully. If you still do not feel comfortable with your understanding of any objective, consider asking your instructor about it.
- Take the Content Self-Evaluation at the end of each workbook chapter, answering each question carefully. Do this in a quiet environment, free from distractions, and allow yourself adequate time to complete the exercise. Correct your self-evaluation by consulting the answers at the back of the workbook, and determine the percentage you have answered correctly (the number you got right divided by the total number of questions). If you have answered most of the questions correctly (85 to 90 percent), review those that you missed by rereading the material on the pages listed in the answer key and be sure you understand which answer is correct and why. If you have more than a few questions wrong (less than 85 percent correct), look for incorrect answers that are grouped together. This suggests that you did not understand a particular topic in the reading. Reread the text dealing with that topic carefully, and then retest yourself on the questions you got wrong. If incorrect answers are spread throughout the chapter content, reread the chapter and re-take the Content Self-Evaluation to assure that you understand the material. If you don't understand why your answer to a question is incorrect, after reviewing the text, consult with your instructor.
- When you have completed *Intermediate Emergency Care: 1985 Curriculum, Third Edition* and its accompanying workbook, prepare for a course test by reviewing both the text in its entirety and your class notes.

If, during your completion of the workbook exercises, you have any questions that either the textbook or workbook doesn't answer, write them down and ask your instructor about them. Prehospital emergency medicine is a complex and complicated subject, and answers are not always black and white. It is also common for different EMS systems to use differing methods of care. The questions you bring up in class, and your instructor's answers to them, will help you expand and complete your knowledge of prehospital emergency medical care.

The authors and Brady Publishing continuously seek to assure the creation of the best materials to support your educational experience. We are interested in your comments. If, during your reading and study of material in *Intermediate Emergency Care: 1985 Curriculum, Third Edition*, you notice any error or have any suggestions to improve either the textbook or workbook, please direct your comments via the Internet at: hiawatha@localnet.com. You can also visit the Brady website at: www.prenhall.com/bledsoe.

GUIDELINES TO BETTER TEST-TAKING

The knowledge you will gain from reading the textbook, completing the exercises in the workbook, listening in your EMT-I class, and participating in your clinical and field experience will prepare you to care for patients who are seriously ill or injured. However, before you can practice these skills, you will have to pass several classroom written exams and your state's certification exam successfully. Your performance on these exams will depend not only on your knowledge but also on your ability to answer test questions correctly. The following guidelines are designed to help your performance on tests and to better demonstrate your knowledge of prehospital emergency care.

1. Relax and be calm during the test.

A test is designed to measure what you have learned and to tell you and your instructor how well you are doing. An exam is not designed to intimidate or punish you. Consider it a challenge, and just try to do your best. Get plenty of sleep prior to the examination. Avoid coffee or other stimulants for a few hours before the exam, and be prepared.

Reread the text chapters, review the objectives in the workbook, and review your class notes. It might be helpful to work with one or two other students and ask each other questions. This type of practice helps everyone better understand the knowledge presented in your course of study.

2. Read the questions carefully.

Read each word of the question and all the answers slowly. Words such as "except" or "not" may change the entire meaning of the question. If you miss such words, you may answer the question incorrectly even though you know the right answer.

EXAMPLE:
The art and science of Emergency Medical Services involves all of the following EXCEPT:

A. sincerity and compassion.
B. respect for human dignity.
C. placing patient care before personal safety.
D. delivery of sophisticated emergency medical care.
E. none of the above

The correct answer is C, unless you miss the "EXCEPT."

3. Read each answer carefully.

Read each and every answer carefully. While the first answer may be absolutely correct, so may the rest, and thus the best answer might be "all of the above."

EXAMPLE:
Indirect medical direction is considered to be:

A. treatment protocols.
B. training and education.
C. quality assurance.
D. chart review.
E. all of the above

While answers A, B, C, and D are correct, the best and only acceptable answer is "all of the above," E.

4. Delay answering questions you don't understand and look for clues.

When a question seems confusing or you don't know the answer, note it on your answer sheet and come back to it later. This will ensure that you have time to complete the test. You will also find that other questions in the test may give you hints to answer the one you've skipped over. It will also prevent you from being frustrated with an early question and letting it affect your performance.

EXAMPLE:
Upon successful completion of a course of training as an EMT-I, most states will

A. certify you. (correct)
B. license you.
C. register you.
D. recognize you as an EMT-I.
E. issue you a permit.

Another question, later in the exam, may suggest the right answer:

The action of one state in recognizing the certification of another is called:

A. reciprocity. (correct)
B. national registration.
C. licensure.
D. registration.
E. extended practice.

5. Answer all questions.

Even if you do not know the right answer, do not leave a question blank. A blank question is always wrong, while a guess might be correct. If you can eliminate some of the answers as wrong, do so. It will increase the chances of a correct guess.

EXAMPLE:
When an EMT-I is called by the patient (through the dispatcher) to the scene of a medical emergency, the medical direction physician has established a physician/patient relationship.

A. True
B. False

A true/false question gives you a 50 percent chance of a correct guess.

The hospital health professional responsible for sorting patients as they arrive at the emergency department is usually the:

A. emergency physician.
B. ward clerk.
C. emergency nurse.
D. trauma surgeon.
E. A and C (correct)

A multiple-choice question with five answers gives a 20 percent chance of a correct guess. If you can eliminate one or more incorrect answers, you increase your odds of a correct guess to 25 percent, 33 percent, and so on. An unanswered question has a 0 percent chance of being correct.

Just before turning in your answer sheet, check to be sure that you have not left any items blank.

Chapter 1

Roles and Responsibilities of the EMT-Intermediate

Review of Chapter Objectives

With each chapter of the workbook, we will identify the objectives and the important elements they describe. You should review them and refer to the pages listed if the elements are not clear.

After reading this chapter, you should be able to do the following:

1. Identify and describe those activities performed by an EMT-Intermediate in the field. pp. 5–8

As with all members of the EMS system, the EMT-Intermediate provides competent medical care and emotional support for the patient, recognizing that he or she may be providing care to some who do not appreciate the service.

2. Define the role of an EMT-Intermediate. pp. 5–8

The EMT-Intermediate must be competent in all the skills of the basic EMT and provide advanced level assessment, the initiation of intravenous lines and fluid administration, advanced airway maneuvers, including endotracheal intubation, and advanced level care of the cardiac, medical, and shock patient.

3. Describe and contrast the difference between an EMT-Basic and EMT-Intermediate training program. pp. 5, 17

Emergency Medical Technician-Basic (EMT-B). This EMS provider is trained to perform a general patient assessment and to provide emergency care such as bleeding control, spinal immobilization, assist in emergency childbirth, patient restraint, and perform CPR. He is also trained in the administration of oxygen and in the use of an automated external defibrillator (AED) and to drive and staff ambulances. The EMT-B also may assist in the administration of certain medications and, in some areas, perform endotracheal intubation.

Emergency Medical Technician-Intermediate (EMT-I). The EMT-I should possess all EMT-B skills and be competent in advanced airway management, intravenous fluid therapy, and certain other advanced skills. In some states, the EMT-I may be trained as a cardiac technician and authorized to administer additional medications.

4. Define the terms "ethics" and "professionalism." pp. 8, 12

Ethics are rules or standards for conduct of a particular group or profession.

Professionalism is the conduct or qualities that characterize a practitioner in a particular field or profession.

©2008 Pearson Education, Inc.

5. **Describe the differences between ethical behavior and legal requirements.** **p. 12**

Ethical behavior—an obligation to care for the patient's emotional well-being
Legal requirements—obligations, as specified by law, to provide for the physical well-being of the patient

6. **State specific activities that are most appropriate to ethical behavior.** **pp. 12–16**

In general, the best guide regarding a question of ethics is "What is in the patient's best interest?" Usually the answer is obvious, but not always. However, in the end, you must act in a manner in which you believe best accommodates the patient's needs and desires.

7. **Identify whether a particular activity is unethical and/or illegal.** **pp. 12–16**

See Objective 6 regarding ethical activities.

Laws frequently describe what is wrong in the eyes of society. Ethics go beyond what is wrong and examines what is right, or good. They are standards that govern the conduct of a specific group. As a result, the law frequently has little or nothing to say about ethical problems.

8. **Identify whether a particular activity is ethical or unethical given certain patient care conditions.** **pp. 12–16**

See Objective 6.

9. **Define the term "profession."** **p. 8**

A profession is a specialized body of knowledge and skills. It is generally self-regulating and has requirements for initial and continuing education.

10. **Define the term "health care professional."** **p. 17**

A health care professional is a person properly trained and licensed or certified as a provider of health care.

11. **Identify whether a particular activity is professional or unprofessional.** **pp. 8–11**

Professionalism is a daily commitment to excellence. Professionals practice their skills to a point of mastery and set high standards for themselves, their crew, their agency, and their system. They critically review their performance and seek ways to improve. Professionals always consider their patient first and give them the utmost respect. Any deviation from this approach is unprofessional.

12. **State certain activities that are most appropriate to professional behavior.** **pp. 8–11**

An EMT-I is responsible for acting in a professional manner both on and off duty. Remember, the community you serve will judge other EMS providers, the service you work for, and the EMS profession as a whole by your actions.

13. **List current state requirements for EMT-Intermediate continuing education.** **p. 18**

Each state establishes criteria to renew or continue certification or licensure. This generally includes refresher training along with skills and knowledge enhancements to permit the EMT-I to operate within the scope of practice. Check with your instructor to determine the exact requirements in your state.

14. **Define and discuss at least three reasons why continuing education is important for the EMT-Intermediate.** **p. 18**

Continuing education is designed to help you maintain basic and advanced knowledge.
Continuing education is designed to help you maintain basic and advanced level skill proficiency.
Continuing education is designed to familiarize you with new procedures and treatments and prepare you through didactic, laboratory, and clinical education prior to their inclusion into your practice.

©2008 Pearson Education, Inc.
Intermediate Emergency Care: 1985, 3rd ed.

15. Define the terms "certification," "licensure," and "registration." **p. 16**

Certification is a process by which an agency or association grants recognition to an individual who meets its qualifications.

Licensure is a process by which a governmental agency grants permission to engage in an occupation based on an applicant's attaining a required competency sufficient to ensure the public's protection.

Registration is the listing of your name and essential information within a particular record of a certifying organization. It may require demonstrating proficiency in skills and/or knowledge.

16. Name and describe current state legislation outlining the scope of prehospital advanced life support. **p. 5**

The roles of the EMT-Intermediate are diverse and are generally outlined in state legislation and local regulations governing the scope of practice of prehospital advanced life support. They include not only patient care, but a variety of other responsibilities before, during, and after an emergency response. Each state, and in some cases locality, has its own scope of practice as described by legislation (medical practice acts and EMS statutes), regulations, and protocols.

17. State the reason it is important to keep one's EMT-Intermediate certification current. **p. 16**

Certification (or licensure) grants the EMT-Intermediate his or her ability to practice. It is essential that he or she assure that all continuing education requirements are completed to maintain certification and the right to practice.

18. State the major purpose of a national association. **p. 17**

Shares ideas and concerns
Speaks with a unified voice to the issues facing emergency medical service
Provides continuing education (newsletters and conferences)

19. State the major purpose of a national registry agency. **p. 17**

Provides national testing of EMT-Basic, EMT-Intermediate, and EMT-Paramedic
Establishes standards for re-registration
Provides basis for interstate reciprocity

20. State the major benefits of subscribing to professional journals. **pp. 18–19**

The major benefits of professional journal subscription include learning of new advances in emergency prehospital care, continuing education, and providing a vehicle for authorship.

21. State the benefits of EMT-Intermediates teaching in their community. **p. 19**

Teaching in your community places you before your "consumers" before they call for help. This gives you an opportunity to develop a positive public image and explain the workings of the system. It will also help you integrate with the other members of the health care system.

Case Study Review

Reread the case study in Chapter 1 and then read the following discussion. As was mentioned in Chapter 1, it is important to review each call that you participate in as an EMT-Intermediate. Similarly, review the case studies preceding each chapter of this text. We will address the important points of scene survey, patient assessment, patient management, patient packaging, and transport. This case study depicts a two-patient trauma call with the opportunity to focus on several elements of your response as an EMT-Intermediate.

©2008 Pearson Education, Inc.

MED-1, with Stephen and Lisa, responds to a drive-by shooting. During the approximately four-minute drive to the scene, Lisa and Stephen discuss their respective roles. They talk about the scene survey, initial assessment and review the signs and symptoms of developing shock. Lisa mentions that they should not approach the area until the police clear them to enter and they are sure the scene is secure.

Once the police direct MED-1 in, the two EMT-Intermediates are joined by EMTs. Lisa and Stephen then each take a shooting victim. Stephen finds a young male with two gunshot wounds. Although the initial assessment detects no suggestion of shock, Stephen will carefully reassess vital signs and the elements of the initial assessment (the ongoing assessment) periodically to monitor his condition. The location of the abdominal wound worries Stephen because the liver is a vascular organ that can bleed profusely and rapidly induce shock. For now, his patient is stable. But Stephen initiates two IVs, just in case the patient's condition changes. Stephen decides that the patient is a candidate for rapid transport directly to the trauma center. He will alert the trauma center of the condition of his patient and his anticipated time of arrival.

Lisa's patient does not exhibit injuries as critical as Stephen's patient. The initial assessment reveals no reason for concern so her attention focuses on the thigh wound. Once the pulse, capillary refill, and motor and sensory function are found to be normal, Lisa bandages the thigh and takes vital signs. Lisa decides to initiate an IV en route to the hospital. Although this patient is stable, Lisa knows that vascular injuries to this area may cause extensive yet hidden hemorrhage. Pressure caused by tissue swelling and hemorrhage may interfere with circulation as well as damage nerves. She will watch this patient closely to assure that his condition does not deteriorate.

The care offered on this call is a good example of what will be expected of you as an EMT-Intermediate. However, not all the roles and responsibilities of an EMT-Intermediate are apparent. Lisa and Stephen have met the requirements of their state and are certified or licensed as EMT-Intermediates. Prior to this call, they assured their ambulance was clean, well maintained, and equipped with the needed supplies and equipment. Their dress is neat and clean, and their manner is professional. Most importantly, Lisa and Stephen take pride in what they do and take special care to meet not only the emergency care needs of their two patients but their emotional needs as well. The actions of Stephen and Lisa will be remembered by the two patients and the bystanders at this incident for a long time to come.

Content Self-Evaluation

Each of the chapters within this workbook includes a short content review. The questions are designed to test your ability to remember what you read. You can find the answers to the questions at the back of this workbook. If you answer any questions incorrectly, review the appropriate pages in the text.

Multiple Choice

______ 1. One of the greatest impacts upon the public's feelings toward the EMS system came from the television program *Emergency*. Which of the following are aspects of that program's presentation of EMS personnel?
- A. clean-cut
- B. respond promptly
- C. calm under stress
- D. skillful and compassionate
- E. all of the above

______ 2. The EMT-Intermediate has a responsibility to become familiar with support services in his or her area.
- A. True
- B. False

______ 3. After leaving the hospital after a call, an EMT-Intermediate is responsible for
- A. restocking the ambulance.
- B. completing the run report.
- C. ensuring that team members are not affected by stress.
- D. reviewing the call with team members.
- E. all of the above

©2008 Pearson Education, Inc.
Intermediate Emergency Care: 1985, 3rd ed.

______ 4. As an EMT-Intermediate and a professional you must set high standards for
A. yourself.
B. your agency.
C. your EMS system.
D. your crew.
E. all of the above

______ 5. Which of the following is not a professional attribute of leadership?
A. inner strength
B. self-confidence
C. accepting of responsibility
D. ability to communicate
E. indecisiveness

______ 6. It is important that you distance yourself from the patient's feelings and place your feelings aside to deal with others.
A. True
B. False

______ 7. Which of the following is an attribute of a professional?
A. empathy
B. self-motivation
C. teamwork
D. self-confidence
E. all of the above

______ 8. As an EMT-Intermediate you are a patient advocate except when
A. faced with a moral dilemma.
B. faced with an ethical dilemma.
C. faced with an uncooperative patient.
D. your safety is threatened.
E. all of the above

______ 9. The rules or standards governing the conduct of members of a particular group or profession are called
A. ethics.
B. morals.
C. licensure.
D. certification.
E. registration.

______ 10. Since EMS is a science, EMT-Intermediates seldom face moral dilemmas.
A. True
B. False

______ 11. As members of the allied health professions, EMT-Intermediates must recognize a responsibility to
A. their patients.
B. society.
C. other health professionals.
D. themselves.
E. all of the above

______ 12. Which of the following means actually "doing good" for the patient?
A. benevolence
B. beneficence
C. autonomy
D. justice
E. nonmaleficence

______ 13. The art and science aspects of emergency medical services involve all of the following except
A. sincerity and compassion.
B. respect for human dignity.
C. placing patient care before personal safety.
D. delivery of sophisticated emergency medical care.
E. scene security.

______ 14. The process by which an organization grants recognition that an individual has met its standards of performance is called
A. licensure.
B. certification.
C. ethics.
D. reciprocity.
E. registration.

©2008 Pearson Education, Inc.

______ 15. Accepting standards established by another agency or state is called
A. licensure.
B. certification.
C. reciprocity.
D. registration.
E. diversification.

______ 16. Upon successful completion of a course of training as an EMT-Intermediate, most states will
A. certify you.
B. license you.
C. register you.
D. recognize you as an EMT-Intermediate.
E. either A or B

______ 17. The organization responsible for testing the various levels of EMTs on a national level is the
A. National Association of EMTs.
B. National Registry of EMTs.
C. National Association of Search and Rescue.
D. National Association of EMS Physicians.
E. State Board of Health.

______ 18. Continuing education is intended to
A. maintain an EMT-Intermediate's initial knowledge.
B. address didactic knowledge only.
C. broaden an EMT-Intermediate's knowledge.
D. A and C
E. none of the above

______ 19. Professional journals provide an EMT-Intermediate with
A. an opportunity to write and publish articles.
B. a source of continuing education material.
C. information on new procedures for the field.
D. all of the above
E. none of the above

______ 20. The EMT-Intermediate will most probably spend more time preparing to perform his or her duties (cleaning and restocking the ambulance, reading and attending continuing education sessions, documenting the last call, etc.) than responding to emergency medical calls.
A. True
B. False

Description

21. List at least three responsibilities of the EMT-Intermediate in preparation for an EMS response.

22. List at least three responsibilities of the EMT-Intermediate during the emergency response.

23. Identify at least five attributes of leadership that an EMT-Intermediate should have.

24. Describe the expectations the public has of the EMS system because of popular television programs depicting EMS personnel at work.

25. List at least three possibilities for continuing education that an EMT-Intermediate might pursue.

©2008 Pearson Education, Inc.
Intermediate Emergency Care: 1985, 3rd ed.

Special Project

Write to the National Registry of EMTs and ask for brochures. Consider becoming nationally registered as an EMT-Intermediate after you complete your training.

The address for the National Registry of EMTs is:

6610 Busch Blvd.
P.O. Box 29233
Columbus, OH 43229
614-888-4484

©2008 Pearson Education, Inc.

Chapter 2

Emergency Medical Services Systems

Review of Chapter Objectives

After reading this chapter, you should be able to do the following:

1. List and define the components of an EMS system. **pp. 25–29**

Prehospital Component
- Citizens who recognize the emergency
- Laypersons trained in CPR and first aid
- Dispatchers
- First responders
- EMT-Basics
- EMT-Intermediates
- EMT-Paramedics
- Fire/Rescue/Hazmat services

Hospital Component
- Emergency and specialty physicians
- Emergency nurses
- Ancillary services
- Rehabilitation services

2. Discuss citizen access and the various mechanisms of obtaining it. **pp. 25, 36–37**

Citizen access to the EMS system comes most often through the telephone or cellular phone by dialing 911. In smaller communities, citizens may be required to dial a seven digit number to access EMS and other emergency services.

3. Define stabilization of patients. **p. 28**

Stabilization refers to the attempts of EMS responders to identify and correct immediate life threats, correct or improve hemodynamic instability, and provide immobilization when necessary.

4. Describe the integration of prehospital care into the continuum of total patient care with the emergency department component of hospital care. **pp. 25–29**

The modern-day emergency medical service system creates a seamless provision of response and care, from the patient's first contact with the dispatcher through the arrival of first responders and basic and advanced life support. That process continues as the patient arrives at the emergency department and receives continually increasing care. From the emergency department, that seamless continuum continues into the hospital and surgery, intensive care, or rehabilitative services.

©2008 Pearson Education, Inc.

5. Describe the development of the EMS system in the United States. **pp. 29–31**

1966 *Accidental Death and Disability: The Neglected Disease of Modern Society*—described the poor state of prehospital care and suggested guidelines for the development of EMS systems
1966 Highway Safety Act—encouraged states to develop EMS systems
1973 Emergency Medical Services System Act—established regional EMS systems
1981 Consolidated Omnibus Budget Reconciliation Act (COBRA)—wiped out federal funding of EMS, except block grants administered by the Department of Transportation
1988 Statewide EMS Technical Assistance Program (NHTSA)—identified regulation and policy, resources management, human resources and training, transportation, facilities, communications, trauma systems, public information and education, medical direction, and evaluation as essential components of the EMS system

6. Explain the oversight duties of an EMS administrative agency. **p. 32**

Regional and Municipal Systems
- Designate who may function within the system
- Develop policies consistent with state requirements
- Develop quality assurance or improvement programs

State Systems
- Allocate funds to regional systems
- Enact legislation concerning the prehospital practice of medicine
- License or certify field providers
- Enforce state regulations
- Appoint regional advisory councils

7. Discuss the role of the physician medical director. **pp. 32–35**

The physician medical director of an EMS system is responsible for all patient care delivered by that system. All care administered by nonphysicians is considered to be given under his or her license and he has oversight over education and training, personnel and equipment selection, clinical protocol development, quality improvement development, and problem resolution, and serves as the chief EMS advocate to the public and health care profession.

8. Discuss the medical community role in overseeing prehospital care. **pp. 32, 33**

Prehospital care is the practice of medicine before a patient arrives at the hospital. Prior to modern day EMS the focus was on rapid transport and little care. As this has changed, the medical community, of which we are a part, bears responsibility to oversee the care provided here. This includes medical direction (both on-line and off-line) as well as quality improvement and assurance.

9. Define and describe medical direction. **pp. 32–35**

Medical direction is the prescription of medical care procedures either directly from a physician via radio, cellular phone, or in person (on-line) or indirectly through protocols, policies, and procedure (off-line). Medical direction is the authorization to practice medicine under the medical director's license.

10. Discuss the role of the EMS physician regarding direct (on-line) and indirect (off-line) medical direction. **pp. 33–34**

General Responsibilities
- Delegates authority to practice medicine in the prehospital setting
- Remains responsible for patient care regardless of whether medical control is direct or indirect

Direct
- Directs communication with medical control physician
- Responsible for patient-delegate care
- Involves EMT/physician interaction

©2008 Pearson Education, Inc.
Intermediate Emergency Care: 1985, 3rd ed.

Indirect
- Training and continuing education
- Medical protocols (non-interaction)
  - Triage
  - Treatment
  - Transport
  - Transfer
- Medical audit/chart review/quality assurance

11. Describe the relationship between an intervener physician on scene, the EMT-I, and the medical direction physician on the radio. **pp. 33, 35**

In the absence of on-line medical direction, a nonaffiliated physician may assume a medical direction role so long as that direction does not differ from established protocols. If it does, the physician must assume full responsibility for patient care and travel with the patient to the emergency department. If there is a medical direction physician on the radio he remains responsible for the actions of the EMS personnel and all of patient care.

12. Define and compare standing orders and protocols as used in prehospital care. **pp. 33–34**

Standing orders—field-care interventions that are completed before contacting the direct medical control physician

Protocols—policies and procedures for all components of an EMS system

13. Explain public involvement in an EMS system, including system access, recognition of an emergency, and initiation of basic life support. **pp. 25, 36–37**

The public should be:

Offered training and information to increase their knowledge of system entry—911, single number, or multi-number entry

Encouraged to take layperson training in first aid and CPR

14. Identify the components of an effective medical and organizational communications system. **pp. 36–38**

Citizen access
Single control center
Organizational communications capabilities
Medical communications capabilities
Hardware (radios, towers, pagers, etc.)
Software (frequencies, protocols, communications plans)

15. Describe the following components of emergency medical dispatching. **pp. 37–38**

a. **System status management**—dynamic use of resources to best meet the needs of the service area and ambulance crews
b. **Interrogation guidelines**—used to ensure that the appropriate information is gathered from the caller
c. **Response protocols**—used to guide the dispatcher in matching the caller's information with the most appropriate unit(s) and personnel for the patient's need
d. **Pre-arrival instructions**—used to communicate care instructions to the caller, assisting him or her in providing patient care
e. **Dispatcher training**—assures both medical and technical preparation for their role

©2008 Pearson Education, Inc.

16. Discuss the difference between initial and continuing education **p. 38**

Your initial education is designed to provide you with the information and skills necessary to meet your state requirements for certification or licensure and prepare you to provide EMT-Intermediate care to your patients. Continuing education is designed to help you maintain those skills and to gain any new knowledge and skills associated with that level of care.

17. Describe the differences and similarities between licensure and certification. **p. 38**

Licensure is specifically extended from a governmental agency (usually the state) to a provider, allowing him to practice a given trade or practice. Certification may be given by other agencies but when certification is given by the state it is effectively a license.

18. Define the four national standard levels of prehospital provider as defined by U.S. DOT curriculum. **p. 38**

First Responder. The first responder is usually the first EMS-trained provider on the scene and is prepared to initially care for and stabilize the patient until personnel with higher levels of training arrive. He is trained to perform a general patient assessment and to provide emergency care such as bleeding control, spinal immobilization, and CPR. He also may assist in emergency childbirth. In some areas, he is trained in the administration of oxygen and in the use of an automated external defibrillator (AED).

EMT-Basic. The EMT-B is prepared to assess, care for, and transport the patient at the basic life support level. He can perform complex immobilization procedures, restrain patients, and drive and staff ambulances. The EMT-B also may assist in the administration of certain medications and, in some areas, perform endotracheal intubation.

EMT-Intermediate. The EMT-I is prepared to assess, care for, and transport the patient using all EMT-Basic skills plus some advanced life support level skills. He can employ advanced airway management, intravenous fluid therapy, and certain other advanced skills. In some states, the EMT-I may be trained as a cardiac technician and authorized to administer additional medications.

EMT-Paramedic. The EMT-P is prepared to assess, care for, and transport the patient using advanced patient assessment, trauma management, pharmacology, cardiology, and other medical skills. He should successfully complete advanced cardiac life support (ACLS) and pediatric advanced life support (PALS) courses offered by the AHA. Basic trauma life support (BTLS) or prehospital trauma life support (PHTLS) course completion is also desirable.

19. Describe how the original American College of Surgeons Essential Equipment List has evolved to its present form and how it relates to local and state laws. **p. 29**

In 1983, the American College of Surgeons, Committee on Trauma recommended a minimum equipment list for basic life support ambulances, while the American College of Emergency Physicians created an advanced life support list in 1988. They collaborated on an updated list in 2000 and partnered with the National Association of EMS Physicians to provide a 2006 edition of the list. It is the standard of the EMS industry and has been adopted by many states.

20. Describe GSA/KKK Ambulance standards. **pp. 39–40**

In 1974 the federal Department of Transportation requested the General Services Administration to develop specifications for ambulance design. The specifications (KKK-A-1822) became the standard for ambulance design and have been updated several times since their introduction.

21. Describe the coordination of patient transfer with ground and air transport services. **pp. 39–40**

Patient transport protocols should:

Take into account the nature of the patient's problem, the severity of the patient's condition, the distance to the various facilities, and the specialty services of the various hospitals

Make efficient use of BLS, ALS, and aeromedical services

©2008 Pearson Education, Inc.
Intermediate Emergency Care: 1985, 3rd ed.

22. Describe the categorization of receiving facilities, and explain how the coordination of resources is attained. **pp. 41–43**

Categorization—allows transportation of patients to appropriate special-service facilities—i.e., burn, trauma, pediatric, perinatal, cardiac, spinal, psychiatric, or poison control centers

Coordination—attained through a central hospital so that the needs of a particular patient are met by the regional system

23. List the components of mutual aid and mass-casualty planning. **p. 43**

Mutual aid agreements
Mass-casualty plans
Coordinated central management agency
Frequent drills

24. Discuss the similarities and differences between quality assurance and continuous quality improvement programs. **pp. 44–46**

Quality assurance—programs that objectively identify problems and continuously monitor the quality of an EMS system or service

Quality improvement—programs that focus on the perceptions of the patient ("the customer") as well as the items evaluated by the quality assurance programs

25. Discuss the value of research in EMS. **pp. 46–47**

Research determines which care procedures and equipment benefit the patient, determines benefit/risk ratio for procedures, determines cost/benefit of sophisticated EMS interventions, and determines if immediate transport or scene care is appropriate.

26. Describe the idea of evidence-based medicine. **p. 47**

Evidence-based medicine is the conscientious, explicit, and judicious use of the current best evidence in making decisions about the care of individual patients. It requires combining clinical experience with the best available clinical evidence from systematic research.

Case Study Review

Reread the case study in Chapter 2, and then read the following discussion. This case study is an overview of the emergency medical services system with a focus on system entry, the contributions that trained bystanders can provide, and the tiered response system.

The call described by this case study is a rather typical trauma emergency and brings to mind several of the important elements of the EMS system and your role as an EMT-Intermediate in that system. Here the bystander comes upon the scene and knows enough to call the 911 center. *Maybe he had a first aid course provided by the local ambulance service that taught him what to do and how to access the region's emergency response system.* There a dispatcher interrogates him to garner enough information to initiate a proper response (fire, EMS, and police).

The response described in this scenario is a tiered response. Two EMTs arrive as first responders and begin the initial emergency medical care at the scene. This assures that emergency medical care arrives quickly to the scene though this is not the ambulance for transport nor the highest level of care available in the system. The second tier of response is the hospital-based EMT-Intermediates who arrive with the ambulance. They quickly transition to assume medical care leadership roles for the two patients. This transition takes place with a smooth exchange of assessment findings. The EMT-Intermediates ask any needed questions and then begin to direct further care. Good EMT-Intermediates will utilize the knowledge and skills of the basic EMTs to assist with the patient care and free them to provide the advanced life support skills and the patient care oversight these patients need.

©2008 Pearson Education, Inc.

As the EMS providers begin to care for the injured, they do so under indirect medical direction. Protocols describe what invasive procedures they can initiate prior to contact with medical direction, such as starting an IV and running the first 250 cc's of fluid. These protocols are well-thought-out long before the first EMS response guided by them. They have been carefully reviewed by the system medical director, who bears responsibility for every patient cared for by the system and is responsible for every action taken by an EMS provider in the system. They are also well known by each care provider in the system as they are the foundation for the care we offer.

Once the initial actions are taken and the assessment concluded, the EMT-Is then participate in direct medical direction by speaking with the physican over the radio. This permits the EMT-Is to continue fluid administration, place an endotracheal tube and stop resuscitation on a patient, now declared dead. The physican providing on-line medical direction by radio or cell phone is acting as the agent of the system medical director.

During the time at the patient's side, the EMT-Is must determine their patient's priority for care and transport. Cardiac arrest in the trauma setting (the female) suggests a hopeless situtation. Here pronouncing the patient dead frees the team to assist in providing care for the other patient. The male patient is seriously injured and the system protocols direct the rapid initiation of the IV lines and the initial administration of fluid (often provided en route to the hospital), permitting the EMT-Is to move quickly to patient transport. Protocols and medical direction consultation will also assure this seriously injured patient is transported to the closest appropriate facility, probably a Level I trauma center.

After the EMT-Intermediates complete the call, it will be reviewed by the system quality improvement committee. Members will examine how the system responded to the needs of the two patients. They will examine the adherence to protocols, the interaction with medical control, the appropriateness of resource utilization, the evaluation of the patient's condition at the scene, and the perceptions from bystanders, care providers, and the surviving patient. This information will be used to determine how well the system functioned and will identify any improvements that could be made. Infrequently, the quality improvement committee directs remediation to individual care providers.

Content Self-Evaluation

Multiple Choice

_____ 1. The system that makes use of several levels of responding emergency medical services personnel—the first responder, EMT, and paramedic—is called
- A. the tiered response system.
- B. a multifaceted system.
- C. an advanced life support system.
- D. a fail-safe system.
- E. volunteer-supplemented system.

_____ 2. The first legislation that addressed emergency medical services in the United States was
- A. the Emergency Medical Services Act.
- B. the Highway Safety Act.
- C. the "White Paper."
- D. Consolidated Omnibus Budget Act.
- E. none of the above

_____ 3. All prehospital medical care provided by the EMT-Intermediate is considered an extension of the medical director's license.
- A. True
- B. False

_____ 4. EMS system funding can come from
- A. tax subsidies.
- B. Medicare, Medicaid.
- C. subscription plans.
- D. user fees.
- E. all of the above

©2008 Pearson Education, Inc.
Intermediate Emergency Care: 1985, 3rd ed.

______ 5. Medical direction provided by on-line radio contact between the EMT-Intermediate and the medical direction physician is known as
A. protocol.
B. direct.
C. indirect.
D. intrinsic.
E. extrinsic.

______ 6. If the nonaffiliated physician at the scene calls for care outside the EMT-I's protocols, he or she must accompany the patient to the hospital.
A. True
B. False

______ 7. Indirect medical direction includes
A. treatment protocols.
B. training and education.
C. quality assurance.
D. chart review.
E. all of the above

______ 8. Protocols standardize field procedures. They should not allow the EMT-Intermediate flexibility to improvise nor adapt to special circumstances.
A. True
B. False

______ 9. The device used by first responders or bystanders to significantly improve the survival rates of patients in cardiac arrest is the
A. transcutaneous pacemaker.
B. esophageal obturator airway.
C. automatic external defibrillator.
D. pulse oximeter.
E. glucometer.

______ 10. The dispatch system that reduces response time by locating ambulances based upon projected call volume is called
A. priority dispatching.
B. system status management.
C. interrogation protocols.
D. medical direction.
E. preplanned dispatching.

______ 11. The dispatch system that interrogates the caller, prioritizes symptoms, selects the appropriate response, and provides the caller with lifesaving instructions is called
A. priority dispatching.
B. system status management.
C. interrogation protocols.
D. medical direction.
E. simplex dispatching.

______ 12. The elements EMS dispatch system includes
A. citizen access.
B. a single control center.
C. medical and operational communications capabilities.
D. hardware and software.
E. all of the above

______ 13. Patients who are transported under the direction of an emergency medical services system should be taken to the closest appropriate medical facility.
A. True
B. False

______ 14. Which of the following groups is responsible for the current minimum equipment list for basic and advanced life support?
A. American College of Emergency Physicians
B. American College of Surgeons
C. National Association of EMS Physicians
D. all of the above
E. none of the above

©2008 Pearson Education, Inc.

_____ 15. An example of hospital specialty service categorization is
- A. a burn center.
- B. a trauma center.
- C. a perinatal center.
- D. a cardiac center.
- E. all of the above

_____ 16. The elements of a mass-casualty plan should include
- A. closely defined geographical boundaries
- B. a flexible communication system.
- C. a central management structure.
- D. B and C.
- E. all of the above

_____ 17. Quality assurance and quality improvement programs look at
- A. response times.
- B. adherence to protocols.
- C. patient survival.
- D. customer perceptions.
- E. all of the above

_____ 18. Quality improvement programs differ from quality assurance programs in that quality improvement also looks at
- A. customer satisfaction.
- B. dispatch procedures.
- C. quality of care.
- D. mortality and morbidity.
- E. none of the above

_____ 19. Many protocols and procedures that EMT-Intermediates use today have evolved without clinical evidence of their usefulness, safety, or benefit to the patient.
- A. True
- B. False

_____ 20. Quality EMS systems are designed with the patient as the highest priority. They begin with a strong administrative agency that structures the system around the patient's needs and grants the medical director ultimate authority in all issues of patient care.
- A. True
- B. False

SEQUENCING

21. Place the steps below in the order in which they would occur in a research project. Number the first step 1, the second step 2, and so on.

_____ A. develop a hypothesis or question to be asked

_____ B. prepare a paper for a magazine

_____ C. collect and analyze data

_____ D. search the literature

DESCRIPTION

22. Identify the purpose of each of the four types of protocols.

Triage: (list at least 1 purpose) _____

Treatment: (at least 2) _____

Transport: (at least 2) _____

Transfer: (at least 1) _____

©2008 Pearson Education, Inc.
Intermediate Emergency Care: 1985, 3rd ed.

23. Identify and describe the four elements of the priority dispatch system.

A. ____

B. ____

C. ____

D. ____

Special Project

Using your knowledge of basic life support, design a research project that investigates the accuracy of blood pressure determination among EMTs.

Hypothesis: Write a hypothesis (a statement that defines what you are trying to prove or disprove).

Literature review: Where would you look for information (search of the literature: magazines, journals, textbooks, etc.)?

Study methods: Explain how you would test your hypothesis (description of what you would do to verify your hypothesis: field study, clinical trial, etc.).

Conclusion: Explain the results of the research, and how it supports or rejects your hypothesis (completed only when the results of the research are known).

©2008 Pearson Education, Inc.

Chapter 3

Medical-Legal Considerations of Emergency Care

Review of Chapter Objectives

After reading this chapter, you should be able to do the following:

1. Discuss the differences between the law, ethical standards, and moral standards. p. 54

An EMT-I's legal responsibility (under the law) to the patient and others is defined by statute, regulation, and common law. Failure to meet this responsibility may result in criminal or civil liability. Ethical responsibilities are those actions expected of an EMT-I by the health care profession and by the public. Moral responsibilities are personal values of right and wrong and are governed by conscience. Legal, ethical, and moral factors guide an individual in his or her actions as an EMT-I.

2. Describe the two general categories of law in the United States, and give examples of each. pp. 54–55

Criminal law—addresses crime and punishment and involves legal action against an individual by the state

Examples: homicide and rape

Civil law—deals with noncriminal matters

Examples: contract disputes, divorce, torts

3. Describe the components of a civil lawsuit. pp. 55–56

Incident. The incident is the event the victim believes caused him injury (damages).

Investigation. The victim's attorney makes a preliminary inquiry into the facts and circumstances surrounding the incident to determine if the case has merit.

Filing of the complaint. The victim (now called the "plaintiff") commences the lawsuit by filing a complaint with the court. The complaint contains information such as the names of the parties, the legal basis for the claim, and the damages sought by the plaintiff. A copy of the complaint is served on those the plaintiff believes caused his injuries (defendants).

Answering the complaint. The attorney for the defendant answers each allegation made in the complaint. The answer is then filed with the court, and a copy is given to the plaintiff's attorney.

Discovery. Before any lawsuit appears before a judge or jury, both parties to an action participate in pretrial discovery. This is the stage of the lawsuit when all relevant information about the incident is shared so that the parties can prepare their trial strategies. Discovery may include:

Deposition is questioning, under oath, of witnesses.

Interrogatory is a set of written questions that requires written responses.

Document production entitles each side to request relevant documents, including the patient care report, hospital medical records, police records, and other records necessary to help prove or defend the lawsuit.

©2008 Pearson Education, Inc.

Trial. At the trial, each side is given the opportunity to present all relevant evidence and testimony from witnesses.

Decision. After deliberations, the judge or jury determines the guilt or liability of the defendant and then decides the amount of damages to award the plaintiff.

Appeal. After the jury's decision is entered by the court, either party may be entitled to an appeal. Generally, grounds for an appeal are limited to errors of law made by the court. Appeals will be heard by a higher-level appellate court.

Settlement. This can occur at any stage of the lawsuit. Generally, the defendant will offer the plaintiff an amount of money that is less than the amount for which he is being sued. The plaintiff may then agree to accept the reduced amount.

4. Define the following terms. **pp. 55–66**

a. **Tort medical liability**—deals with civil wrongs committed by one individual against another, such as a malpractice **p. 55**
b. **Duty to act**—the obligation to respond to a situation **p. 61**
c. **Negligence**—deviation from accepted standard of care **pp. 61–62**
d. **Informed consent**—consent obtained only after the patient understands the nature, extent, and potential risks of treatment; required prior to beginning prehospital care **p. 63**
e. **Expressed consent**—occurs when a patient verbally, nonverbally, or in writing, gives permission to receive medical treatment **p. 63**
f. **Implied consent**—presumed from a patient who is unable to provide informed consent either due to inability to communicate or mental impairment **p. 63**
g. **Assault**—any action that places a person in fear of immediate bodily harm **p. 66**
h. **Battery**—act of unlawfully touching another person without his or her consent **p. 66**
i. **Abandonment**—termination of a health care provider-patient relationship without assurance that equal or greater care will continue **p. 66**
j. **False imprisonment**—intentional and unjustifiable detention of a person against his or her will **p. 66**
k. **Libel**—act of injuring someone's name or character by false or malicious writing **p. 66**
l. **Slander**—act of injuring someone's name or character by false or malicious spoken words **p. 66**

5. Discuss the medical practice act and its implications in prehospital care. **p. 56**

Medical practice act—state legislation that sets the standards for the practice of medicine
Implications—allows the EMT-Intermediate to perform as an agent under the license of a physician

6. Explain what is meant by the term "delegation of authority." **p. 56**

The EMT-Intermediate functions as the agent of medical control, or an authorized physician.

7. Describe the purpose and limitations of Good Samaritan Laws. **p. 57**

Purpose—provide protection against negligence proceedings for those who render care at an emergency scene without compensation, offer their services in good faith, and are not negligent

Limitations—the constitutionality of Good Samaritan laws is being challenged and often does not apply to those who are paid for their services

8. Explain the need to know state motor vehicle laws that apply to emergency vehicles. **p. 57**

Provisions extend special privileges and place certain responsibilities on the operator of an authorized emergency vehicle. As an EMT-I, you will need to know both the privileges and responsibilities of driving an emergency vehicle under your state's laws.

9. Discuss the major provisions contained in the Health Insurance Portability and Accountability Act (HIPAA). **pp. 57–58**

The Health Insurance Portability and Accountability Act (HIPAA) of 1996 changed the methods EMS providers use to file for insurance and Medicare payments and adds important new layers of

©2008 Pearson Education, Inc.
Intermediate Emergency Care: 1985, 3rd ed.

privacy protection for EMS patients. Furthermore, EMS providers must develop administrative, electronic, and physical barriers to unauthorized disclosure of patients' protected health information. HIPAA provides both civil and serious criminal penalties for violations of privacy. The requirements of HIPAA are detailed, and every EMS provider must become familiar with them.

10. Explain the purpose of a "living will, durable power of attorney for health care," and a "do not resuscitate" order. **pp. 58–60**

Living will—legal document by which a patient specifies the kinds of medical treatment he or she wishes to receive in cases of serious injury or illness

Durable power of attorney for health care—legal document that designates another person to make health care decisions for a patient

Do not resuscitate order—order written by a physician directing that resuscitation should be withheld; when in doubt of a DNR's authenticity, provide resuscitation

11. Discuss the concept of "standard of care" as it applies to prehospital care. **p. 60**

The standard of care is the standard against which an EMT-Intermediate will be judged to determine negligence.

The standard of care is the care a similarly trained and experienced EMT-Intermediate would be expected to provide under similar circumstances.

12. List and describe the four components required to prove negligence in a malpractice proceeding. **pp. 61–62**

Duty to act—that an EMT-Intermediate had a legal obligation to care for a patient

Breach of duty—that the EMT-Intermediate failed to meet the expected standard of care

Damages—that the victim was injured or harmed

Proximate cause—that actions taken by the EMT-Intermediate were the direct or indirect cause of harm experienced by the patient

13. Discuss the concept of res ipsa loquitur. **pp. 61–62**

Literal meaning—"the thing speaks for itself"

Legal meaning—that the damages would not have occurred in the absence of somebody's negligence; that the instruments of damage were under the defendant's control at all times; that the patient did nothing to contribute to his or her injury

14. Discuss the significance of obtaining expressed consent. **p. 63**

Expressed consent is the most common type of consent. It occurs when a person, verbally, nonverbally, or in writing, grants permission to treat. Often, the act of the patient requesting an ambulance is considered an expression of a desire to be treated.

15. Describe the extent to which force and restraint may be used to protect the EMT, patient, and a third party. **pp. 67–68**

The use of force to restrain a patient may be necessary when the patient is violent or poses a danger to him- or herself or to others. Then only such force and restraint should be used as is required. In conditions where force and restraint are necessary to care for a patient, the police should be involved.

16. Discuss the special considerations necessary at a crime or accident scene. **p. 68**

Your responsibility at the crime scene is first to ensure your safety and that of your patient and then to ensure the health of the victim (your patient). If the patient is not obviously dead, initiate resuscitation and care directed at his or her injuries. Limit any movement of articles around the patient and at the scene and, if possible, document what you moved and from what location you moved it. Do not cut through clothing where objects entered the body; remove the clothing without cutting it or by cutting around the openings.

©2008 Pearson Education, Inc.

17. Discuss the significance of accurate documentation and record keeping. **p. 69**

Documentation establishes what was found and what was done at the emergency scene. It must be completed promptly, thoroughly, objectively, and accurately. At the same time, the confidentiality of the information obtained must be maintained. The documentation will become a part of the patient's medical record and help guide continuing patient care. It will also become a record of what you did at the emergency scene and during transport should your actions ever come into question. It may also become a legal document in a court of law when someone feels he has been injured (damaged) by someone else.

18. List several methods of protecting yourself from malpractice liability. **p. 69**

Practice good prehospital care
Provide care for the patient as you would wish to be cared for
Document all emergency medical responses completely and appropriately
Purchase and maintain malpractice insurance

Case Study Review

Reread the case study in Chapter 3 and then read the following discussion. This call represents a realistic emergency medical response that has many elements of interest from a medical-legal point of view. It identifies a number of situations that may put you, as an EMT-Intermediate, at risk of malpractice if you do not employ proper legal principles.

En route to the scene, the EMT-Intermediates of Ambulance 6 prepare for a full cardiac arrest. They ready and check the oxygen, airway equipment, suction, and the defibrillator. They also review their roles in the impending resuscitation and their system's cardiac arrest protocols. For example, they might plan to initiate resuscitation by invoking implied consent. The patient will be unable otherwise to give consent, and hence they assume the patient would consent if indeed he could.

Upon arrival, EMT-Intermediates observe that the patient has severe respiratory problems, rather than a cardiac arrest. They also face family members with different desires about how to proceed. The two EMTs must sort out the legalities while attending to the patient's needs. The daughter requests that he be allowed to die, while the patient's wife asks for aggressive resuscitation. The only circumstance where an EMT-Intermediate would not resuscitate is when they find a valid "do not resuscitate" order. Such an order is prescribed by state law and varies across the nation. When in doubt, an EMS team should resuscitate.

In this case, someone requested an ambulance—a clear call for help. Secondly, the spouse of the patient requests care. Further, a "do not resuscitate" order is not available. The EMT-Intermediates' decision to resuscitate this patient is appropriate.

Another legal consideration in this scenario is patient consent. The EMT-Intermediate assessing the patient must determine the patient's level of consciousness and ability to give consent. If the patient is found to be alert, the EMT-Intermediate must explain what care they will provide and give the patient the opportunity to decline such care. If the patient is unresponsive, consent is implied. If the patient then becomes conscious and alert, he may refuse care and the crew of Ambulance 6 would have to cease care. They would also need to explain the possible consequences of halting care (withdrawal of consent). It would also be necessary to have the patient sign a written release form and have it witnessed by someone other than the ambulance crew.

In this case, the EMT-Intermediates placed an endotracheal tube, which is an invasive advanced life support procedure. Such a procedure is permitted only through delegation of authority from the medical control physician to the prehospital care provider. They may employ such a procedure via a standing order or after direct communication with the physician via radio. Failure to get the appropriate permission for the procedure or performing advanced skills beyond the local protocol may expose the care providers to charges of practicing medicine without a license.

After this call, the EMT-Intermediates will document the call on the run report. They must be accurate and keep all information confidential. The use of slang, derogatory labels, or subjective statements in the report may expose the care providers to charges of libel—the act of injuring a person's character or

©2008 Pearson Education, Inc.
Intermediate Emergency Care: 1985, 3rd ed.

reputation by malicious or false writings. The report may also be examined in a court of law to determine what care was given and if it was appropriate. Poor documentation may call into question the quality of care given. Complete, accurate, and appropriate documentation will substantiate complete, accurate, and appropriate care.

To extend this case, consider this scenario:

Both the EMT-Intermediates attending this patient have their own malpractice insurance. The company they work for has a blanket policy covering a potential lawsuit. However, when they investigated the coverage the EMTs found that individuals were not well covered. Also, the policy did not cover the EMT-Intermediates while off duty or while working for the rural services where they volunteer. Their personal malpractice insurance is inexpensive and affords them some peace of mind. You might do well by investigating your own coverage.

Content Self-Evaluation

Multiple Choice

______ 1. The type of law where society takes action against an individual for wrongdoing is
- A. civil law.
- B. tort law.
- C. criminal law.
- D. malfeasance.
- E. negligence.

______ 2. An EMT-Intermediate may become involved in the legal system because he or she will be called
- A. as a witness in a criminal offense.
- B. to testify in a civil matter.
- C. to defend himself or herself in a malpractice suit.
- D. to testify in a contract dispute.
- E. all of the above

______ 3. The principle allowing an EMT-Intermediate to function in the field under the auspices and license of a physician is called
- A. res ipsa loquitur.
- B. medical control.
- C. the Good Samaritan principle.
- D. delegation of authority.
- E. none of the above

______ 4. The Good Samaritan law was designed to protect EMS personnel against legal liability resulting from negligent care.
- A. True
- B. False

______ 5. Generally, which circumstances require an EMT-Intermediate to report an incident to law enforcement officials?
- A. child or elderly abuse
- B. rape or sexual abuse
- C. a shooting
- D. physical assault
- E. all of the above

______ 6. You respond to a home where a patient has a "do not resuscitate" order. You are obligated to provide advanced life support to the limit of your training and ability.
- A. True
- B. False

______ 7. The principle of providing the same level of treatment as any other similarly trained individual would provide in a similar situation is called
- A. negligence.
- B. standard of care.
- C. duty to act.
- D. an act of omission.
- E. proximate cause.

©2008 Pearson Education, Inc.

_____ 8. In a malpractice suit, the plaintiff must prove all of the following EXCEPT
A. the EMT-Intermediate had a duty to act.
B. the party was damaged or injured.
C. the EMT-Intermediate failed to meet the standard of care.
D. actions by the EMT-Intermediate caused some of the damages.
E. the party was slandered.

_____ 9. The principle of law where the damages could not have occurred without negligence is called
A. malfeasance.
B. malpractice.
C. nonfeasance.
D. res ipsa loquitur.
E. none of the above

_____ 10. The permission to provide care after a patient understands the benefits and risks of treatment is called
A. the patient's right to know.
B. informed consent.
C. duty to act.
D. implied consent.
E. none of the above

_____ 11. Once a patient has given consent for care, he or she cannot refuse further care until evaluated by a physician.
A. True
B. False

_____ 12. A patient's refusal to receive care and/or be transported should be
A. recorded in the run report.
B. signed by the patient.
C. witnessed by someone other than the EMS crew.
D. B and C only
E. all of the above

_____ 13. Caring for a patient without obtaining the proper consent is grounds for charges of
A. assault and battery.
B. malpractice.
C. negligence.
D. res ipsa loquitur.
E. B and C

_____ 14. Recording false and malicious information on a patient's run report might subject an EMT-Intermediate to legal action because of
A. libel.
B. medical control policy violation.
C. malpractice.
D. slander.
E. violation of a medical practice act.

_____ 15. At the possible crime scene, you should do all of the following EXCEPT
A. remove clothing by cutting through holes.
B. move only what you must.
C. remove clothing by cutting around holes.
D. enter scene only when safe.
E. provide lifesaving care.

©2008 Pearson Education, Inc.
Intermediate Emergency Care: 1985, 3rd ed.

Description

16. Compare and contrast negligence and res ipsa loquitur as they apply to the EMT-Intermediate.

____

____

____

17. List three potential patient conditions in which care can be given even though patient consent cannot be obtained.

____

____

____

18. Reread the case study for this chapter, and briefly record the essential information that should be written in the narrative run report.

____

____

____

Special Project

List your state's requirements for licensure of an EMT-Intermediate ambulance service.

Personnel Requirements:

How many persons must respond with the ambulance?

What training must they have?

Vehicle Requirements:

What type of vehicle is required?

Equipment Requirements:

What emergency care equipment is required?

What radio equipment is required?

©2008 Pearson Education, Inc.
Intermediate Emergency Care: 1985, 3rd ed.

Chapter 4

Medical Terminology

Review of Chapter Objectives

After reading this chapter, you should be able to do the following:

1. **Define and describe the function of the following word parts:**

   a. **Combining form**—conveys the essential meaning of a word; the word to which a suffix, prefix, or both is attached **p. 75**

   b. **Suffix**—one or more syllables affixed to the beginning of a combining word to modify its meaning **p. 76**

   c. **Prefix**—one or more syllables affixed to the end of a combining word to modify its meaning **p. 77**

2. **Identify and define common prefixes and suffixes. p. 77**

   The addition of prefixes and suffixes modifies the meaning of the combining form. A suffix is a syllable that is attached to the end of a combining form to modify its meaning, creating a new word. A prefix is a syllable that is attached to the beginning of a combining form and, like a suffix, modifies its meaning, creating a new word. Occasionally, a medical word may have two prefixes or suffixes, one right after the other. Not every medical word will contain a prefix or a suffix; they are optional word parts.

3. **Identify and define common combining forms. p. 76**

   Every medical word contains a combining form, which is the foundation of the word and gives the word its medical meaning. A combining form has two parts: a *root* (which contains the medical meaning) and a *combining vowel.* The combining vowel (usually *o*, but occasionally *a, e,* or *i*) helps join the root to another word part and is necessary in order to make the whole word pronounceable.

4. **Discuss the importance of correct understanding, use, pronunciation, and spelling of medical terms. p. 75**

   Medical terminology is the specialized language used in all fields of medicine—including EMS. To communicate effectively with other members of the health care team, you must be able to speak, write, use, and understand this language. A knowledge of the basic components of medical terms will help you understand the language used not only in this and other textbooks, but in classroom lectures, continuing education sessions, periodicals, and any other medium in which information is shared. Knowledge of medical terminology will also facilitate competent, professional communication with physicians, nurses, and other health care personnel.

©2008 Pearson Education, Inc.

5. Describe the characteristics of the following sectional planes of the human body: pp. 78–80

a. Frontal plane (coronal plane) divides the body vertically into a dorsal or posterior (back) and a ventral or anterior (front) section, and parallels the head-to-toe axis of the body.
b. Transverse plane lies perpendicular to the head-to-toe axis of the body, dividing it into superior (upper) and inferior (lower) sections.
c. Sagittal plane also parallels the head-to-toe axis of the body, but divides the body into left and right portions.
d. Midsagittal plane divides the body down the midline into equal left and right halves.

6. Describe the characteristics of the following anatomical locations: pp. 79–81

a. **Midline**—line extending down the center of the body when viewed from the front, dividing it into equal left and right halves
b. **Medial**—toward the midline of the body
c. **Lateral**—away from the midline of the body
d. **Midaxillary line**—line extending down the body when viewed from the side, passing through the mid-armpit and ankle
e. **Superior**—above; at a higher level
f. **Inferior**—below; at a lower level
g. **Cephalic**—toward the head
h. **Caudal**—toward the coccyx
i. **Proximal**—toward the torso
j. **Distal**—away from the torso
k. **Midclavicular line**—vertical line through the center of each clavicle

7. Describe the characteristics of the following anatomical postures: pp. 81–83

a. **Supine**—lying horizontal with the face up
b. **Prone**—lying horizontal with the face down
c. **Recumbent**—lying on the side, either right or left
d. **Fowler's position**—sitting position with the back elevated between 45 and 60 degrees from horizontal
e. **Trendelenburg position**—supine with feet higher than head

8. Describe the characteristics of the following anatomical movements: pp. 81–84

a. **Flexion**—decreasing the angle of a joint and bringing two body parts closer together
b. **Extension**—increasing the angle of a joint and moving two body parts away from one another
c. **Abduction**—movement of a body part away from the midline
d. **Adduction**—movement of a body part toward the midline
e. **Circumduction**—swinging of a body part in a circular motion. Combines successive movements of flexion, abduction, flexion, and adduction
f. **Medial rotation**—twisting of the arm so that the thumb turns inward, toward the midline.
g. **Lateral rotation**—twisting of the arm so that the thumb turns outward, away from the midline

Case Study Review

Reread the case study in Chapter 4 and then read the following narrative. This case study highlights the importance of the language of medicine as you care for a patient and interact with the medical community.

©2008 Pearson Education, Inc.
Intermedite Emergency Care: 1985, 3rd ed.

Along with the extensive experience of Shelly and Emily comes an extensive understanding of medical terminology and the language of medicine. With just a little understanding of combining forms, suffixes and prefixes, Stephen will soon be able to decipher much of what is being said. For example: polyuria, polyphasia and polydipsia all have the same prefix—"poly," meaning frequent. When joined with the combining forms listed above they mean frequent urination, frequent eating, and frequent drinking.

As Stephen listens to the patient report, he hears common terms like "hyper" (meaning above normal), "hypo" (meaning below normal) and "tachy" (meaning rapid). He hears them combined with combining forms that sound somewhat familiar: cardic (heart), glycemic (sugar) and pneic (breathing). With time, these terms will become more and more familiar and Stephen's ability to use the language of medicine will increase.

Stephen will need to get a pocket medical dictionary to help him with this new language. It will come in handy whenever he hears a new word. It will also become very helpful as he records information on the prehospital care report. There it is critical that medical terms and abbreviations be spelled and used correctly.

In addition to the language of medicine, Stephen will need to master the use of anatomical terms. During his career as an EMT-Intermediate, he will need to describe where signs and symptoms are found on the human body. This will involve using sectional planes and anatomical locations to help specify the exact location of a patient complaint or visible indication of injury.

Medical Term Dissection

Identify the meaning of the prefex, combining form, and suffix for each of the following medical terms. (For those prefexes, combining forms, and suffixes not identified in your text, look up the word in a medical dictionary and remember, not all terms have both prefixes and suffixes.)

Prefix	*Combining Form*	*Suffix*
1. myasthenia		
2. cephalgia		
3. percuss		
4. cyanosis		
5. hyperflexion		
6. pathology		
7. tachypnea		
8. rhinorrhea		
9. dysuria		
10. hypertrophy		
11. osteocyte		
12. hypoxemia		
13. hepatomegaly		
14. abduct		
15. otoscope		
16. perinatal		
17. antecubital		
18. dissect		
19. epicardium		
20. postpartum		
21. intervertebral		
22. neuroplasty		
23. hemothora		
24. polyphagia		

©2008 Pearson Education, Inc.
Intermediate Emergency Care: 1985, 3rd ed.

Anatomical Locations

Match the term with the corresponding description.

25. medial	A. above, at a higher level
26. cephalic	B. twisting outward
27. abduction	C. toward the coccyx
28. extension	D. toward the torso
29. proximal	E. toward the head
30. superior	F. movement away from the midline
31. caudal	G. toward the midline
32. lateral	H. increasing a joint angle
33. lateral rotation	I. away from the midline
34. distal	J. away from the torso

Special Project

The use of a medical dictionary is essential to learning the language of medicine. It will help you understand medical terminology and use it properly. It is also essential to use the dictionary to assure proper spelling as you prepare written patient reports. Locate the following medical terms in a medical dictionary.

acromegaly	bathophobia	blastocyte
cathartic	cynanthropy	dipsomania
ergotherapy	hypoglossal	leukocytogenesis
monomorphic	prodromal	serotonin

©2008 Pearson Education, Inc.
Intermedite Emergency Care: 1985, 3rd ed.

Chapter

5

Documentation

Review of Chapter Objectives

After reading this chapter, you should be able to do the following:

1. Identify the general principles regarding the importance of EMS documentation and ways in which documents are used. **pp. 91–93**

The principal EMS document, the prehospital care report (PCR), is the sole permanent written record of the response, assessment, care, and transport offered during an emergency call. It is a medical document conveying details of care and patient history that remains a part of the patient record as well as a legal document that may be reviewed in a court of law. The PCR may also be reviewed by medical direction to determine the appropriateness of your actions during the call and used by your service to bill the patient for services. Lastly, the PCR may be used by researchers to determine the effectiveness of care measures in improving patient outcomes.

2. Explain the role of documentation in agency reimbursement. **p. 92**

Good documentation is essential for ambulance agencies that bill for services they provide. The PCR provides the name and address of the patient as well as the nature and circumstances of injury and illness. It also includes the care and transport provided. Without this information, the service may not be able to obtain reimbursement for services rendered and, ultimately, to afford to provide the vehicle, equipment, and personnel necessary to provide prehospital emergency care.

3. Identify and properly use medical terminology, medical abbreviations, and acronyms. **pp. 95–101**

Medical terminology is the very precise and exact wording used to describe the human body and injuries or illnesses. Proper use of this terminology turns the PCR into a medical document. However, if terms are misspelled or misused, they may distract from the document and confuse the reader about the patient's condition and the care he either has had or should receive. Carry a pocket dictionary, and only use words when you are sure of both their spelling and usage. The same holds true of medical abbreviations. They must be applied properly and have the same meaning to both the writer and reader. EMS systems should use a standardized set of abbreviations and acronyms to assure standard and efficient documentation.

4. Demonstrate how to properly record direct patient or bystander comments. **p. 102**

Direct statements by patients and bystanders must be recorded exactly as they were made and the key phrases placed in quotation marks. Treating the information this way is highly important because it identifies that the information is directly from the source, not an interpretation. Identify clearly the source of any quotation you include in a PCR.

©2008 Pearson Education, Inc.

5. **Demonstrate proper document revision and correction.** **pp. 104–105**

Everyone makes mistakes during a health care career and during the process of care documentation. When this happens, it is essential to make corrections in such a way that there is no appearance of impropriety. If an error is made, draw a single line through the error and enter the correction and your initials. If the error is noted after the report is turned in, write a narrative addendum explaining both the nature of the error and the needed correction and assure that the addendum is included with all copies of the PCR. Correct errors as soon as possible after they are discovered.

6. **Identify and eliminate extraneous or nonprofessional information.** **p. 105**

The ambulance call should be documented in a brief and professional way. The PCR describing it may be scrutinized by hospital staff, the medical direction physician, quality improvement committees, supervisors, lawyers, and the news media. Any derogatory comments, jargon, slang, biased statements, irrelevant opinions, or libelous statements will distract from the seriousness of the document and from acceptance of the preparer's professionalism.

7. **Describe the differences between subjective and objective elements of documentation.** **pp. 105–107**

Subjective information is information that you obtain from others or is your opinion that is not based on observable facts. It includes the patient's, family's, or bystander's description of the chief complaint and symptoms, medical history, and nature of the illness or mechanism of injury.

Objective information is information you obtain through direct observation, palpation, auscultation, percussion, or diagnostic evaluation of your patient. It includes the vital signs and the results of the physical exam, including such things as glucose level determination and cardiac dysrhythmia interpretation and pulse oximeter readings.

8. **Describe the special documentation considerations concerning patient refusal of care and/or transport.** **pp. 110, 112–113**

Be careful in the documentation of a patient who refuses care and/or transport. While a conscious and mentally competent patient has the right to refuse care, his doing so may pose legal problems for care providers. Document the nature and severity of the patient's injuries, any care you offered, any care he refused, and document carefully the assessment criteria you used to determine the patient was capable of making the decision to refuse care or transport. Also document the patient's reasons for refusing care and your efforts to convince him to change his mind. If possible, have the refusal of care and your explanation to the patient of the consequences of care refusal signed by the patient and witnessed by family or bystanders or police. Advise the patient to seek other medical help, like his family physician, and to call EMS again if he changes his mind or his condition worsens.

9. **Describe the special considerations concerning mass-casualty incident documentation.** **p. 114**

Often a mass-casualty situation calls for an atypical EMS response and unusual documentation procedures. Care providers rarely stay with a patient from the beginning to the end of prehospital care, and the time spent at a patient's side is very much at a premium. Hence documentation must be efficient and incremental. Document your assessment findings and any interventions you perform at the patient's side quickly and clearly. Many agencies or systems have their own forms such as triage tags that simplify the documentation procedure.

10. **Describe the potential consequences of illegible, incomplete, or inaccurate documentation.** **p. 115**

A legible, complete, and accurate PCR is essential to call documentation. The information in it must be easy to read thanks to both good penmanship and conscientious attention to detail. The report must describe all the pertinent information gathered at the scene and en route to the hospital as well as all actions taken by you and others in the care of the patient. Failure to create a thorough,

©2008 Pearson Education, Inc.
Intermediate Emergency Care: 1985, 3rd ed.

readable PCR reduces the information available to other caregivers and may reduce their ability to provide effective care. The document you produce also reflects on your ability to provide assessment and care and your professionalism in general.

11. Explain the confidential nature of an EMS report. **p. 115**

Confidentiality is a patient right and breaching it can result in severe consequences. Do not discuss or share patient or call information with anyone not involved in the care of the patient. The only exceptions—as necessary—are administration, which may need information for billing; police agencies carrying out a criminal investigation; requests for the information under subpoena from a court; and quality assurance committees that may need the information (with the patient's name blocked out) for system review and improvement or for research.

Case Study Review

Reread the case study in Chapter 5 and then read the following discussion. This case study identifies some of the important considerations regarding the prehospital care report and its potential to support (or incriminate) a care provider who is called into a court of law. The scenario emphasizes the importance of good documentation as described in Chapter 5.

We seldom realize the importance others may place on our prehospital documentation. In this case study, Tom Brewster is surprised when, three years after a call, he is summoned to give a legal deposition about it. While this example speaks to legal reasons for review of documentation, Tom might just as well have been asked about the quickness of the ambulance response, the time he and his crew spent on scene, or specific aspects of the care he provided. While attorneys may represent the most feared interrogators to most EMT-Is, the EMS system medical director, quality improvement personnel, or administrative personnel might also ask for details of some incident months or years in the past. For these reasons, your accurate and thorough documentation of the emergency scene and the assessment and care you provide is of great importance to you and your service.

Tom was asked about his recall of the events of the call and the comments made by the patient. His prehospital care report provided enough information to prompt Tom to remember the incident, the patient, and the care he gave. He was fortunate that his documentation provided this information and that he could piece together the events of that response. It is likely that the patient's attorney would challenge Tom's recall after three years. Documentation of the patient's statement that he "fell asleep" would be a factor critical in determining the reason for the crash (ruling out medical causes). Tom was apparently thorough in gathering the patient history and recording it on the PCR because he was able to recall that there was no history of either diabetes or heart disease. Tom further benefited from performing a routine but complete patient assessment, including glucose testing and ECG monitoring.

This case study emphasizes the importance of preparing a prehospital care report that describes exactly what happened and exactly what you did. Had Tom used sloppy penmanship or subjective statements or failed to provide complete information, the patient's attorney would have been able to challenge Tom's objectivity and accuracy. As things stood, the report supported Tom's recall and evaluation of the patient's condition.

Content Self-Evaluation

Multiple Choice

______ 1. The prehospital care report is likely to be reviewed by which of the following?
- A. researchers
- B. EMS administrators
- C. lawyers
- D. medical professionals
- E. all of the above

______ 2. Which of the following is NOT an appropriate purpose for reviewing a prehospital care report?
A. to identify a chronological account of the patient's mental status
B. to learn about what calls other prehospital care providers had
C. to help detect patient improvement or deterioration
D. to identify what bystanders and family may have said at the scene
E. to determine baseline assessment findings

______ 3. The prehospital care report may yield information that the quality improvement committee may use to identify problems with individual EMT-Is or with the EMS system.
A. True
B. False

______ 4. The prehospital care report should contain all of the following EXCEPT
A. a description of your patient's condition when you arrived.
B. your opinions about the patient's attitude or social/economic situation.
C. a description of your patient's condition after interventions.
D. the medical status of your patient upon arrival at the emergency department.
E. response time to the call.

______ 5. If you have doubts about the spelling of a term when completing a PCR, use a phonetically close spelling; doing this may still convey the right meaning and will not reflect poorly on your professionalism.
A. True
B. False

______ 6. Which of the following is NOT a time commonly recorded on the prehospital care report?
A. call received
B. dispatch time
C. arrival at the patient's side
D. arrival at the scene
E. departure from the scene

______ 7. Since your watch, the dispatch clock, and other timing devices are not often synchronized, it is important to record all times on the PCR care report from one clock or watch when possible or to indicate when different clocks are used.
A. True
B. False

______ 8. Which of the following is NOT an example of a pertinent negative?
A. no shortness of breath in a myocardial infarction patient
B. no history of epilepsy in seizing patient
C. clear breath sounds in a congestive heart failure patient
D. a blood pressure of 90/60
E. no jugular vein distention in a congestive heart failure patient

______ 9. The recommended way of indicating the exact words spoken by a patient or bystander is to
A. underline the passage.
B. draw one line through the center of the word or passage.
C. begin and end the passage with quotation marks.
D. place the passage in parentheses.
E. none of the above

______ 10. All of the following describe good documentation EXCEPT
A. complete.
B. altered.
C. accurate.
D. objective.
E. legible.

©2008 Pearson Education, Inc.
Intermediate Emergency Care: 1985, 3rd ed.

______ 11. The PCR is created by the EMT-I as a personal record of what happened at the scene and during transport and thus its legibility to others is not important.
A. True
B. False

______ 12. The benefit of check boxes on a prehospital care report is that they
A. assure common information is recorded for every call.
B. eliminate the need for a patient narrative.
C. address every chief complaint.
D. speed the completion of the narrative.
E. all of the above

______ 13. When should the prehospital care report be completed?
A. at the end of the day
B. at the end of your duty shift
C. once back at quarters
D. shortly after leaving the hospital
E. upon or shortly after transferring patient care at the hospital

______ 14. Whenever possible, have all members of your crew read or reread the prehospital care report before you submit it.
A. True
B. False

______ 15. What is the best way to add additional information to the prehospital care report after it has been submitted to the hospital?
A. Search and make changes on all copies.
B. Change only the original report.
C. Create an addendum and add it to all reports.
D. Never add additional material to the report once distributed.
E. Send a memorandum to medical direction.

______ 16. Use of professional jargon in the PCR is an indicator of the writer's professionalism.
A. True
B. False

______ 17. Which of the following is the best example of a subjective and possibly libelous statement?
A. "The patient smelled of beer."
B. "The patient walked with a staggering gait."
C. "The patient used abusive language and spoke with slurred speech."
D. "The patient was drunk and obnoxious."
E. None of the above is a potentially libelous statement.

______ 18. Which of the following is a part of the subjective patient information?
A. chief complaint
B. past medical history
C. history of the current medical problem
D. patient description of what happened
E. all of the above

______ 19. The portion of your narrative report that contains your general impression of the patient is the
A. subjective narrative.
B. objective narrative.
C. assessment/management plan.
D. SOAP plan.
E. none of the above

©2008 Pearson Education, Inc.

______ 20. You should document a pediatric assessment in head-to-toe order, even though you may have performed it from toe-to-head.
A. True
B. False

______ 21. Which of the following is true about the body systems method of assessment?
A. It focuses on body systems rather than body areas.
B. It usually addresses only the system(s) affected.
C. It is best suited to screening and preadmission exams.
D. It can be a comprehensive approach to documentation.
E. all of the above

______ 22. The term that describes what you believe to be the patient's most likely problem is the
A. definitive assessment.
B. clinical diagnosis.
C. assessment object.
D. field diagnosis.
E. none of the above

______ 23. The management portion of your documentation should include which of the following?
A. any interventions
B. the results of ongoing assessments
C. any changes in the patient's condition
D. the patient's condition when care is transferred at the emergency department
E. all of the above

______ 24. Which of the following is NOT a part of the subjective information recorded on the PCR?
A. vital signs
B. past medical history
C. review of systems
D. chief complaint
E. none of the above

______ 25. Which of the following are elements of the objective information recorded on the PCR?
A. your general impression of the patient
B. the results of any diagnostic tests
C. the results of the physical exam
D. vital signs
E. all of the above

______ 26. Which of the following formats records the chief complaint, history, assessment, treatment, and transport information in that order?
A. SOAP format
B. CHART format
C. Patient management format
D. Call incident format
E. none of the above

______ 27. The most significant feature of the patient management format of documentation is that it
A. documents the chronological sequence of events and actions.
B. focuses exclusively on assessment findings.
C. uses a free-flowing narrative style.
D. is most frequently used for patients with minor injuries/problems.
E. none of the above

______ 28. The call incident format for documenting an emergency response is best suited for which type of patient?
A. the unresponsive medical patient
B. the responsive medical patient
C. the trauma patient with no significant mechanism of injury
D. the trauma patient with a significant mechanism of injury
E. both B and C

©2008 Pearson Education, Inc.
Intermediate Emergency Care: 1985, 3rd ed.

______ 29. In obtaining a patient refusal against medical advice, it is important to
A. determine that the patient is alert, oriented, and competent to make the decision.
B. clearly explain to the patient the risks of not receiving care.
C. try to convince the patient to obtain care.
D. explain that if the condition worsens the patient should call for the ambulance or otherwise seek immediate care.
E. all of the above

______ 30. If your ambulance call is canceled en route to the scene, you should
A. simply return to base.
B. write canceled on the front of the PCR.
C. note the canceling authority and time of cancellation on the PCR.
D. secure the name of the patient as well as any other information.
E. none of the above

Matching

Write the letter of the word or phrase in the space provided next to the appropriate abbreviation.

A. shortness of breath
B. acute myocardial infarction
C. positive end-expiratory pressure
D. normal sinus rhythm
E. nausea/vomiting
F. do not resuscitate
G. breath sounds/blood sugar
H. premature ventricular contraction
I. not applicable
J. nitroglycerin
K. intraosseous
L. weight
M. sexually transmitted disease
N. against medical advice
O. congestive heart failure
P. chief complaint
Q. left lower quadrant
R electrocardiogram
S. to keep open
T. central nervous system
U. intracranial pressure
V. jugular vein distention
W. treatment
X. motor vehicle crash
Y. year old

______ 31. CC
______ 32. y/o
______ 33. wt
______ 34. CNS
______ 35. SOB
______ 36. n/v
______ 37. AMI
______ 38. CHF
______ 39. ICP
______ 40. MVC
______ 41. STD
______ 42. NTG
______ 43. LLQ
______ 44. BS
______ 45. ECG
______ 46. JVD
______ 47. n/a
______ 48. AMA
______ 49. DNR
______ 50. PEEP
______ 51. Tx
______ 52. IO
______ 53. TKO
______ 54. NSR
______ 55. PVC

©2008 Pearson Education, Inc.

Special Projects

Documentation: Radio Report/Prehospital Care Report

The preparation of both the radio message to medical direction and the written run report are two of the most important tasks you will perform as an EMT-I. Read the following information, compose your initial and updated radio messages, and then complete the run report for this call.

The Call

At 1832, medic rescue unit 21 is paged through dispatch and is en route to a one-car collision at the corner of Elm and Wildwood Lane. One patient is reported unconscious, and the fire department is also en route. You and your partner, Mike Grailing (an EMT-I), arrive with the ambulance at 1845 and find that there are wires down, fuel spilling from the gas tank, and window glass around the scene. Bystanders state that "the car swerved wildly, then hit the power pole." You notice there are no skid marks. You stand by, awaiting arrival of the fire department and the securing of the scene.

Once the scene is safe, your partner employs a jaw thrust with cervical precautions and applies cervical immobilization, while you apply the cervical collar (1850) and begin the assessment. You notice a break in the car's windshield and a small contusion on your patient's forehead. He is unconscious, has a strong pulse, and displays some respiratory wheezing and stridor. Assessment of the neck reveals a small welt but no other apparent injuries. The pupils are equal and reactive. Oxygen is administered at 12 liters per minute via nonrebreather mask, the patient awakens, and initial vitals (including a respiratory rate of 30 with audible wheezes, BP of 110/76, a strong pulse of 90, and oxygen saturation of 94 percent) are taken at 1852. The ECG displays normal sinus rhythm.

The patient awakes and asks, "What happened?" He states that he thinks he was stung by a bee. Two years ago he had a similar sting and reaction and has a kit at home that his physician prescribed for him. He is experiencing itching, and there are noticeable hives. He says he feels like "I have a lump in my throat."

Based upon protocol, you initiate the IV run TKO with lactated Ringer's solution in the right forearm using a 16-gauge over-the-catheter needle while the patient is being immobilized and moved to a long spine board.

Medical direction is contacted and you call in the following:

____

____

____

____

____

____

____

____

____

____

Orders for 0.3 mg epinephrine SQ (1:1,000) and 50 mg Benadryl IM are received and the medications are administered at 1855. Just prior to moving the patient to the ambulance, the patient is monitored and found to have the following vitals: BP 118/88, pulse 78 strong and regular, respirations 20 and regular with clear breath sounds, an ECG showing normal sinus rhythm, and a pulse oximetry reading of 99 percent.

©2008 Pearson Education, Inc.
Intermediate Emergency Care: 1985, 3rd ed.

The patient history, which is taken at the scene and during transport, reveals that the patient's name is William Sobeski, his age is 28, and he lives at 2145 East Brookline Drive in the city of Rochester. The patient denies any allergy, except to bee stings. He was stung by a bee two years ago and was rushed to the emergency department because he "couldn't catch his breath." He denies any headache, visual disturbances, and any numbness and tingling. He also denies taking any prescribed medications and has not eaten since noon. The patient requests Community Hospital because his sister works there. En route, vitals are BP 122/78, pulse of 68 strong and regular, respirations 22 and regular, and a pulse oximetry reading of 98 percent, all taken at 1902.

Contact medical direction and provide the following update:

ETA 10 Minutes

The final vitals, taken just before arrival, are BP 122/80, pulse 86, oxygen saturation of 98 percent, and respirations 24 and regular with no wheezes. The ECG still displays normal sinus rhythm, and the patient is conscious and oriented. He states that the feeling of a lump in the throat is gone.

The trip is uneventful, and the patient is delivered to the emergency department at 1925. The patient care responsibilities are transferred to the staff, and the attending physician is given the final patient update. The vehicle is restocked, cleaned, and you are ready for service at 1955.

©2008 Pearson Education, Inc.

Using the information contained in this narrative, complete the run report below.

Date / /	Emergency Medical Services Run Report		Run # 911
Patient Information	Service Information		Times
Name:	Agency:		Rcvd :
Address:	Location:		Enrt :
City: St: Zip:	Call Origin:		Scne :
Age: Birth: / / Sex: [M][F]	Type: Emrg[ ] Non[ ] Trnsfr[ ]		LvSn :
Nature of Call:			ArHsp :
Chief Complaint:			InSv :

Description of Current Problem:	Medical Problems
	Past / Present
	[ ] Cardiac [ ]
	[ ] Stroke [ ]
	[ ] Acute Abdomen [ ]
	[ ] Diabetes [ ]
	[ ] Psychiatric [ ]
	[ ] Epilepsy [ ]
	[ ] Drug/Alcohol [ ]
	[ ] Poisoning [ ]
	[ ] Allergy/Asthma [ ]
	[ ] Syncope [ ]
	[ ] Obstetrical [ ]
	[ ] GYN [ ]
	Other:
Trauma Scr: Glasgow:	

On Scene Care:	First Aid:
	By Whom?

02 @ L : Via	C-Collar :	S-Immob. :	Stretcher :

Allergies/Meds:	Past Med Hx:

Time	Pulse	Resp.	BP S/D	LOC	ECG
:	R: [r][i]	R: [s][l]	/	[a][v][p][u]	
Care/Comments:					
:	R: [r][i]	R: [s][l]	/	[a][v][p][u]	
Care/Comments:					
:	R: [r][i]	R: [s][l]	/	[a][v][p][u]	
Care/Comments:					
:	R: [r][i]	R: [s][l]	/	[a][v][p][u]	
Care/Comments:					

Destination:	Personnel:	Certification
Reason:[ ]pt [ ]Closest [ ]M.D. [ ]Other	1.	[P][E][O]
Contacted: [ ]Radio [ ]Tele [ ]Direct	2.	[P][E][O]
Ar Status: [ ]Better [ ]UnC [ ]Worse	3.	[P][E][O]

©2008 Pearson Education, Inc.
Intermediate Emergency Care: 1985, 3rd ed.

Compare the radio communication and run report form that you prepared against the example in the Answer Key section of this Workbook. As you make this comparison, keep in mind that there are many "correct" ways to communicate this body of information. Ensure that the information you have recorded contains the major points of your assessment and care and enough other material to describe the patient and his condition to the receiving physician and anyone else who might review the form. Remember that this document may be the only record of your assessment and care for this patient. When you are done, it should be a complete account of your actions.

Crossword Puzzle

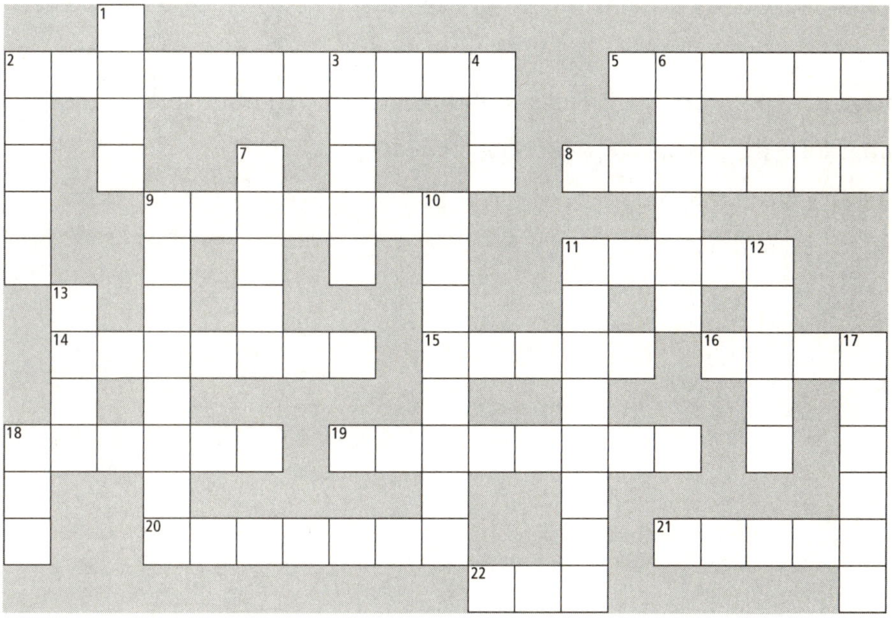

Across

2. A rapid heartbeat
5. A wound
8. High-pitched respiratory sounds
9. Related to the heart
11. ______ complaint: the reason the patient called EMS
14. Fluid buildup in the abdomen
15. Written defamation of another person
16. Type of respirator used when treating a suspected tuberculosis patient
18. Involuntary response to a stimulus
19. Acute alteration in mental function
20. Loud, high-pitched inspiratory wheeze
21. Elements of the head assessment (abbr.)
22. Advanced life support (abbr.)

©2008 Pearson Education, Inc.

Down

1. Repeat a verbal order
2. ______ volume: normal respiratory volume
3. Basic EMS communication device
4. Against medical advice (abbr.)
6. Vomitus
7. Sound indicating turbulent blood flow
9. Light, popping nonmusical inspiratory sounds
10. Type of phone service used by many EMS systems
11. Grating sensation or sound
12. ______ diagnosis; prehospital evaluation of the patient's condition and its causes
13. Questionnaire used for suspected alcoholic patients
17. Severity of an injury or illness
18. Review of the systems (abbr.)

©2008 Pearson Education, Inc.
Intermediate Emergency Care: 1985, 3rd ed.

Chapter

6 EMS Communications

Review of Chapter Objectives

After reading this chapter, you should be able to do the following:

1. Describe the sequence of an EMS event. **p. 121**

Occurrence—illness or injury that provides the need for the EMS response
Detection—recognition that there is a need for the EMS response
Notification and response—call to appropriate EMS personnel and direction of units to the scene
Treatment and preparation—phase in which the patient is assessed, managed, and prepared for transport
Transport and delivery—loading, transport, continuation of care, and the delivery of the patient to the emergency department
Preparation for the next event—cleaning and restocking of the ambulance, completion of paperwork, notification of EMS dispatch that the EMS unit is back in service

2. Describe the five communications phases of an EMS response. **pp. 122–124**

Notification—notification of an emergency situation by a citizen, municipal worker, etc.
Dispatch—alerting and sending the appropriate EMS personnel to the scene
Medical communications—transmission of the results of patient assessment to the medical command physician and a request for permission to employ care procedures
Hospital arrival—phase of communication in which an EMT-Intermediate verbally informs the medical direction physician of what was found in the field, what was revealed by a pertinent patient history, what care steps were offered and what results came of that care
In service—notification to the dispatcher that the unit has been restocked, cleaned, and is back in service

3. Define the following terms.

a. **Base station**—principal transmitter and receiver of an EMS system; located close to the antenna and is usually operated by a remote unit found in the dispatch center **p. 124**
b. **Mobile two-way transmitter/receiver**—vehicle mounted radio unit with a lower transmission power than the base station **p. 125**
c. **Portable radio**—handheld radio unit with less power and range than the mobile radio **p. 125**
d. **Repeater**—radio base station modified to retransmit a radio broadcast so the area covered by the EMS radio system can be increased; normally located strategically within the service area and tied to the dispatch center by either a telephone or radio link **p. 125**
e. **Voting**—process by which the repeater station receiving the strongest incoming signal is chosen to rebroadcast that signal **p. 125**
f. **Remote console**—unit designed to control the base station from a location some distance away **pp. 125, 127**

©2008 Pearson Education, Inc.

g. **Encoder**—electronic device that generates unique signals or tones within a radio transmission; signals can be recognized by another radio's decoder **p. 127**

h. **Decoder**—electronic device that listens to radio transmissions and recognizes only those signals for which it is encoded **p. 127**

4. Describe the advantages of a repeater system over a nonrepeater system. p. 125

A repeater system permits a communications network to be dependable over a large service area or over terrain that otherwise would limit communications.

It often allows communications even though one tower may be inoperative and offers greater assurance that weak transmissions from a mobile or portable unit will be heard.

5. List the two types of sound wave transmission. p. 129

Amplitude modulation—modification of a radio transmission by varying the amplitude of the signal; referred to as AM; has a relatively poor quality of transmission, though its range is good

Frequency modulation—modification of a radio transmission by varying the frequency of the signal; referred to as FM; has very good quality of transmission, though its range is less than that of AM

6. Define the following terms.

a. **Hertz**—number of cycles of electrical activity per second in a radio signal **p. 129**

b. **Band**—group of radio frequencies close together in the electromagnetic spectrum **p. 129**

c. **Biotelemetry**—process of transmitting physiological data, such as an electrocardiogram, usually by radio **p. 129**

d. **Modulator**—device that electronically transforms electrical impulses into sound waves that may be transmitted **p. 129**

e. **Demodulator**—device that recognizes a specific modulated transmission and converts it back to electrical impulses **p. 129**

f. **Trunking**—computer-assisted radio system that maximizes the use of available radio channels **p. 131**

7. Describe the 10 "Med Channels" and their usage. p. 131

Med Channels—ultra high frequency (UHF) channels designated as medical communications channels; duplex pairs designed for advanced life support service

Usage—channels one through eight are for paramedic/medical control communications; nine and ten are reserved for EMS dispatch

8. Describe the most common causes of interference in biotelemetry communications. p. 129

Muscle tremors, loose electrodes, 60 Hz interference (from other electrical sources)
Fluctuations in transmitter power
Transmission of voice and telemetry simultaneously

9. Discuss the importance of communications equipment maintenance. p. 132

Protects fragile, expensive equipment and ensures that it operates when needed
Proper maintenance requires:

- Regular cleaning
- Proper repair of malfunctions
- Frequent recharging of batteries
- Storage of spare batteries

10. Describe briefly the functions and responsibilities of the Federal Communications Commission p. 132

The Federal Communications Commission is responsible for the overall operation and regulation of radio service. It approves equipment, allocates frequencies, licenses transmitters, licenses repair personnel, monitors the system, and spot-checks station records.

©2008 Pearson Education, Inc.
Intermediate Emergency Care: 1985, 3rd ed.

11. Define briefly the role of the EMS dispatcher. **pp. 132–133**

Responsible for gathering information from the caller
Instructs the caller in limited first aid procedures
Directs the appropriate resources (EMS, fire department, police, etc.) to the right location
Monitors the response to a call by the responding units
Monitors and coordinates general radio communications

12. List important caller information that must be obtained from a caller by the EMS dispatcher. **p. 133**

The location and nature of the emergency. (The responding unit may be dispatched as soon as these facts are known.)
An appropriate call-back number, in case of accidental telephone disconnection.
Information that will help determine the need for specific additional resources.

13. Describe how the information necessary to initiate an EMS response is obtained. **pp. 132–133**

Access of the EMS system by the victim, a relative or friend of the victim, a bystander, or another member of the public safety service system, like a police officer.
Interrogation of the caller by the dispatcher to determine the nature of the call, the exact location, and any other pertinent information.

14. Describe the purpose of EMS radio codes and give examples of local radio codes. **p. 133**

Designed to communicate a large amount of information quickly and accurately.
Allows transmission of information in a format not readily understood by the public.
Example: 10 Codes "10-4"—acknowledgement/understood.

15. List radio techniques that improve clarity and efficiency. **pp. 133–134**

Listen before using a channel to ensure it is not in use.
Key the transmitter button for one second before speaking.
Speak close into the microphone or directly across it.
Speak clearly and slowly.
Speak in a normal pitch.
Do not convey emotion.
Keep the message brief.
Use a standard format for message composition.
Protect patient privacy.
Confirm reception of the message.
Repeat important information back to sender.
Write down important information.
Do not use slang, salutations, or profanity.
Obtain confirmation that your message was received and understood.

16. Describe the structure and importance of the verbal communication of patient information to medical direction and hospital staff. **pp. 134–135**

Communication of patient information to the hospital or to medical direction is a fundamental component of the EMS system. Verbal communications, which may occur via radio, cell phone, or land line, provide the hospital with information to prepare for patient care upon arrival. In addition, these communications also initiate medical orders for patient treatment in the field.

A standard format for transmission of patient assessment information enables efficient use of the medical communications system, permits the physician to assimilate information quickly about the patient's condition, and assures that medical information is complete. A medical report (verbal or written) should include:

1. Unit call name and name or number of the EMT-Intermediate
2. Description of the scene

©2008 Pearson Education, Inc.

3. Patient's age, sex, and weight
4. Patient's chief complaint
5. Patient's primary problem
6. Associated signs and symptoms
7. Brief history of the present illness
8. Pertinent past medical history, including surgeries, medications, and medication allergies
9. Physical exam findings, including:
    - Level of consciousness (AVPU system)
    - Vital signs
    - Pertinent physical exam findings
    - ECG (if applicable)
    - Trauma score and Glasgow Coma Scale score (if applicable)
      (Other pertinent observations, including significant positive and negative findings)
10. ALS skills and treatments performed on standing orders
11. Other treatment given
12. Response to treatment
13. Request for orders
14. Estimated time of arrival at the hospital
15. Name of private physician

17. List the important components of the patient prehospital care report. **pp. 135–136**

Unit designation, personnel, and level of certification
Scene description
Patient's name, age, sex, height, weight
Patient's chief complaint/primary problem
Associated signs and symptoms
Brief history of current medical problem
Pertinent past medical history
Findings of physical exam—vital signs, level of consciousness, ECG, trauma score, Glasgow Coma Scale, etc.
Treatment rendered, time rendered, and results of care
Estimated time of arrival
Name of private physician

18. Prepare and present a sample patient medical report on a simulated patient. **pp. 134–136**

As you prepare a patient care report, assure it accurately records the circumstances surrounding the medical or trauma emergency. Assure the document is complete, accurate, neat, and easy to read. The document you prepare should clearly describe what you saw, heard, and found at the emergency scene.

19. Describe the importance of written medical protocols. **p. 134**

Written medical protocols define specific pre-approved care steps that may be given for certain patient conditions. They expedite care at the scene.

20. Name five uses of the written EMS form. **pp. 135–136**

The patient report becomes a medical record of the patient's prehospital care.
The patient report becomes a legal record of the patient's prehospital care.
It may document a patient's refusal of care and transport.
It may also be used for medical audits, quality improvement, data collection and billing purposes.
The EMT-I's defense against malpractice.

21. Prepare an EMS form based on a simulated patient. **pp. 135–136**

(See Special Projects)

©2008 Pearson Education, Inc.
Intermediate Emergency Care: 1985, 3rd ed.

Case Study Review

Reread the case study in Chapter 6 and then read the following discussion. This case review highlights some important aspects of radio communications during an EMS response and shows the value that state-of-the-art communications have in emergency medical service.

An accident along Interstate Highway 20 demonstrates the various elements of an EMS communications system and the valuable service such a system provides. A cellular phone brings the report of the accident through the universal entry number 911. Because Duane is in an unfamiliar area, dialing 911 saves both precious time and brings Duane in contact with a trained dispatcher who has access to all the public safety services. Since Duane's cellular phone is not tied to a specific location like a telephone, the dispatcher must ask specific questions about the location.

The dispatcher asks predetermined questions to identify quickly the pertinent information she needs to direct the appropriate personnel and equipment to the right location and to determine the medical dispatch priority. She activates a predesignated response, electronically alerting EMS, fire, police, and rescue services. The computer-aided dispatch (CAD) system also provides each responding service with printed dispatch information, thereby eliminating any confusion regarding street names and directions.

Finally, the dispatcher returns to the caller to advise him to stay off the highway. If this were a medical call or had occurred on a safer stretch of roadway, she would likely provide Duane with pre-arrival emergency medical care instructions and may try to gain more information regarding the incident.

Ambulance 15 arrives first at the scene. The senior EMT-Intermediate assumes the role of incident commander. She does a quick scene survey, advises incoming units of the situation, and directs them to a staging area. Due to the multiple-agency response, her most effective means of communication would be a handheld portable radio, operating on the mutual aid frequency. As soon as a fire officer arrives, the senior EMT-Intermediate would relinquish scene command so she could focus on patient assessment and care. As higher level EMS personnel (the paramedics) arrive, the EMT-Intermediates give a quick patient status report and relinquish primary patient care responsibilities.

The paramedic in each ambulance uses the radio to contact the trauma center and alert them to the crash, the number of injured, the nature and severity of injuries, and the estimated time of arrival at the emergency department. They provide further information on the patients as they depart the scene en route to the trauma center. This communication is possible through the use of a system-wide repeater system. If the signal from the ambulance is too weak to reach the distant trauma center, the ambulance radio will activate a remote tower that will then retransmit the signal to the hospital's remote receiver.

Upon arrival at the emergency department, the EMT-Intermediate gives a verbal patient report to the trauma team. This report is followed by complete documentation of the call on the prehospital care report (PCR). This form includes such information as the mechanism of injury, chief complaint, results of the initial and rapid trauma assessments, serial vital signs, pertinent patient history, and care provided at the scene and en route to the hospital. It will become part of the patient's permanent record, a document for quality improvement, and a legal record of the findings and actions of the EMS personnel on this call.

Content Self-Evaluation

Multiple Choice

_____ 1. As an EMT-Intermediate, you will likely communicate with which of the following people?
- A. patient, family, and bystanders
- B. the emergency medical dispatcher
- C. other responding personnel
- D. medical direction physicians
- E. all of the above

©2008 Pearson Education, Inc.

______ 2. The main transmitter of an EMS radio system is generally located close to the antenna and is called the
A. remote console.
B. repeater.
C. base station.
D. satellite receiver.
E. encoder module.

______ 3. The normal range for the mobile transmitter, without a repeater, is about
A. 5 miles.
B. 10 to 15 miles.
C. 25 miles.
D. 50 to 100 miles.
E. 125 miles.

______ 4. The device that receives a radio signal and retransmits the message at a higher power level is the
A. portable radio.
B. mobile radio.
C. repeater.
D. remote console.
E. none of the above

______ 5. The device that activates a radio to receive and recognize messages containing a certain signal or tone is called a(n)
A. remote receiver.
B. satellite receiver.
C. encoder.
D. decoder.
E. none of the above

______ 6. Mobile data terminals are a part of which system?
A. simplex
B. multiplex
C. trunking
D. duplex
E. digital

______ 7. The type of radio transmission that is strictly "line of sight" and less subject to atmospheric interference is called amplitude modulation (AM).
A. True
B. False

______ 8. The process of sending data such as an ECG over the radio is called
A. simplex transmission.
B. biotelemetry.
C. amplitude modulation.
D. duplex transmission.
E. trunking.

______ 9. A system that automatically routes transmissions to the next available frequency is called
A. band management.
B. frequency assessment.
C. trunking.
D. frequency encoding.
E. frequency modulation.

______ 10. The Federal Communications Commission (FCC) is responsible for which of the following?
A. frequency allocation
B. establishing technical standards
C. licensing repair personnel
D. licensing radio systems
E. all of the above

______ 11. All of the following are appropriate for good EMS communications except to
A. speak close to the microphone.
B. speak directly into or across the microphone.
C. talk in a normal tone.
D. speak without emotion.
E. explain everything in detail.

______ 12. If the portable radio you are using does not transmit from your location, attempt to
A. move to higher ground.
B. touch the antenna to something metal while transmitting.
C. move toward a window or away from structural steel.
D. A and C
E. all of the above

©2008 Pearson Education, Inc.
Intermediate Emergency Care: 1985, 3rd ed.

______ 13. One of the more important skills of an EMT-Intermediate is to gather essential patient information, organize it, and relay it to the medical direction physician.
A. True
B. False

______ 14. Which of the following should be addressed by state or local protocols?
A. care steps for all major medical emergencies
B. patients who refuse care
C. non-EMS physicians on the scene
D. "do not resuscitate" orders
E. all of the above

______ 15. The written run report may become
A. a record of the patient's initial condition.
B. a legal record of prehospital care.
C. the source of essential information for billing, etc.
D. documentation of a patient's refusal of care.
E. all of the above

SEQUENCING

16. Place the following sequence of events in prehospital care in the order in which they would occur. Number the first event 1, the second event 2, and so on.
______ A. treatment and preparation for transport
______ B. preparation for the next event
______ C. occurrence and detection
______ D. notification and response

DESCRIPTION

17. List at least two responsibilities of the Federal Communications Commission.

18. List at least three responsibilities of the EMS dispatcher.

Special Project

The authoring of both the radio message to the receiving hospital and the written run report are two of the most important tasks you will perform as an EMT-Intermediate. Read the following paragraphs, compose a radio message, and complete the run report for this call.

The Call

At 3:15 P.M., your ambulance, Unit 89, is paged out to an unconscious person at the local baseball field on a very hot (97°), humid Saturday. You are accompanied by EMT-Intermediate Steve Phillips, your partner for the day.

You arrive on scene at 3:22 to find a young male collapsed at third base. You find him to be unconscious, perspiring heavily, and with skin cool to the touch. You remove a pillow under the boy's head, placed there by bystanders. The airway is clear, breathing adequate, and the pulse rapid and bounding. One bystander says, "He was playing ball and just collapsed." Another young bystander

©2008 Pearson Education, Inc.

identifies himself as the victim's brother and states that "nothing like this has happened before." He identifies his brother as 13-year-old John Thompson. He lives about a mile away.

The rest of the assessment reveals no signs of trauma. Blood pressure is 136/98, pulse 92 and strong. The ECG traces normal sinus rhythm. Respirations are 24 and normal in depth and pattern (at 3:27). The young boy responds to painful stimuli, but not to verbal command or his name. You note pupils to be equal and slow to react. You apply oxygen at 4 liters by nasal cannula, and move the patient into the shade.

You contact the receiving hospital and call in the following report:

____

____

____

____

____

Expected ETA is 20 minutes.

Medical control at the receiving hospital orders you to start an IV line with normal saline at a TKO rate. You repeat the orders to medical control and then begin your care. Your first IV attempt on the right forearm is unsuccessful; the second attempt on the left forearm gets a flashback and infuses well. You retake vitals. The patient is now responding to verbal stimuli, the BP is 134/96, pulse 90, ECG reads NSR, respirations 24. The patient is loaded on the stretcher at 3:37 and moved to the ambulance.

You contact medical control and provide the following update:

____

____

____

____

____

ETA 10 Minutes

En route vitals (3:45) are BP 132/90, ECG reads NSR, pulse 88, respirations at 24. The patient is now conscious and alert, although he cannot remember the incident. The trip is uneventful, and you arrive at the hospital at 3:57. You transfer the responsibility for the patient to the emergency physician. You then restock and wipe out the ambulance and report it back in service at 4:15. You now sit down to write the run report.

Complete the run report on the following page from the information contained in the narrative of this call.

(Compare the radio communication and run-report form that you prepared against the example in the answer key section of this workbook. As you make this comparison, keep in mind that there are many "correct" ways to communicate this body of information. Ensure that you have recorded the major points to describe the patient and his condition at all stages of the run.)

©2008 Pearson Education, Inc.
Intermediate Emergency Care: 1985, 3rd ed.

Date / /	Emergency Medical Services Run Report	Run # 912

Patient Information	Service Information	Times
Name:	Agency:	Rcvd :
Address:	Location:	Enrt :
City: St: Zip:	Call Origin:	Scne :
Age: Birth: / / Sex: [M][F]	Type: Emrg[ ] Non[ ] Trnsfr[ ]	LvSn :
Nature of Call:		ArHsp :
Chief Complaint:		InSv :

Description of Current Problem:

Trauma Scr: Glasgow:

Medical Problems

Past		Present
[ ]	Cardiac	[ ]
[ ]	Stroke	[ ]
[ ]	Acute Abdomen	[ ]
[ ]	Diabetes	[ ]
[ ]	Psychiatric	[ ]
[ ]	Epilepsy	[ ]
[ ]	Drug/Alcohol	[ ]
[ ]	Poisoning	[ ]
[ ]	Allergy/Asthma	[ ]
[ ]	Syncope	[ ]
[ ]	Obstetrical	[ ]
[ ]	GYN	[ ]

Other:

On Scene Care:	First Aid:
	By Whom?

02 @ L : Via	C-Collar :	S-Immob. :	Stretcher :

Allergies/Meds:	Past Med Hx:

Time	Pulse	Resp.	BP S/D	LOC	ECG
:	R: [r][i]	R: [s][l]	/	[a][v][p][u]	
Care/Comments:					
:	R: [r][i]	R: [s][l]	/	[a][v][p][u]	
Care/Comments:					
:	R: [r][i]	R: [s][l]	/	[a][v][p][u]	
Care/Comments:					
:	R: [r][i]	R: [s][l]	/	[a][v][p][u]	
Care/Comments:					

Destination:	Personnel: Certification
Reason:[ ]pt [ ]Closest [ ]M.D. [ ]Other	1. [P][E][O]
Contacted: [ ]Radio [ ]Tele [ ]Direct	2. [P][E][O]
Ar Status: [ ]Better [ ]UnC [ ]Worse	3. [P][E][O]

©2008 Pearson Education, Inc.
Intermediate Emergency Care: 1985, 3rd ed.

Chapter 7

Human Body Systems

Review of Chapter Objectives

After reading this chapter, you should be able to do the following:

1. Describe the cell membrane, cytoplasm, and organelles typical of eukaryote cells. pp. 141–142

Cell Membrane—The cell membrane is the outer covering that encircles and protects the cell. It is semipermeable, and maintains electrolyte and fluid balance and the transfer of enzymes, hormones, and nutrients into and out of the cell.

Cytoplasm—Cytoplasm is the thick, viscous fluid that fills and gives shape to the cell. Substances dissolved in the cytoplasm include electrolytes, proteins, glucose (sugar), and lipids (fatty substances).

Organelles—Organelles perform specific functions within the cell and include the nucleus, the endoplasmic reticulum, the Golgi apparatus, mitochondria, lysosomes, and peroxisomes.

2. Identify and discuss the seven major functions of cells. p. 142

Movement is performed by muscle cells.

Conductivity is the function of nerve cells that creates and transmits an electrical impulse in response to a stimulus.

Absorption is a function of cells of the intestines (and kidneys), which take in nutrients (water and electrolytes) that pass through the body.

Secretion is performed by glands that produce substances such as hormones, mucus, sweat, and saliva.

Excretion is a function all cells perform as they break down nutrients and expel wastes.

Respiration is the function by which cells take in oxygen and release carbon dioxide.

Reproduction is the process by which cells enlarge, divide, and reproduce themselves.

3. Define the terms *tissue* and *organ*. pp. 142, 144

Tissue refers to a group of cells that perform a similar function.

An organ is a group of tissues functioning together. For example, the pancreas consists of epithelial tissue, connective tissue, and nervous tissue that contribute to digestion and the transport and metabolism of glucose.

4. List and define the four basic types of tissue found in the human body. pp. 142–143

Epithelial tissue lines internal and external body surfaces and protects the body. In addition, certain types of epithelial tissue perform specialized functions such as secretion, absorption, diffusion, and filtration. Examples of epithelial tissue are skin, mucous membranes, and the lining of the intestinal tract.

Muscle tissue has the capability of contraction when stimulated. There are three types of muscle tissue: (1) Cardiac muscle, which is tissue found only within the heart. It has the unique

©2008 Pearson Education, Inc.

capability of spontaneous contraction without external stimulation. (2) Smooth muscle is the muscle found within the intestines and encircling blood vessels. Smooth muscle is generally under the control of the involuntary, or autonomic, component of the nervous system. (3) Skeletal muscle is the most abundant muscle type. It allows movement and is mostly under voluntary control.

Connective tissue is the most abundant tissue in the body. It provides support, connection, and insulation. Examples of connective tissue include bones, cartilage, and fat. Blood is also sometimes classified as connective tissue.

Nerve tissue is tissue specialized to transmit electrical impulses throughout the body. Examples of nerve tissue include the brain, spinal cord, and peripheral nerves.

5. Identify and describe the five body cavities commonly recognized in the human. pp. 143–144

The **cranial cavity** is the hollow spherical portion of the skull that houses the brain.

The **spinal cavity** is the hollow tube-like cavity within the vertebral column. It is continuous with the cranial cavity, and also is referred to as the spinal canal, which contains the spinal cord. As the cranial and spinal cavities contain the brain and the spinal cord, we can say that the central nervous system is enclosed within these cavities.

The **thoracic cavity** is formed by the ribcage and the inferior border by the diaphragm. The heart, great vessels, lungs, mainstem bronchi, and esophagus are contained within the thoracic cavity as is the mediastinum.

The **abdominal cavity** is formed by the diaphragm superiorly, the spine posteriorly, the abdominal wall laterally and anteriorly, and the pelvic bones inferiorly. The abdominal cavity contains organs of the digestive and urinary systems and is lined with a serous membrane called the peritoneum.

The **pelvic cavity**, which is continuous with the abdominal cavity, is bordered by the pelvic bones (ilium, ischium, sacrum, coccyx, and pubis) and contains portions of the digestive, urinary, and reproductive systems.

6. Describe the structure and function of the following organ systems.

a. Skeletal system pp. 145–152

Bone tissue is alive and requires a constant supply of blood and nutrients to survive. The major structures of the long bones include the diaphysis (the central shaft area) the epiphysis (the bone end), the metaphysis (the transitional area between the two), and the medullary canal (the central space in the bone).

The skeleton consists of about 206 bones and is divided between the axial and appendicular skeletons. The appendicular skeleton consists of the appendages—the clavicle and scapula, humerus, radius/ulna, carpals, metacarpals, and phalanges of the upper extremity and the pelvis, femur, tibia/fibula, tarsals, metatarsals, and phalanges of the lower extremity. The axial skeleton consists of the facial bones and cranium of the skull, the 33 bones of the vertebra column, and the 12 rib pairs joining the sternum and forming the thorax.

The skeletal system is responsible to protect vital organs, allowing for efficient movement, storing of salts and other materials, and the production of red blood cells.

b. Muscular system pp. 152–153

There are about 700 muscles divided among three types—skeletal, smooth and cardiac. The cardiac muscle is most specialized with properties of automaticity (able to initiate contraction on its own), emitting an electrical charge (excitability) and able to conduct electrical impulses (conductivity). Smooth muscle is involuntary and responsible for such things as moving food through the digestive system and controlling the size of blood vessels. Skeletal muscle is under our conscious control and makes up the majority of muscle mass in the human body.

c. Integumentary system pp. 154–155

The integumentary system, or skin, is comprised of two layers, the dermis and epidermis. The epidermis provides protection against trauma, the entry of infectious or toxic agents and waterproofs the exterior of the body. It is made up of predominately dead cells. The dermis consists of connective tissue capillaries, glands, and nerves. It is very flexible and helps in either radiating heat away or conserving it.

©2008 Pearson Education, Inc.
Intermediate Emergency Care: 1985, 3rd ed.

Beneath the dermis is a layer of tissue called the subcutaneous layer. It consists of fatty tissue that insulates against both trauma and heat loss.

d. Nervous system **pp. 155–164**

The nervous system is divided into two subsystems, the central nervous system and the peripheral nervous system. The central nervous system consists of the brain and spinal cord and is responsible for higher functions (the brain) and communication between the central and peripheral nervous system (the spinal cord). The major portion of the brain, the cerebrum is responsible for higher thought and body function control while the cerebellum is responsible for sensory and motor coordination and balance. The brainstem controls major body functions like blood pressure, heart, and respiratory rate and temperature. The brain and spinal cord are protected by the cranium and vertebral column and three layers of connective tissue, called the meninges.

The peripheral nervous system consists of the 12 cranial nerves and the nerve roots that branch from the spinal cord. They innervate virtually every portion of the body. The peripheral nervous system is divided into the sympathetic and parasympathetic nervous systems. The sympathetic nervous system basically increases activity, and during extreme stimulation induces the fight or flight response. The parasympathetic nervous system is responsible for controlling vegetative and regenerative function.

e. Cardiovascular system **pp. 165–176**

The cardiovascular system is a fluid transport system responsible for moving oxygen and nutrients to body cells and removing carbon dioxide and wastes from the cells. It consists of the heart, blood vessels, and blood. The heart is a closed-fist-sized, muscular pump, located in the central thorax. It has four chambers (two atria and two ventricles) separated from one another by valves and separated left to right by the septum. Its electrical system causes it to contract between 60 and 100 times per minute, pumping about 70 mL of blood with each contraction.

That cardiac output is delivered to the vascular system consisting of arteries, capillaries, and veins. The arteries direct blood to the various organs. Smaller arteries, called arterioles, then regulate the actual blood flow to the tissues. The capillaries are the vessels through which the actual exchange of oxygen, nutrients, waste products, and carbon dioxide takes place. The blood then returns to the heart through the veins.

The blood is a slurry of fluid, called the plasma, and the cells. The plasma comprises about 55% of the blood volume and consists of water, electrolytes, and proteins. The vast majority of blood cells are red blood cells that contain hemoglobin (an iron compound), which carries the oxygen from lungs to the cells. White blood cells help fight infection and platelets assist with clotting.

f. Lymphatic system **pp. 191–193**

The lymphatic system is a valveless system of ducts that draw fluid away from the interstitial space and return it to the circulatory system. Nodes in the system have resident white blood cells that assist the immune system. The lymphatic system also helps with the absorption of fats from digestion and includes the spleen, a vascular organ associated with disease immunity.

g. Respiratory system **p. 177**

The respiratory system brings oxygen into the lungs, where it fills the hemoglobin of the red blood cells and then takes carbon dioxide out. It consists of the airway, lungs, and bellows system. The airway is a tube through which air moves during respiration. It consists of the mouth and nose, throat (pharynx), larynx, trachea, bronchi, and bronchioles. The lungs are filled with microscopic balloon-shaped chambers (alveoli) where the actual oxygen/carbon dioxide exchange takes place. The bellow system controls the volume of the skeletal thorax through the contraction and relaxation of the muscles between the ribs (intercostal muscles) and the diaphragm. This changing volume moves air in and out through the airway and into and out of the alveoli.

h. Gastrointestinal system **pp. 177–182**

The gastrointestinal system is a 25-foot-long muscular tube that moves food through it while subjecting that food to various digestive fluids. It also is responsible for absorbing nutrients and ultimately expelling the undigested residue. It consists of the esophagus, stomach, small intestine (duodenum, jejunum, and ileum), large bowel, rectum, and anus. It and many abdominal organs are covered by the peritoneum.

©2008 Pearson Education, Inc.

i. Genitourinary system **pp. 183–187**

The genitourinary system consists of the two kidneys, the ureters, the bladder, and the urethra. The kidneys filter blood to assist in the regulation of water and electrolytes in the blood and assist in blood pressure regulation. They excrete water, electrolytes, and waste materials as urine. The ureters carry these waste products to the bladder for storage until the urine is released through the urethra.

j. Reproductive system **pp. 188–189**

The female has two ovaries located in the lower abdominal cavity that produce the female hormones and release an egg every 28 days. This egg travels through one of two hollow tubes (the fallopian tubes) to the uterus. If the egg is fertilized by a sperm, it will attach to the uterus wall and begin the development of a fetus. The uterus is a thick muscular organ, designed to accept the developing fetus and support its development for the next 280 days. At the lower end of the uterus is the cervix, a valve-like structure that holds the fetus within the uterus until delivery begins. The fetus will move down the birth canal (the vagina) during delivery.

The male has two testes that are responsible for the development of sperm and produce the male hormones. The sperm travels from each testicle through paired epididymis and the vas deferens to the prostrate. There the sperm is mixed with fluid to form semen. During intercourse, the semen is ejaculated through the male urethra.

k. Endocrine system **pp. 189–191**

The endocrine system consists of eight glands: the hypothalamus, pituitary, thyroid, parathyroid, thymus, pancreas, adrenal, and gonads. These structures secrete chemical messengers (hormones) into the bloodstream. The hypothalamus links the nervous and endocrine system. The pituitary gland is controlled by the hypothalamus and regulates the function of the other endocrine glands. The thyroid gland is located in the anterior neck and regulates body metabolic rates and calcium levels. The parathyroid glands are located laterally to the thyroid and also control calcium levels. The thymus sits just beneath the sternum and promotes the maturation of the immune cells. The pancreas produces and secretes insulin and glycogen to control the blood glucose levels. Adrenal glands secrete epinephrine and norepinephrine, the principle hormones of the sympathetic nervous system, as well as hormones responsible for regulation of fluid and salt balance and metabolism.

l. Special sensory system **pp. 193–196**

The ears provide both hearing and positional sense functions while the eyes provide for sight. The nose senses odors; the tongue, taste; and the skin senses pain, pressure, and temperature.

7. Identify the four quadrants of the abdomen, and list the organs contained in each. **pp. 187–188**

Right upper quadrant (RUQ): most of the liver, gallbladder, small intestine, large intestine, right kidney

Left upper quadrant (LUQ): part of the liver, stomach, small intestine, large intestine, spleen, left kidney, large intestine, pancreas

Right lower quadrant (RLQ): appendix, small intestine, large intestine, right ovary, uterus, urinary bladder, ureter

Left lower quadrant (LLQ): small intestine, large intestine, left ovary, uterus, urinary bladder, ureter

8. Describe the difference between ventilation and respiration. **pp. 177–181**

Respiration is the actual exchange of oxygen and carbon dioxide between the air in the alveoli and the capillary and the capillary and the body cell. Ventilation is the mechanical process that moves air in and out of the lungs. Ventilation is necessary for respiration to occur.

9. Define the terms joint, cartilage, ligament, and tendon. **p. 147**

A **joint** is a relatively sophisticated structure where bones are held together and, in most cases, can move. Numerous types of joints exist in the body, and are classified by the amount of movement they permit.

Cartilage is a continuous collagen extension of the underlying bone and covers a portion of the epiphyseal surface. Cartilage is very slippery and somewhat compressible, permits relatively friction-free joint movement, and absorbs some of the shock associated with activity, such as walking.

©2008 Pearson Education, Inc.
Intermediate Emergency Care: 1985, 3rd ed.

A **ligament** is a band of connective tissue that holds bones together at a joint. It stretches and permits motion at the joint while holding the bone ends firmly in position. The ends of the ligaments attach to the joint ends of each of the associated bones.

Tendons connect muscles to bones.

Case Study Review

Reread the case study in Chapter 7 and then read the following discussion. This case study demonstrates the important link between understanding the anatomy and physiology of the human body and the assessment and care of the prehospital patient.

Michelle, Sean, and Mark are asked to respond to a "reported unconscious diabetic." Sean and Mark know from their past training and experience that a diabetic problem is related to the body's control of blood and cellular sugar (glucose) levels and that this control is provided by the endocrine system and specifically the pancreas. They will direct much of their assessment to determine if the problem is truly due to diabetes, although they will also assure the other body systems are functioning properly.

The patient displays confusion because the brain cannot store glucose and suffers early when the blood glucose falls. The patient becomes diaphoretic as the sympathetic portion of the autonomic nervous system is activated. Blood is diverted to more critical organs from the integumentary system, resulting in the cool clammy skin. Hypertension is a problem associated with the cardiovascular system and may or may not have a bearing on this patient's condition. Her blood pressure of 128/78 would be considered normal; however in light of preexisting hypertension, they will probably consider this patient somewhat hypotensive.

The team also quickly examines the effectiveness of the patient's other body systems. The respiratory system is providing breaths at a normal rate and volume, with the lungs clear of edema. The heart is pumping an adequate volume of blood (full pulse), at an appropriate regular rate (at 92) and the heart demonstrates normal electrical activity on the ECG. These systems are working well together as the blood arriving at the fingertip reveals a hemoglobin saturation of 97%. The peripheral nervous system seems to be operating well as there are no distal sensory or motor deficits noted. This information suggests that the patient's problem may indeed be caused by an endocrine problem, and most likely, hypoglycemia.

As Sean checks the blood glucose level, the problem is confirmed. The reading of 32 mg/dL is very low and explains the confusion and the patient's other signs. In this patient, the pancreas does not normally produce adequate amounts of insulin. The patient takes supplemental insulin to help the body compensate. However, with the stress of infection the pancreas increases its production of insulin and the body consumes glucose more quickly. When the patient takes her insulin, her blood glucose drops and she now shows the signs and symptoms of hypoglycemia.

The understanding that Sean possesses regarding human body systems is very helpful in making sense of the various disease processes. It forms the basis to understand an individual disease, its impact on the human body, its presentations (signs and symptoms), and the care steps that might be beneficial.

Content Self-Evaluation

Multiple Choice

______ 1. The fundamental unit of the human body is
- A. the cell.
- B. tissue.
- C. the organ.
- D. the organism.
- E. DNA.

©2008 Pearson Education, Inc.

_____ 2. One of the three main elements of a typical cell is the
A. cell membrane.
B. cilia.
C. leukocyte.
D. eosinophil.
E. basophil.

_____ 3. The characteristic ability of a cell membrane to selectively permit material to pass through it is called
A. diffusiveness.
B. imperviousness.
C. semipermeability.
D. cytoplasmicism.
E. isotonicism.

_____ 4. The thick viscous fluid that fills the cell and gives it shape is called
A. ribosome.
B. lysosome.
C. cytoplasm.
D. protoplasm.
E. C or D

_____ 5. The tissue type that covers the internal and external body surfaces is
A. epithelial.
B. smooth muscle.
C. nerve.
D. connective.
E. skeletal muscle.

_____ 6. The tissue type that is mostly under voluntary control is
A. epithelial.
B. cardiac muscle.
C. nerve.
D. connective.
E. skeletal muscle.

_____ 7. The tissue type that provides support and insulation is
A. epithelial.
B. cardiac muscle.
C. nerve.
D. connective.
E. skeletal muscle.

_____ 8. Which of the following cavities contains elements of the central nervous system?
A. abdominal
B. cranial
C. spinal
D. thoracic
E. B and C

_____ 9. Which of the following is located within the thorax?
A. the heart
B. both lungs
C. the esophagus
D. the trachea
E. all of the above

_____ 10. The structure that separates the chest cavity from the abdominal cavity is the
A. mediastinum.
B. peritoneum.
C. perineum.
D. diaphragm.
E. vena cava.

_____ 11. The body organ system that produces most body heat is the
A. muscular system.
B. gastrointestinal system.
C. genitourinary system.
D. endocrine system.
E. lymphatic system.

_____ 12. The body organ system that is important in fighting disease and filtration is the
A. muscular system.
B. gastrointestinal system.
C. genitourinary system.
D. endocrine system.
E. lymphatic system.

_____ 13. Which of the following is NOT a function performed by the musculoskeletal system?
A. vital organ protection
B. a portion of the immune response
C. storage of material necessary for metabolism
D. produces red blood cells
E. efficient movement against gravity

©2008 Pearson Education, Inc.
Intermediate Emergency Care: 1985, 3rd ed.

______ 14. The central portion of a long bone is called the
A. diaphysis.
B. epiphysis.
C. metaphysis.
D. cancellous bone.
E. compact bone.

______ 15. The region at both ends of the long bones is called the
A. diaphysis.
B. epiphysis.
C. metaphysis.
D. cancellous bone.
E. compact bone.

______ 16. The covering of the shaft of the long bones that initiates the bone repair cycle is the
A. periosteum.
B. peritoneum.
C. perforating canal.
D. osteocyte.
E. epiphysis.

______ 17. Bands of strong material that stretch and hold the joint together while permitting movement are the
A. bursae.
B. tendons.
C. ligaments.
D. cartilage.
E. metaphyses.

______ 18. A large (actually the largest) opening in the cranium is the
A. auditory canal.
B. orbit of the eye.
C. foramen magnum.
D. tentorium.
E. transverse foramen.

______ 19. The vertebral column is made up of how many vertebrae?
A. 24
B. 33
C. 43
D. 45
E. 54

______ 20. The region of the vertebral column that has 12 vertebrae is the
A. cervical.
B. thoracic.
C. lumbar.
D. sacral.
E. coccygeal.

______ 21. How many rib pairs are floating ribs?
A. 1
B. 2
C. 3
D. 6
E. 8

______ 22. The muscular system consists of about how many muscles?
A. 100
B. 200
C. 300
D. 500
E. 700

______ 23. The outermost layer of the skin is the
A. epidermis.
B. subcutaneous tissue.
C. cutical.
D. dermis.
E. sebum.

______ 24. Which of the following glands secrete sebum?
A. sudoriferous glands
B. sebaceous glands
C. subcutaneous glands
D. adrenal glands
E. none of the above

______ 25. The transitional area between the end and central portion of the long bone is called the
A. diaphysis.
B. epiphysis.
C. metaphysis.
D. cancellous bone.
E. compact bone.

©2008 Pearson Education, Inc.

______ 26. The cerebellum is the center of conscious thought and perception.
A. True
B. False

______ 27. The layers of the meninges, from the cerebrum to the skull, occur in which sequence?
A. dura mater, pia mater, arachnoid
B. dura mater, arachnoid, pia mater
C. arachnoid, pia mater, dura mater
D. arachnoid, dura mater, pia mater
E. pia mater, arachnoid, dura mater

______ 28. The space between the pia mater and the arachnoid membrane is the
A. epiarachnoid space.
B. epidural space.
C. subarachnoid space.
D. subdural space.
E. cerebral space.

______ 29. The somatic nervous system primarily innervates the
A. cardiac muscle.
B. glands.
C. skeletal muscle.
D. smooth muscle.
E. respiratory system.

______ 30. The _____ nervous system is mediated by acetylcholine, epinephrine, and norepinephrine.
A. autonomic
B. parasympathetic
C. somatic
D. sympathetic
E. central

______ 31. Acetylcholine is the neurotransmitter of which nervous system?
A. adrenergic
B. afferent
C. parasympathetic
D. sympathetic
E. central

______ 32. From innermost to outermost, the three tissue layers of the heart are
A. the endocardium, the pericardium, and the myocardium.
B. the endocardium, the myocardium, and the syncytium.
C. the endocardium, the myocardium, and the pericardium.
D. the myocardium, the epicardium, and the pericardium.
E. the epicardium, the myocardium, and the endocardium.

______ 33. The relaxation phase of the cardiac cycle is called diastole.
A. True
B. False

______ 34. The layer of the meninges that is strong and lines the interior of the cranium is the
A. pia mater.
B. falx cerebri.
C. arachnoid.
D. dura mater.
E. tentorium.

______ 35. The blood vessel that returns blood to the atria from the body is the
A. aorta.
B. inferior vena cava.
C. superior vena cava.
D. pulmonary vein.
E. B and C

______ 36. The blood supply to the left ventricle, interventricular septum, part of the right ventricle, and the heart's conduction system comes from the two branches of the left coronary artery, which are the
A. anterior descending artery and the circumflex artery.
B. anterior descending artery and the posterior descending artery.
C. circumflex artery and the posterior descending artery.
D. circumflex artery and the marginal artery.
E. marginal artery and the posterior descending artery.

©2008 Pearson Education, Inc.
Intermediate Emergency Care: 1985, 3rd ed.

______ 37. The sympathetic receptor in the heart that increases heart rate and contractility is
A. alpha 1.
B. alpha 2.
C. beta 1.
D. beta 2.
E. none of the above

______ 38. Stimulation of the heart by the sympathetic nervous system results in
A. negative inotropic and chronotropic effects.
B. negative chronotropic and dromotropic effects.
C. positive chronotropic and dromotropic effects.
D. positive inotropic and chronotropic effects.
E. positive inotropic and dromotropic effects.

______ 39. The major determinants of blood volume are red blood cell mass and
A. erythropoietin levels.
B. plasma volume.
C. total body water.
D. stem cell percentage.
E. bone marrow volume.

______ 40. The component of the red blood cell that is responsible for transporting oxygen is the
A. basophil.
B. granulocyte.
C. hemoglobin.
D. neutrophil.
E. lymphocyte.

______ 41. The inner layer of the arteries and veins is which of the following?
A. lumen
B. tunica intima
C. tunica media
D. tunica adventitia
E. Purkinje

______ 42. The blood cells responsible for blood clotting are
A. red blood cells.
B. white blood cells.
C. lymphocytes.
D. platelets.
E. monocytes.

______ 43. The delicate vascular organ that performs some immune functions is the
A. spleen.
B. small bowel.
C. pancreas.
D. gallbladder.
E. liver.

______ 44. Which of the following correctly lists the order in which air passes through airway structures during inspiration?
A. trachea, larynx, laryngopharynx, nasopharynx
B. nasopharynx, trachea, laryngopharynx, larynx
C. nasopharynx, laryngopharynx, larynx, trachea
D. laryngopharynx, nasopharynx, larynx, trachea
E. trachea, laryngopharynx, larynx, nasopharynx

______ 45. The point at which the trachea divides into the two mainstem bronchi is called the
A. hilum.
B. parenchyma.
C. vallecula.
D. carina.
E. pleura.

______ 46. The mainstem bronchus that leaves the trachea at almost a straight angle is the right mainstem bronchus.
A. True
B. False

______ 47. The right lung has only two lobes because the heart's greatest mass is on the right.
A. True
B. False

©2008 Pearson Education, Inc.

______ 48. The muscle(s) of respiration responsible for reducing the distance between ribs and helping lift the thorax is (are) the
A. intercostal muscles.
B. diaphragm.
C. sternocleidomastoid muscles.
D. scalene.
E. rectus abdominis.

______ 49. At the beginning of and during most of expiration, the pressure within the thorax is
A. less than the environmental pressure.
B. more than the environmental pressure.
C. equal to the environmental pressure.
D. first lower than and then higher than the environmental pressure.
E. first higher than and then lower than the environmental pressure.

______ 50. The tissue covering each lung and the interior of the thorax is the
A. hilum.
B. parenchyma.
C. vallecula.
D. carina.
E. pleura.

______ 51. Which aspect of the respiratory cycle is passive?
A. inspiration
B. expiration
C. neither A nor B
D. both A and B
E. both A and B, but only during stress

______ 52. The amount of oxygen in the air is approximately
A. 21 percent.
B. 4 percent.
C. 0.4 percent.
D. 0.04 percent.
E. 0.10 percent.

______ 53. Which of the following will reduce the carbon dioxide levels in the blood?
A. administration of bicarbonate
B. administration of antacids
C. hyperventilation
D. high-flow oxygen
E. hypoventilation

______ 54. Which of the following statements is TRUE regarding the digestive tract?
A. It is a 25-foot-long hollow tube.
B. It churns food.
C. It introduces digestive juices.
D. It propels food through it.
E. all of the above

______ 55. In what order does digesting food pass through the digestive tract?
A. duodenum, ileum, jejunum, colon
B. duodenum, jejunum, ileum, colon
C. jejunum, ileum, colon, duodenum
D. ileum, jejunum, colon, duodenum
E. colon, jejunum, ileum, duodenum

______ 56. The movement of digesting material through the digestive system occurs through a process called
A. peristalsis.
B. chyme.
C. peritonitis.
D. emulsification.
E. evisceration.

______ 57. The solid organ of the abdomen responsible for detoxifying blood is the
A. spleen.
B. small bowel.
C. pancreas.
D. gallbladder.
E. liver.

______ 58. Which of the following abdominal organs is found in the left upper quadrant?
A. spleen
B. gallbladder
C. appendix
D. sigmoid colon
E. liver

©2008 Pearson Education, Inc.
Intermediate Emergency Care: 1985, 3rd ed.

______ 59. Which of the following abdominal organs is found in the right lower quadrant?
A. spleen
B. gallbladder
C. appendix
D. sigmoid colon
E. liver

______ 60. Which of the following abdominal organs is found in all of the abdominal quadrants?
A. pancreas
B. gallbladder
C. appendix
D. sigmoid colon
E. small bowel

______ 61. The major functions of the urinary system include all of the following EXCEPT
A. maintenance of blood volume.
B. control of development of white blood cells.
C. regulation of arterial blood pressure.
D. maintenance of the balance of electrolytes.
E. removal of many toxic wastes from the blood.

______ 62. A muscular tube that forms the most distal part of the female reproductive system is the
A. ureter.
B. urethra.
C. vagina.
D. vulva.
E. fallopian tube.

______ 63. Sperm cells are eliminated from a man's body after they move out of the testicles and pass through the following structures in first-to-last sequence.
A. vas deferens, epididymis, urethra
B. ureter, epididymis, vas deferens, urethra
C. epididymis, vas deferens, urethra
D. epididymis, vas deferens, prostate gland, urethra
E. vas deferens, epididymis, prostate gland, urethra

______ 64. The gland that is the connection between the endocrine system and the central nervous system is the
A. pituitary.
B. hypothalamus.
C. thymus.
D. pineal.
E. thyroid.

______ 65. The hormones epinephrine and norepinephrine are secreted by the adrenal medulla.
A. True
B. False

______ 66. The structure responsible for our positional sense is the
A. ossicle.
B. cochlea.
C. semicircular canals.
D. sinuses.
E. vitreous humor.

______ 67. Which of the following is the opening through which light travels to contact the light-sensing tissue in the eye?
A. retina
B. aqueous humor
C. vitreous humor
D. pupil
E. iris

______ 68. Which of the following is the light-sensing tissue in the eye?
A. retina
B. aqueous humor
C. vitreous humor
D. pupil
E. iris

______ 69. The white of the eye is the
A. sclera.
B. conjunctiva.
C. cornea.
D. aqueous humor.
E. vitreous humor.

©2008 Pearson Education, Inc.

_____ 70. The delicate, clear tissue covering the pupil and iris is the
A. sclera.
B. conjunctiva.
C. cornea.
D. aqueous humor.
E. vitreous humor.

©2008 Pearson Education, Inc.
Intermediate Emergency Care: 1985, 3rd ed.

Chapter 8

General Patient Assessment and Initial Management

Review of Chapter Objectives

After reading this chapter, you should be able to do the following:

1. **Understand the importance of a step-by-step approach to high-quality prehospital intermediate life support.** **pp. 204–205**

   Assures a thorough and complete assessment that identifies all significant patient problems and symptoms
   Enables an EMT-Intermediate to correct life-threatening situations and to establish the priorities of care
   Assures continuity of care through communication to the emergency department

2. **Identify the information gathered in each phase of patient assessment.** **pp. 205–258**

   Review of dispatch information
   - Location of the call
   - Nature of the call
   - Equipment that may be needed
   - Other units that may be responding

   Scene size-up/environmental safety
   - Hazards to personal and patient safety (standard precautions)
   - Mechanism of injury
   - Number of patients
   - Additional resources needed

   Initial assessment
   - Rapid identification of life-threatening injuries/problems
   - Rapid correction of life-threatening injuries/problems
   - Determination of the priority for transport

   Focused exam and history
   - Head-to-toe evaluation for the signs of injury
   - Verbal questioning for symptoms
   - Inspection, palpation, auscultation, and percussion

   Vital signs
   - Pulse rate and quality
   - Respiratory rate, depth, and effort
   - Blood pressure
   - Temperature—core and peripheral

Patient history
History of previous illness
Past medical history
Medications
Allergies
Personal physician

3. Describe the type of information that can be obtained from a careful evaluation of the dispatcher's information. **pp. 205–206**

Type of run (medical vs. trauma)
Seriousness
Multiple patient incidents
Hazardous material incidents
Crime scenes
Patient age and sex
Chief complaint and significant history
Scene survey/environmental safety

4. Recognize hazards/potential hazards associated with the medical and trauma scene. **pp. 206–213**

During the scene size-up, you must examine the scene before you arrive at the patient's side. It is a time to evaluate and prepare for hazards including blood, fluids, airborne pathogens, and other conditions that may threaten your life or health. These conditions include the hazards of fire, structural collapse, traffic, unstable surfaces, electricity, broken glass, or jagged metal. Hazardous materials can involve chemical spills, radiation, and toxic environments. Finally, scene hazards can also include violent, disturbed, or unruly bystanders or patients. These hazards are not limited to the trauma scene but may be found at many medical scenes as well.

5. Identify unsafe scenes and describe methods for making them safe. **pp. 207–213**

Your responsibility at the emergency scene is to recognize hazards, including fire, structural collapse, traffic, unstable surfaces, electricity, broken glass, jagged metal, and hazardous materials and then act appropriately to protect yourself, other rescuers, and your patient. Unless you are specially trained and equipped to handle a specific hazard, do not enter the scene. In most cases, you will rely on the fire department, rescue service, police department, power company, hazmat team, or other specially trained personnel to secure the scene before you enter. If there is ever a question of whether a scene is safe or unsafe, do not enter the scene.

6. Discuss common mechanisms of injury/nature of illness. **pp. 214–216**

Trauma is induced by a mechanism of injury through which forces enter the body and do physical harm. Common mechanisms include blunt trauma—for example, vehicle crashes (auto, recreational, watercraft, and bicycle), pedestrian vs. vehicle impacts, falls—and penetrating trauma—for example, gunshot and knife wounds. Medical problems have a related cause called the nature of the illness. The scene can provide evidence as to the nature of the illness. Examples include the presence of nebulizers, which suggest asthma, drug paraphernalia, which suggest overdose, and medications, which suggest preexisting cardiac or other problems.

7. Discuss the reason for identifying the total number of patients at the scene. **p. 214**

Determining the number of patients at a scene is important to assure that the needed resources are summoned to the scene and that every patient is cared for. At each and every scene, you should ask yourself, "Could there be others who are injured or ill?" While at the trauma scene it is common to find a patient wandering among the bystanders; the medical scene can have "hidden patients" too. The wife of a cardiac arrest patient, for example, may herself become a patient because of the emotional stress of the incident. Knowing the number of patients can help you gauge whether on-scene resources are adequate or whether you need to request that additional

©2008 Pearson Education, Inc.
Intermediate Emergency Care: 1985, 3rd ed.

units and manpower be dispatched to the scene. The earlier this request is made, the quicker those resources will arrive.

8. Organize the management of a scene following size-up. p. 212

The management of the scene following the scene size-up includes requesting both the appropriate units and personnel to manage scene hazards and the appropriate number and care levels of ambulances and personnel to treat the patients. You must also take the necessary steps to assure overall scene safety and to protect yourself, the patient, other scene personnel, and bystanders. The scene size-up also prepares you to manage the care of the patient by helping you recognize the mechanism of injury and anticipate injuries (index of suspicion) or by recognizing the nature of the illness.

9. Explain the reasons for identifying the need for additional help or assistance during the scene size-up. pp. 206–211

Multiple patients at the emergency scene can rapidly overwhelm your ability to provide effective care. If you wait until you are at a patient's side before calling for additional help, you may be distracted from making the call and delay an effective response. In cases where the number of patients far outstrips your ability to provide care, you may need to initiate a mass casualty response.

10. Summarize the reasons for forming a general impression of the patient. p. 217

The initial general impression of your patient takes into account the patient's age, gender, race, and other factors that will help you determine the seriousness of the problem and establish your priorities for patient care and transport. As you learn more about the patient through the initial assessment and the focused history and physical assessment, you will refine and improve on the accuracy and depth of the general impression. As you develop your general impression of the patient early in the assessment process, you can also begin to establish a rapport with him or her, explaining why you are there, what will be happening to him or her, and giving the patient the opportunity to refuse care.

11. Discuss methods of assessing mental status/levels of consciousness in the adult, infant, and child patient. pp. 218–219

Initially determine the patient's mental status by categorizing him according to the AVPU system. Using this method, the patient is classified either Alert, responsive to Verbal stimuli, responsive to Painful stimuli, or Unresponsive. You can further refine the evaluation by questioning the patient to determine orientation to place, time, and person and by differentiating his or her response to pain into purposeful and purposeless movement and decerebrate and decorticate posturing categories. An alert response for the infant or child is difficult to assess because of that patient's limited speech capabilities. Evaluate pediatric patients for activity and curiosity, being aware that the quiet child is often a seriously ill or injured one.

12. Describe the A, B, and C of the initial assessment. pp. 216, 219–227

Airway and cervical spine control—Ensures that the trauma patient's spine is stabilized and that the airway is maintained and clear of obstruction (In the unconscious patient, this may involve patient positioning or include basic and advanced airway procedures such as oral airway or endotracheal tube placement.)

Breathing—Ensures that respirations are adequate in volume and rate (Breathing may be assisted with supplemental oxygen or provided by bag-valve mask.)

Circulation—Determines if capillary refill is more than 3 seconds, if the skin is cool and clammy, if pulses are rapid and weak, or if distal pulses are absent (If such signs suggest shock, elevate the patient's legs and consider the use of PASG. Stop any obvious and severe hemorrhage.)

©2008 Pearson Education, Inc.

13. Explain the reason and process for prioritizing a patient for care and transport. pp. 227–228

At the conclusion of the initial assessment, you must determine your patient's priority, which will indicate how to proceed with assessment, care, and transport. With a seriously ill or injured patient, perform a rapid head-to-toe assessment. With a stable medical or trauma patient, perform a focused history and physical exam. You will also need to determine the priority for transport—either immediate transport with care rendered en route or with most care provided at the scene followed by transport.

14. Discuss the reasons for reconsidering the mechanism of injury. pp. 228–229

After the initial and rapid trauma assessments or focused history and physical exam, you have gathered enough information about your patient to determine if the mechanism of injury (and your resulting index of suspicion for associated injuries) agree with your assessment findings. If they do, maintain your priority for care and transport. If they do not agree, reevaluate your index of suspicion and the physical findings and possibly adjust your patient's priority. If you do alter your patient's priority, always err on the side of precaution.

15. Explain why patients should receive a rapid trauma assessment. pp. 229–230

Every patient with a significant mechanism of injury, an altered level of consciousness, or multiple body-system traumas should receive the rapid trauma assessment. These patients are likely to have serious internal injuries and/or hemorrhage. However, the signs and symptoms of serious injury and shock are often hidden by other, more gruesome or painful injuries or by the body's compensatory mechanisms. Without maintaining a high index of suspicion for serious injury and evaluating the patient via the rapid trauma assessment, you are likely to overlook the patient with serious and life-threatening injury.

16. Discuss medical identification devices/systems. p. 233

Examine the patient's wrists, ankles, and neck for medical alert jewelry reflecting preexisting medical conditions such as diabetes, epilepsy, allergies, use of medications, and the like. Also check the wallet or purse for such information. This information may help you and the emergency department in prescribing care for the patient.

17. Describe physical examination of the trauma patient. pp. 229–235

The physical assessment of the trauma patient begins during the initial assessment with the check of the ABCs and then branches to either the rapid trauma assessment or focused history and physical exam. The patient with a serious mechanism of injury, altered mental status, or multi-system trauma receives a rapid trauma assessment, a fast, systematic physical exam evaluating body regions where serious or life-threatening problems are likely to occur. This assessment is a rapid evaluation of the critical structures and regions of the head (HEENT), neck, chest, abdomen, pelvis, extremities, posterior body, and vital signs. The patient with isolated trauma has an assessment directed at the areas of expected injury or patient complaint.

18. Describe the elements of the rapid trauma assessment and discuss their evaluation. pp. 230–235

Each region of the body is inspected, palpated, and, as appropriate, auscultated and percussed to identify the signs of injury (DCAP-BTLS and crepitation). For each region, the specific assessment considerations include the following:

Evaluate the head for any signs of serious bleeding and deformity from skull fracture. Also check for discharge from the ears and nose, for the stability of the facial bones, and for the patency of the airway.

Evaluate the neck for lacerations involving the major blood vessels and serious hemorrhage and possible air embolism. Examine the jugular veins for abnormal distention and palpate the position and any unusual motion of the trachea. Also examine for subcutaneous emphysema and then any evidence of spinal trauma.

©2008 Pearson Education, Inc.
Intermediate Emergency Care: 1985, 3rd ed.

Evaluate the chest for signs of respiratory distress, including use of accessory muscles and retractions, and any signs of open wounds. Also observe the motion of the chest. Chest excursion should be bilaterally equal and symmetrical. Palpate for signs of clavicular or costal fracture and subcutaneous emphysema. Erythema may be present, but the frank ecchymotic discoloration of a contusion takes time to develop. Auscultate the lungs at the mid-axillary line for bilaterally equal breath sounds.

Evaluate the abdomen for exaggerated abdominal wall motion, and inspect and palpate for signs of injury, noting rigidity, guarding, tenderness, and rebound tenderness.

Evaluate the pelvis for signs of injury and apply pressure directed posteriorly and medially to the iliac crests and pressure directed posteriorly to the symphysis pubis to check for pelvic instability.

Evaluate the extremities for signs of injury, distal circulation, and innervation.

Evaluate the posterior body for signs of injury, and be especially watchful for potential signs of spinal injury.

Evaluate vital signs, first to establish a baseline, and then to obtain other readings to compare to that baseline. Evaluate direct pupil response to light during the rapid trauma assessment, but evaluate the other pupillary responses during more specific and directed evaluation.

Gather a patient history while you perform the rapid trauma assessment. This should include the elements of the SAMPLE assessment (Signs/Symptoms, Allergies, Medications, Past medical history, Last oral intake, and Events preceding the incident).

19. Identify cases when the rapid assessment is altered or suspended to provide patient care. pp. 230–233

The rapid trauma assessment is interrupted to provide patient care whenever you identify any life-threatening condition that can be quickly addressed. Just as you would suction the airway when you find it full of fluids during the initial assessment, you might provide pleural decompression during the rapid trauma assessment when you notice a developing tension pneumothorax. You might also administer oxygen to a patient who begins to display dyspnea and accessory muscle use during your chest examination. Other examples might include employing the PASG for the patient with the early signs of shock compensation and an unstable pelvic fracture found during the pelvic assessment or immediate provision of spinal immobilization upon noticing a neurologic deficit during the extremity exam.

20. List the steps in conducting a patient history. pp. 236–238

Introductions
Chief complaint
History of present illness
Past medical history
Family and social history

21. Identify the questions that should be asked for a pertinent patient history. pp. 235–237

Chief complaint/history of present illness (OPQRST)

Onset: What were you doing when the problem began? Did it start slowly or quickly?

Provocative and palliative factors: What events, actions, or circumstances might be related to the onset of pain or discomfort? What circumstances either increase or decrease the pain or discomfort of the chief complaint?

Quality of the chief complaint: How is the pain described by the patient? Is it gnawing, cramping, dull, sharp, etc.?

Region, radiation, and recurrence of symptoms: What is the exact location of the pain or discomfort? Is it moving or radiating?

Severity of symptoms: How severe is the pain as assessed by the patient's description and his or her reaction to it?

Time of symptoms: How long has the discomfort or pain affected the patient? Is it an acute problem or one that developed over time?

©2008 Pearson Education, Inc.

Past Medical History (SAMPLE)
S = Signs and symptoms
What signs or symptoms do you have?
A = Allergies
What substances or medications is the patient allergic to, and could they be contributing factor?
M = Medications
What prescribed medications is the patient using, what are they for, and could they be contributing to the current problem?
P = Past Medical History
What preexisting medical problems does the patient have? Are they pertinent to the current problem?
L = Last eaten
What did you last eat and drink?
E = Events
What were you doing when this began?

22. Explain responses for compiling a family/social history. **p. 238**

Identify heredity and lifestyle factors that may be related to or contributing to the patient's problem, such as smoking, substance abuse, or a family history of cardiac or hypertension disease.

23. Describe physical examination of the medical patient. **pp. 238–241**

The medical patient physical exam evaluates the head, ears, eyes, nose, and throat (HEENT), chest, abdomen, pelvis, extremities, posterior surface, and vital signs discreetly, looking for illness or disease signs. The exam may be modified to meet the specific patient complaints of chest pain, respiratory distress, altered mental status, and acute abdomen. The medical patient exam may also include pulse oximetry, cardiac and glucose level monitoring as well as venous blood sampling.

24. Discuss the reason for performing a focused history and physical exam. **p. 228**

The focused history and physical exam is the third step (following the scene size-up and initial assessment) of the patient assessment process. It is an assessment directed at the areas where the signs of serious injury or illness are expected. It also draws upon a quick history to identify information supporting a specific diagnosis and elements critical to the continued care of the patient. The focused history and physical exam takes you quickly toward determining the nature of the illness or the existence of serious and specific injuries. It is performed in different ways for trauma patients with significant injuries or mechanisms of injury, trauma patients with isolated injuries, responsive medical patients, and unresponsive medical patients.

25. Cite some of the differences in assessing the trauma and medical patient. **pp. 228–242**

Trauma patient—assessed through the primary survey to determine whether he or she would be best served by rapid transport or on-scene care; need to examine mechanism of injury, the signs or symptoms of serious internal or external injury, and the status of airway, breathing, and circulation

Medical patient—assessed to determine any immediate life threat—such as ectopic pregnancy—which may demand immediate transport; need to determine the problem affecting the patient through signs, symptoms, and patient history, since the mechanism of injury may not be apparent

26. Describe the methods of conducting a prehospital physical examination. **pp. 248–250**

Inspection—observation of the patient's body for signs of injury or disease such as deformities, contusions, lacerations, discolorations, bleeding, etc.

Palpation—feeling of a patient's body for deformities, temperature variation, crepitus, masses, guarding, tenderness, etc.

Auscultation—listening through a stethoscope to breath sounds generated by the patient, such as crackles and wheezes

©2008 Pearson Education, Inc.
Intermediate Emergency Care: 1985, 3rd ed.

27. Identify the steps in conducting a head-to-toe physical examination. **pp. 250–255**

Head—examination of the ears, eyes, facial bones, nose, and mouth for signs of injury or medical problems, including:
- Battle's sign
- Bilateral periorbital ecchymosis (raccoon eyes)
- Cerebrospinal fluid (CSF) drainage
- Pupillary size, response, and tracking
- Instability
- Swelling, discoloration, hemorrhage, wounds

Neck—examination of the neck for the following:
- Jugular vein distention
- Tracheal deviation
- Crepitus
- Swelling, discoloration, hemorrhage, wounds

Chest and upper back—examination of the chest and upper back for the following:
- Symmetry, bilateral excursion
- Retraction, paradoxical movement, sucking chest wounds
- Crackles, wheezes, diminished or unequal breath sounds
- Respiratory rate, depth, and pattern
- Instability, crepitus
- Swelling, discoloration, hemorrhage, wounds

Abdomen and lower back—examination of the abdomen and lower back for the following:
- Symmetry, pulsation
- Diaphragmatic breathing
- Tenderness, rebound tenderness, guarding, or distention
- Swelling, discoloration, hemorrhage, wounds
- Evisceration

Pelvis—examination of the pelvis for the following:
- Crepitus, instability
- Swelling, discoloration, hemorrhage, wounds
- Genitalia—examination of the genitalia for the following:
  - Swelling, discoloration, hemorrhage, wounds, discharge

Lower extremities—examination of the lower extremities for the following:
- Distal pulse, capillary refill, neurologic deficit
- Instability, crepitus
- Swelling, discoloration, hemorrhage, wounds

Upper extremities—examination of the upper extremities for the following:
- Distal pulse, capillary refill, neurologic deficit
- Instability, crepitus
- Swelling, discoloration, hemorrhage, wounds

28. Discuss the evaluation of the four prehospital vital signs. **pp. 242–246**

Blood pressure—suggests the effectiveness of the circulatory system (In adults, systolic blood pressure above 140 mmHg or diastolic above 90 mmHg suggest hypertension.)

Pulse—irregularities in rate and strength may suggest stress, shock, head injury, or other problems (A normal pulse rate is between 60 and 100 beats per minute. Children have a faster heart rate, while well-conditioned athletes have slower rates.)

Respirations—rate, volume, and pattern used to determine the effectiveness and efficiency of respiratory effort (Normal respirations in the adult occur at 12 to 20 breaths per minute, with each breath moving about 500 mL of air. In the child, the rate is faster, while the volume of each breath is lower.)

Skin condition—provides indication of the body's ability to generate and dissipate heat to maintain a standard internal environment at 37°C (The skin should be pink, warm, and dry to the touch.)

©2008 Pearson Education, Inc.

29. Describe the components of the ongoing assessment, and discuss the rationale for repeating the initial assessment. **pp. 255–258**

The components of the ongoing assessment include reassessment of the pertinent elements of the initial assessment, focused history and physical exam or rapid trauma assessment, and vital signs and include:

Mental status. Quickly reevaluate the patient's mental status to determine AVPU status or level of orientation.

Airway patency/breathing rate and quality. Perform a quick check of airway patency and breathing rate, volume, and quality to assure respiration is adequate.

Pulse rate and quality. Quickly reevaluate the pulse rate, strength, and regularity to assure they remain within normal limits.

Skin condition. Quickly check the skin for moisture, temperature, and capillary refill to monitor distal perfusion.

Vital signs. Reassess blood pressure and temperature (along with pulse and respiration) and compare to baseline findings to determine whether the patient's condition is improving, deteriorating, or remaining the same.

Focused assessment. Quickly reevaluate the signs of injury/illness to identify any changes. This may include reevaluating pertinent negatives to rule out an evolving problem.

Effects of interventions. Repeat the ongoing assessment soon after any major intervention to determine the intervention's impact on the patient's condition.

Transport priorities. Based upon the findings of the ongoing assessment, either confirm or modify the patient's priority for care and transport.

The initial assessment, with its examination of mental status and evaluation of the airway, breathing, and circulation, contains crucial elements of continuing patient assessment. These components of the initial assessment can quickly tell you when the patient is suffering from a life-threatening or serious problem and can help you monitor the patient's need for care. For this reason, these components are an integral part of any ongoing assessment.

30. Describe trending of assessment components. **p. 258**

Trending of the elements of the ongoing assessment—comparing of sequential findings—will suggest whether your patient's condition is improving, deteriorating, or remaining the same. This information prompts you to modify your priorities for patient care and transport, and may ultimately cause you to modify your field diagnosis.

Case Study Review

Reread the case study in Chapter 8 and then read the following discussion. This case study examines an assault and applies the elements of response that have been addressed within this chapter. Included in this case study are the dispatch information, scene survey, primary assessment, determination of the need for rapid transport or on-scene care, and some of the steps of immediate patient stabilization as called for by the primary survey.

Wendy and Sean listen carefully to the dispatch information as they prepare to respond. They note the "unfriendly" part of town and agree that they will not arrive at the scene until the police secure it. The nature of the call, "assault," tells them to expect trauma: a gunshot, knife wound, or blunt trauma from a fist fight. Wendy accesses the trauma kit and reviews the regional trauma protocols and identifies the location of the nearest trauma center while Sean drives to the scene. As they follow the police into the scene they know it will be secure shortly. However, they are very cautious as these types of calls can become dangerous very quickly.

There is excitement at the scene as the EMT-Intermediates arrive. However, the assessment process drilled into Wendy and Sean during their training and few years of experience ensures that they will follow an organized and ordered step-by-step assessment process. They will employ the scene size-up and initial assessment and then determine the patient's need for immediate care and transport.

©2008 Pearson Education, Inc.
Intermediate Emergency Care: 1985, 3rd ed.

Wendy assumes responsibility for the initial assessment, while Sean stabilizes the head and neck. Wendy clears the airway with suction and inserts the oral airway. She then moves to the next primary assessment step: breathing. The patient is breathing with rapid, shallow breaths. Wendy exposes the chest and discovers a sucking chest wound. She quickly seals the wound while Sean begins ventilation with a bag-valve mask and oxygen flowing at 15 l per minute.

Wendy notices that the patient's radial pulse is strong. This sign suggests the patient's circulatory status is stable for now. Through her experience, Wendy knows that the body compensates well for blood loss, especially in younger patients. She continues to monitor both the vital signs and the patient's level of consciousness for any signs of deterioration.

Wendy relays the findings of her initial assessment to paramedic John Scanlon. She tells him of the sealed pneumothorax, the absence of breath sounds on the right side, the patient's circulatory status, and his level of consciousness. The patient's level of consciousness and the penetrating chest injury both require immediate transport to the trauma center.

Content Self-Evaluation

Multiple Choice

_____ 1. Which of the following is not a phase of assessment?
A. review of the dispatch information
B. the vital signs
C. detailed physical assessment
D. ongoing assessment
E. initial assessment

_____ 2. After the scene size-up and if necessary, you should inform the dispatcher of
A. the nature of the medical or trauma emergency.
B. what resources you need.
C. the phone number at which you can be reached.
D. what actions you and your crew are taking.
E. all of the above except C

_____ 3. The scene size-up should include all of the following except
A. identification of mechanism of injury.
B. identification of hazards.
C. assessment of the patient for life-threatening problems.
D. locating all potential patients.
E. determination of any additional assistance needed.

_____ 4. Which of the following is NOT a component of the scene size-up?
A. standard precautions
B. general impression of the patient
C. location of all patients
D. mechanism of injury/nature of the illness analysis
E. scene safety

_____ 5. Which of the following standard precaution devices will you employ with every patient you treat?
A. latex or vinyl gloves
B. protective eyewear
C. face mask
D. gown
E. B and C

_____ 6. Whenever you plan to intubate a patient, you should wear
A. latex or vinyl gloves and a gown.
B. protective eyewear, a gown, and a face mask.
C. latex or vinyl gloves, protective eyewear, and a face mask.
D. protective eyewear and a gown.
E. latex or vinyl gloves.

©2008 Pearson Education, Inc.

_____ 7. The HEPA respirator is designed to filter out which of the following pathogens that may be encountered when providing prehospital emergency care?
A. tuberculosis
B. small pox
C. anthrax
D. the flu
E. tetanus toxoid

_____ 8. The intent of the safety analysis portion of the scene survey is to assure the safety of
A. the patient.
B. bystanders.
C. fellow responders.
D. yourself.
E. all of the above

_____ 9. To properly handle a scene safety issue, you must be
A. properly trained.
B. properly equipped.
C. properly clothed.
D. prepared to attempt rescue procedures in which you have not been trained.
E. A, B, and C

_____ 10. Potential hazards to rule out before entering the scene include all of the following EXCEPT
A. fire.
B. electrocution.
C. contamination with blood.
D. structural collapse.
E. broken glass and jagged metal.

_____ 11. When called to a shooting or domestic disturbance, until the police arrive and secure the scene you should remain
A. outside the neighborhood.
B. outside the residence.
C. just down the street.
D. at the door but don't enter.
E. either B or C

_____ 12. At which of the following incidents would you NOT expect to discover more than one patient in your scene size-up?
A. a two-car accident
B. a carbon monoxide poisoning in a home
C. a car crash in which a child seat and diaper bag are visible
D. a fall out of a tree
E. a hazardous materials spill in a high-school chemistry lab

_____ 13. You should delay the call for additional ambulances until you begin your initial assessment because you will not have enough information to determine the needs of the scene until then.
A. True
B. False

_____ 14. The two important functions that must begin immediately in the mass-casualty situation are
A. triage and incident command.
B. rescue and triage.
C. fire fighting and rescue.
D. incident command and extrication.
E. incident command and scene isolation.

_____ 15. The responsibilities of incident command at a disaster scene include all of the following EXCEPT
A. performing a scene size-up.
B. triaging initial patients for care.
C. determining the need for additional resources.
D. radioing for additional equipment and personnel.
E. directing incoming crews.

©2008 Pearson Education, Inc.
Intermediate Emergency Care: 1985, 3rd ed.

______ 16. The responsibilities of the triage person at the disaster scene include all of the following EXCEPT
A. determining a patient's priority for immediate transport.
B. determining a patient's priority for delayed transport.
C. performing simple, but lifesaving procedures.
D. providing intensive care on salvageable patients.
E. all of the above

______ 17. The mechanism of injury analysis examines
A. body locations affected.
B. strength of the crash forces.
C. direction of the crash forces.
D. nature of the crash forces.
E. all of the above

______ 18. The index of suspicion is best defined as
A. patient priority for care based on the MOI.
B. anticipation of the nature of forces involved in an accident.
C. anticipation of injuries based upon the MOI.
D. anticipation of degree of injury based on the patient's appearance.
E. none of the above

______ 19. The nature of the illness is determined from information you receive from
A. the patient.
B. the patient's family.
C. bystanders.
D. scene clues.
E. all of the above

______ 20. The initial assessment includes all of the following EXCEPT
A. forming a general impression of the patient.
B. stabilizing the cervical spine as needed.
C. immobilizing of fractures.
D. assessing the airway.
E. assessing the circulation.

______ 21. The general patient impression is based upon all of the following EXCEPT
A. blood pressure.
B. mechanism of injury.
C. chief complaint.
D. the environment.
E. your instincts.

______ 22. The first step of the initial assessment is
A. airway assessment.
B. breathing assessment.
C. forming a general impression.
D. airway assessment with cervical spine stabilization.
E. cervical spine stabilization.

______ 23. During the initial assessment, the cervical spine should be stabilized
A. after the airway is established.
B. just before you attempt artificial ventilation.
C. immediately, if suggested by the MOI.
D. after the circulation check.
E. as the last step of the initial assessment.

______ 24. The major goal of the primary assessment is to
A. score the patient's condition.
B. identify care delivered in the "Golden ten minutes."
C. determine whether trauma-center care is needed.
D. correct life threats and determine the need for immediate transport.
E. identify the signs and symptoms of shock.

©2008 Pearson Education, Inc.

______ 25. A patient who is disoriented and confused would be classified as which of the following under the AVPU system?
A. A
B. V
C. P
D. U
E. cannot be determined with the information at hand

______ 26. Stridor can usually be caused by all of the following EXCEPT
A. infection.
B. gastric distress.
C. foreign body.
D. severe swelling.
E. allergic reaction.

______ 27. Which of the following might cause wheezing?
A. asthma
B. bronchitis
C. emphysema
D. broncholitis
E. all of the above

______ 28. A patient with abnormally deep respirations is said to be
A. hyperpneic.
B. tachypneic.
C. eupneic.
D. bradypneic.
E. hypopneic.

______ 29. Which of the following is the normal respiratory rate for the adult?
A. 8 to 10
B. 12 to 20
C. 16 to 24
D. 20 to 24
E. none of the above

______ 30. Retractions in upper airway obstruction may involve which of the following?
A. diaphragm
B. intercostals spaces
C. above the clavicles
D. above the sternum
E. all except A

______ 31. Which of the following can affect capillary refill in the adult?
A. smoking
B. medications
C. cold weather
D. chronic conditions
E. all of the above

______ 32. The focused history and physical exam is conducted differently for the four different categories of patients. Which of the following is an example of a patient who does NOT fit into one of those categories?
A. responsive medical patient
B. unresponsive medical patient
C. pediatric patient with altered consciousness
D. trauma patient with an isolated injury
E. trauma patient with a significant mechanism of injury

______ 33. Which of the following is NOT a mechanism of injury that calls for rapid transport to the trauma center?
A. ejection from a vehicle
B. vehicle rollover
C. severe vehicle deformity in a high-speed crash
D. fall from less than 20 feet
E. bicycle collision with loss of consciousness

______ 34. The decision to provide rapid transport of a patient to the trauma center is predicated upon either the mechanism of injury or the
A. blood pressure reading.
B. physical signs of trauma.
C. pulse oximetry reading.
D. ongoing assessments.
E. none of the above

©2008 Pearson Education, Inc.
Intermediate Emergency Care: 1985, 3rd ed.

______ 35. If you arrive at your patient's side only moments after the accident, he or she may not have lost enough blood to demonstrate the signs of shock.
A. True
B. False

______ 36. Which of the following body regions is examined during the rapid trauma assessment?
A. head
B. neck
C. pelvis
D. thorax
E. all of the above

______ 37. The "B" of DCAP-BTLS stands for
A. burns.
B. bumps.
C. blemishes.
D. bilateral injury.
E. bruises.

______ 38. Which of the following is NOT represented within the DCAP-BTLS mnemonic?
A. contusions
B. abrasions
C. burns
D. crepitus
E. swelling

______ 39. To assure adequate air exchange for the patient with a flail chest, you should
A. perform a needle decompression.
B. apply a large dressing with tape.
C. apply oxygen only.
D. perform an endotracheal intubation.
E. cover the wound with an occlusive dressing.

______ 40. You find that a patient is able to move a limb, but the limb is cool, pale, and without a pulse. This is consistent with
A. neurologic compromise.
B. vascular compromise.
C. both a vascular and neurologic compromise.
D. spinal injury.
E. peripheral nerve root injury.

______ 41. With a patient who has a crushing injury to his index finger received when it was caught in a closing door, which form of patient assessment would be most reasonable?
A. the rapid trauma assessment and a quick history
B. the rapid trauma assessment and a detailed history
C. a quick history and a physical exam focused on the injury
D. a detailed patient history and a physical exam focused on the injury
E. a detailed physical exam

______ 42. The pain or discomfort that caused the patient to call you to his or her side is called the
A. presenting problem.
B. differential diagnosis.
C. field diagnosis.
D. chief complaint.
E. present illness.

______ 43. A patient statement that "deep breathing makes my chest hurt" represents which element of the OPQRST-ASPN mnemonic for investigation of the chief complaint?
A. O
B. P
C. R
D. S
E. PN

______ 44. The jugular veins in a patient with normal cardiovascular function remain full or distended up to which of the following degrees of patient tilt?
A. 15 degrees
B. 30 degrees
C. 45 degrees
D. 60 degrees
E. 90 degrees

©2008 Pearson Education, Inc.

_____ 45. In a patient who displays hyperresonance to percussion, you should suspect
A. pleural effusion.
B. pulmonary edema.
C. pneumonia.
D. emphysema.
E. none of the above

_____ 46. Examine a patient for unusual pulsation of the descending aorta
A. just right of the umbilicus.
B. just left of the umbilicus.
C. along a line from the umbilicus to the middle symphysis pubis.
D. just beneath the zyphoid process.
E. anywhere in the abdomen.

_____ 47. Accumulation of fluid within the abdominal cavity is common in patients with
A. hypovolemia.
B. aortic aneurysm.
C. emphysema.
D. gastric ulcer disease.
E. cirrhosis of the liver.

_____ 48. If you hear bilateral crackles on inspiration when auscultating a patient's chest, you should suspect
A. congestive heart failure.
B. bronchospasm.
C. asthma.
D. chronic obstructive pulmonary disease.
E. all of the above

_____ 49. A patient in whom unequal pupils are a normal condition displays
A. Cullen's sign.
B. anisocoria.
C. consensual response.
D. accommodation.
E. Bell's palsy.

_____ 50. Which of the following is a discoloration over the flanks suggesting intraabdominal bleeding?
A. Cullen's sign
B. Starling's sign
C. bilateral periorbital ecchymosis
D. Grey-Turner's sign
E. none of the above

_____ 51. Vital signs provide the assessing EMT-I with
A. a window into what is happening with the patient.
B. an objective capsule of the patient's clinical status.
C. possible indications of severe illness.
D. possible indications of the need to intervene.
E. all of the above

_____ 52. The width of a blood pressure cuff should be at least
A. 10% of the width of the arm.
B. 20% of the width of the arm.
C. 30% of the width of the arm.
D. 120% of the width of the arm.
E. 140% of the width of the arm.

_____ 53. You might expect the resting pulse rate of an athlete to be about
A. 30 to 50.
B. 40 to 50.
C. 60 to 100.
D. 70 to 140.
E. 80 to 100.

_____ 54. Normal tidal volume is about what volume of air?
A. 100 ml
B. 200 ml
C. 400 ml
D. 500 ml
E. 1,000 ml

©2008 Pearson Education, Inc.
Intermediate Emergency Care: 1985, 3rd ed.

______ 55. A pulse oximetry reading of 88 percent would indicate the need for
A. aggressive airway and ventilatory care.
B. only the administration of blow-by oxygen.
C. only some repositioning of the patient's head.
D. no care at this point.
E. careful monitoring of the patient for further deterioration.

______ 56. EMT-Is employ the complete detailed physical assessment at the scene
A. rarely.
B. occasionally.
C. frequently.
D. rarely in trauma patients, frequently in medical patients.
E. frequently in trauma patients, rarely in medical patients.

______ 57. Which injury is likely to cause cerebrospinal fluid to flow from the ear canals?
A. skull fracture
B. ear trauma
C. pressure injury
D. increasing intracranial pressure
E. all of the above

______ 58. Kussmaul's respirations may be due to which of the following?
A. excessive carbon dioxide
B. a diabetic problem
C. severe acidosis
D. head injury
E. all of the above

______ 59. Serial ongoing assessments will facilitate
A. reassessment of the patient.
B. revision of the field diagnosis.
C. changes in the management plan.
D. documentation of the effects of interventions.
E. all of the above

______ 60. Which of the following is indicative of shock?
A. falling blood pressure, falling pulse rate
B. falling blood pressure, rising pulse rate
C. rising blood pressure, falling pulse rate
D. rising blood pressure, rising pulse rate
E. none of the above

LISTING

List the components of patient assessment in the order they would be performed in the field.

61. ______________________________

62. ______________________________

63. ______________________________

64. ______________________________

65. ______________________________

Special Project

The authoring of radio messages to medical control is one of the most important tasks that you will perform as an EMT-Intermediate. Read the following information. Then compose an initial and an updated radio message that you might send to medical control.

©2008 Pearson Education, Inc.
Intermediate Emergency Care: 1985, 3rd ed.

The Call

At 6:32 P.M., dispatch pages medic rescue unit 21 and sends the unit to a one-car accident at the corner of Elm and Wildwood Lane. One patient is reported unconscious. The fire department is also en route.

You and your partner, Mike Grailing, arrive with the ambulance at 6:45 and find that there are wires down, fuel spilling from the gas tank, and window glass around the scene. Bystanders state that the car swerved wildly, then hit the power pole. You notice there are no skid marks. You await arrival of the fire department, which will secure the scene.

Once the scene is safe, you and your partner approach. The patient is sitting behind the driver's seat with his eyes closed. He is unrestrained. Your partner employs a jaw thrust with cervical precautions and cervical immobilization. You now begin the assessment. You notice a break in the car's windshield and a small contusion on your patient's forehead. He is unconscious, has a strong pulse, and displays minor respiratory wheezing and stridor. Assessment of the neck reveals a small welt but no other apparent injuries. The pupils are equal and reactive. Oxygen is administered at 12 L per minute via nonrebreather mask, and initial vitals (respiratory rate of 24 with audible wheezes, BP of 110/76, strong pulse of 90, and oxygen saturation of 94%) are taken at 6:52. The ECG displays normal sinus rhythm.

The patient awakens and asks, "What happened?" He thinks he was stung by a bee. Last year he had a similar reaction to a bee sting and has a kit at home that his physician prescribed for him. The patient complains of itching. You notice hives starting to form.

Based upon protocol, you initiate the IV run T.K.O. with lactated Ringer's solution in the right forearm using a 16-gauge over-the-catheter needle while the patient is being immobilized and moved to a long spineboard.

Medical control is contacted, and you call in the following:

____

____

____

____

Just prior to movement to the ambulance (6:59), the patient is monitored and found to have the following vitals: BP 118/88, pulse 78 strong and regular, respirations 20 and regular with clear breath sounds, an ECG showing a normal sinus rhythm, and a pulse oximetry reading of 99%.

The patient history, which is taken at the scene and during transport, reveals that the patient is William Sobeski. He is 28 years old and lives at 2145 East Brookline Drive in the city of Rochester. The patient denies any allergy except to bee stings. He was stung by a bee a year ago and was rushed to the emergency department because he "couldn't catch his breath." He denies any headache, visual disturbances, and any numbness and tingling. He also denies taking any prescribed medications other than that prescribed for bee stings. He has not eaten since noon. He requests Community Hospital because his sister works there.

Contact medical control and provide the following update:

____

____

____

____

©2008 Pearson Education, Inc.
Intermediate Emergency Care: 1985, 3rd ed.

Chapter 9

Advanced Airway Management, Oxygenation, and Ventilation

Review of Chapter Objectives

After reading this chapter, you should be able to do the following:

1. Describe the anatomy of the upper airway, including:

Mouth (**oral cavity**)—single cavity that serves as an auxiliary air passage; posterior upper surface includes the soft palate, which moves upward and closes off the passages from the nose to the pharynx during swallowing **p. 269**

Nose—hollow, two-sided chamber lined with mucous membranes; warms, filters, and humidifies air as it enters the respiratory system; openings include the nares, or nostrils **pp. 268–269**

Pharynx (**throat**)—functions as the transitional area (passage) for food and air between the nose and mouth and between the esophagus and larynx **p. 269**

Epiglottis—flap-like structure covering the opening of the trachea (glottis); closes during swallowing to prevent food or fluids from entering the trachea and respiratory system **p. 269**

Larynx—tubular structure ("Adam's apple") that begins the lower airway; consists of the thyroid and cricoid cartilages, the vocal cords, the arytenoid folds, and the upper portion of the trachea **pp. 269–270**

2. Name the three regions of the pharynx. **p. 269**

Nasopharynx
Oropharynx
Laryngopharynx (or hypopharynx)

3. Identify the relationship between the larynx and the tongue, pharynx, epiglottis, esophagus, and vocal cords. **pp. 269–270**

Tongue—found well above the larynx
Pharynx—airway chamber found directly above the larynx
Epiglottis—flap of tissue that covers the glottic opening of the larynx
Esophagus—found directly posterior to the larynx
Vocal cords—found within the larynx; form the glottic opening

4. Discuss the following functions of the respiratory system.

Mechanics of ventilation (exchange of gases between a living organism and its environment) **pp. 273–275**

Lungs expand as the thoracic cage expands due to the contraction of the diaphragm, intercostal muscles, and other accessory muscles.
The elastic recoil of the lungs and gravity cause inspired air to be moved out of the lungs.

Pulmonary circulation **pp. 275–276**
Right ventricle pumps blood depleted of its oxygen into the pulmonary artery.
Blood is directed to the respective lungs through the right and left pulmonary arteries, which then divide ultimately to the pulmonary capillaries.
Blood returns through the pulmonary veins to the left atrium.
Gas exchange in the lungs
Air brought into the lungs contains 21 percent oxygen and very little carbon dioxide. **pp. 275–277**
Exhaled air contains about 14 percent oxygen and 5 percent carbon dioxide.
Diffusion of the respiratory gases **p. 277**
Oxygen in the inspired air diffuses across the alveolar space and then through the alveolar wall and the pulmonary capillary membrane where the oxygen attaches to the hemoglobin.
Carbon dioxide diffuses from the blood plasma in the reverse direction.

5. Describe oxygen transport in the blood, and cite factors that affect it. pp. 277–278

Oxygen is transported by hemoglobin found in the red blood cells. As it passes a well-oxygenated alveolus, 97 percent of the red blood cells are saturated. Very little oxygen is carried in or by the plasma of the blood. As the oxygenated blood passes the body's cells, the hemoglobin releases the oxygen.

Factors that affect oxygen saturation and transport include the following:

Inadequate alveolar ventilation—reduction of available oxygen at the alveolar level; may be caused by low oxygen levels in the air, respiratory muscle paralysis, chronic obstructive pulmonary disease (COPD), asthma, or pneumothorax
Decreased alveolar diffusion—caused by pulmonary edema, a condition in which fluid enters the space between the interior of the alveoli and the capillary; commonly increases the distance the oxygen must diffuse and hampers effective exchange
Ventilation/perfusion mismatch—results from lack of air exchange in some of the alveoli (as in atelectasis); unoxygenated blood from these alveoli mixes with the oxygenated blood from other areas of the lung. (Note: If the circulation is obstructed to some of the alveoli, such as in pulmonary embolism, a significant amount of blood is prevented from reaching the alveolar/capillary membrane.)

6. Discuss carbon dioxide transport in the blood and list factors that affect it. pp. 278–279

Approximately 70 percent of the carbon dioxide in the blood is transported as bicarbonate, 20 percent is transported attached to the hemoglobin, and about 1 percent is dissolved in the plasma.

Factors that affect carbon dioxide transport include the following:

Increased CO_2 production—produced by actions such as fever, muscle exertion, shivering, and metabolic acidosis
Decreased CO_2 elimination—caused by decreased alveolar ventilation from conditions such as drug induced respiratory depression, airway obstruction, COPD, and impairment of respiratory muscles

7. Describe the neurological control of respiration. p. 279

Control of respiration by the involuntary nervous system through the use of stretch receptors in the tissue of the lungs and through chemoreceptors that monitor the oxygen and carbon dioxide levels in the blood and the pH of the cerebrospinal fluid
Increase in the stimulus to breathe from an increase in CO_2, a decrease in oxygen, or a decrease in pH
Decrease in stimulus to breathe from a stretching of the lung tissue (such as a deep breath)

8. Describe the various measures of respiratory function and give the average normal values for each. pp. 280–281

Tidal volume (VT)—average volume of air inspired (or expired) with each breath, about 500 mL

©2008 Pearson Education, Inc.
Intermediate Emergency Care: 1985, 3rd ed.

Dead space volume (VD)—portion of the tidal volume that does not reach the alveoli and is unavailable for gas exchange, about 150 mL

Alveolar volume (VA)—amount of air that reaches the alveoli with each breath, about 350 mL

Minute volume (Vmin)—amount of air moved by the respiratory system with each breath (tidal volume) 3 respiratory rate

Functional reserve capacity (FRC)—maximum amount of air a person can move between a maximum inhalation and a maximum exhalation, about 4.5 liters

9. Describe the common causes of airway obstruction, and detail the special considerations of each. pp. 281–282

Tongue—most common cause of airway obstruction; in the unconscious person, lack of muscle tone allows the tongue to rest against the posterior pharynx, and thereby obstructs the airway.

Foreign body—large, poorly chewed food and aspirated objects; most common cause of airway obstruction in children; often presents with the victim grasping his or her throat

Trauma—physical injury to structures of the upper airway; can be caused by objects such as teeth, tissue, or blood or by collapse of the airway due to penetrating trauma

Laryngeal spasm or edema—spasm of glottis (smallest portion of the airway) due to anaphylaxis, epiglottitis, and inhalation of toxic substances, superheated steam, or smoke; edema due to trauma

Aspiration—caused by aspirated vomitus, blood, teeth, etc.

10. Describe assessment of the airway and the respiratory system. pp. 283–290

A continual, ongoing assessment

During initial assessment, focus directed at detecting any potentially life-threatening airway problems. (Note: If the patient is not conscious, alert, and speaking, the airway and respiration are closely evaluated. The rate, depth, and symmetry of respiration are noted, as is the presence of any unusual respiratory sounds.)

During focused exam and history, focus directed at the finer details of respiratory evaluation, such as monitoring skin color, auscultation of breath sounds, checking for abnormal breathing sounds, palpation of the thorax, and using pulse oximetry and/or capnography

11. Discuss pulse oximetry and capnography, and describe the prehospital use of both. pp. 288–290

Pulse oximetry—noninvasive monitoring of the arterial oxygenation of the skin; reflection of the oxygen delivery to the end organs provides oxygen saturation of the hemoglobin

End-tidal CO_2 detection (capnography)—accomplished either by a disposable device or an electronic sensor affixed to an endotracheal tube; measures the amount of CO_2 in the exhaled gas; disposable units change color while electronic detectors register a reading. (Note: In prehospital care, the presence of CO_2 reflects proper endotracheal tube placement. However, in patients without effective circulation the CO_2 levels may be very low.)

12. Discuss the various oxygen administration devices used in prehospital care, and describe the advantages and disadvantages of each. pp. 292–294

Nasal cannula—provides oxygen concentrations between 24 and 44 percent at liter flow rates of 1 to 6 liters per minute; well tolerated by the patient, but administers only low concentrations of oxygen

Simple face mask—delivers oxygen at 40 to 60 percent concentrations with oxygen flow rates of 8 to 12 liters per minute; delivers moderate levels of oxygen, but muffles patient speech and may cause feelings of confinement

Nonrebreather mask—delivers 80 to 100 percent oxygen with flow rates of 10 to 15 liters per minute; delivers high concentrations of oxygen, but it muffles patient speech and may feel confining (preferred oxygen-delivery device for the hypoxic patient)

Venturi mask—delivers precise oxygen levels of 24, 28, 35, or 40 percent; ideal for the patient who needs a closely titrated oxygen flow

©2008 Pearson Education, Inc.

13. Describe the procedures used to open the airway manually. **pp. 294–297**

Head-tilt/chin-lift (preferred technique in the non-trauma patient)—places one hand on the forehead gently tilting the head back, while the other hand is on the mandible, displacing it anteriorly

Jaw thrust (or the triple-airway maneuver)—places both hands on the lateral mandible, displacing it inferiorly and anteriorly (Note: If spinal injury is suspected, the head should not be tilted backwards.)

Jaw lift—places the rescuer's thumb into the mouth where the jaw and tongue are grasped between the thumb and fingers and are displaced anteriorly; requires care to ensure that the patient does not clench his or her teeth against the rescuer's thumb (Note: Do not tilt the head with this maneuver if spinal injury is suspected.)

14. Describe the indications and application of cricoid pressure (Sellick maneuver) for airway control and in endotracheal intubation. **pp. 295–297, 319**

Sellick maneuver (also called cricoids pressure) is used to prevent gastric insufflations and regurgitation. It is also used during endotracheal intubation to align the airway for better visualization. The cricoids cartilage is located and gentle downward pressure is applied. This will compress the esophagus and prevent air travel down it during ventilation and the passage of gastric contents upward. Moving this cartilage slightly in a posterior direction will also make the glottis easier to visualize during endotracheal intubation attempts.

15. Discuss the indications, contraindications, and methods of performing suctioning. **pp. 297–299**

Suctioning—use of pressures less than atmospheric to draw fluids and semifluids out of the airway

Indications—should be used any time it can effectively remove material from the airway

Contraindications—avoid continuous suctioning; draws against the patient's ventilation attempts and generally interrupts ventilation in the apneic patient

Methods—can be provided by electric or mechanical devices

16. Discuss indications, contraindications, and methods for insertion of the following airways.

Oropharyngeal airway—designed to maintain an airway by displacing the tongue anteriorly; should not be used for patients who are conscious or have an intact gag reflex; positioned by displacing the tongue forward with a tongue blade and inserting the oral airway along the base of the tongue (Note: The oral airway (or endotracheal tube) should be used when the patient is ventilated by any mechanical device.) **pp. 300–303**

Nasopharyngeal airway—soft rubber tube that is lubricated and inserted posteriorly in the largest nostril; designed to be inserted into the nasopharynx in the unconscious or semiconscious patient; indicated in the semiconscious patient who requires airway management or in cases when an oral airway is indicated (Note: The nasal airway should be used with care in the patient with possible skull fracture.) **pp. 304–306**

17. Discuss indications, contraindications, and methods for use for the following devices.

Pocket mask—provides some protection against direct contact with the patient and the patient's exhaled air; sealed to the patient's face with the rescuer's hands during ventilation **pp. 307–308**

Bag-valve device—provides positive-pressure ventilation; sealed to the patient's face by one of the rescuer's hands, while the other hand squeezes the bag; best used for the intubated patient because the volume of air and the pressure delivered to the patient are low (Note: If the patient is not intubated, the air exchanged may not be enough to sustain life. Any time a BVM is used, it should have the oxygen reservoir attached and oxygen flowing at 12 to 15 liters per minute.) **pp. 308–309**

Demand valve resuscitator—ventilates the patient with a flow of oxygen when a button or bar is pushed; can be used with face masks, EOA, EGTA, PTL airways, or endotracheal tubes; provides the patient with 100% oxygen (Note: The pressures at which it delivers oxygen may cause gastric insufflation or lung tissue damage. It is not recommended for patients who are intubated or the pediatric patient.) **pp. 309–310**

©2008 Pearson Education, Inc.
Intermediate Emergency Care: 1985, 3rd ed.

Automatic ventilator—provides a patient with ventilation with 100% oxygen at a rate and volume determined by the user; recent advances in technology make automatic ventilators compact and dependable for field use (Note: These devices are not recommended for children under the age of 5 years and are dependent upon a good airway.) **pp. 310–311**

18. Describe the visual landmarks for direct laryngoscopy. pp. 269–270, 318–319, 321

To insert an endotracheal tube, it is necessary to place the patient in the sniffing position and then insert the laryngoscope into the mouth to lift the tongue and mandible anteriorly so the vocal cords can be visualized. If a curved laryngoscope blade is used, the tip must be placed in the vallecula, which when lifted anteriorly, will help move the epiglottis away from the glottic opening. If a straight blade is used, the epiglottis is actually lifted along with the tongue and jaw as the structures are moved anteriorly to expose the glottic opening. Once the glottic opening is exposed, the vocal cords can be seen. Pass the ET tube cuff about 1–2 cm past the vocal cords. If you cannot visualize the vocal cords, the procedure may not be successful.

19. Describe the methods of assessing, confirming, and securing correct placement of an endotracheal tube (ETT). pp. 322–324

The most reliable method of confirming proper ETT placement is direct visualization of its passage through the vocal cords. Following ETT placement, watch to be sure that the patient's chest rises with ventilations. If the ETT is misplaced in the esophagus, the chest will not rise. You should auscultate for breath sounds. Their equal presence over both sides (apices and bases) of the chest and their absence over the epigastrium help to confirm proper ETT placement. It is important to assure proper ETT placement. Verify and document at least three different indicators of proper placement. These may include:

- Visualization of the tube passing between the cords.
- Presence of bilateral breath sounds.
- Absence of breath sounds.
- Positive end-tidal CO_2 change on capnography.
- Verification of endotracheal placement by an esophageal detector device.
- Presence of condensation inside the ETT.
- Absence of vomitus inside the ETT.
- Absence of phonation, or vocal sounds, once the tube is placed.

Traditionally ETT have been secured by adhesive tape. It is strongly advised that a commercially available and sterile tube restraint be used to tie the tube in place and keep the ETT from moving from its original position.

20. Describe the considerations for and use of the following airway devices

Pharyngeo-tracheal lumen airway (PTL)—two-tube device, one tube of which isolates the oro- and nasopharynx while a second tube and cuff seals off either the trachea or esophagus; lumen of the tube allows ventilation if trachea is intubated (Note: While the PTL airway has many applications, it can be difficult to determine whether the distal tube is located in the esophagus or trachea.) Determine which tube is in the trachea and use it to ventilate the patient. **pp. 330–333**

Laryngeal mask airway (LMA)—a tube with a mask structure attached that is negotiated, blindly, into the larynx. There the mask isolates the trachea and allows ventilation. **pp. 333–336**

Esophageal tracheal combitube airway (ETC)—similar to the PTL airway, except that it is designed to be inserted into either the trachea or esophagus; occludes the passageway and the oral pharynx, isolating the trachea from the esophagus (Note: As with the PTL, EOA, and EGTA, the biggest drawback to this device is that the user must determine which tube the airway is in to assure the patient will be adequately ventilated.) **pp. 336–338**

Cobra perilaryngeal (PLA) airway—similar to the LMA but with a slightly different mask design. It displaces soft tissue away from the glottic opening. **pp. 338–339**

King LT airway—a single lumen airway inserted into the esophagus. It isolates the glottis opening using two balloons, one to seal the esophagus and the other to seal the proximal airway. **p. 339**

©2008 Pearson Education, Inc.

Case Study Review

Reread the case study in Chapter 9 and then read the following discussion. The EMT-Intermediates in this case study deal with a patient in full cardiac arrest. While many aspects of intermediate emergency care are involved, the focus of this study is airway care and ventilation.

John and Linda respond to a full cardiac arrest with a step-by-step team approach. They move deliberately through the ABCs of CPR and then progress into advanced life support procedures. John opens the airway and then determines that the patient is in respiratory arrest. Before moving on, he assures that an oral airway is inserted and then attempts ventilation using a bag-valve mask with 100 percent oxygen. His ventilations meet with resistance so John attempts to visualize the obstruction and performs a finger sweep to remove it. His attempts are unsuccessful.

Linda determines that the patient has a strong pulse and begins to set up the equipment for intubation. When the finger sweep fails to remove the obstruction, she uses the laryngoscope to visualize the airway. In this case, it is hard to clearly see the entire airway so Linda initially displaces the larynx posteriorly, bringing the anatomical structures and the obstruction into view. Once the obstruction is clearly in view, John holds the larynx in position while Linda grasps and removes the piece of meat with the McGill forceps. John begins to ventilate Travis at 12 times per minute with the bag-valve mask and 100% oxygen. Linda notes good chest rise and fall with each of John's ventilations and hears breath sounds bilaterally. The pulse oximeter reads very low, as expected after a period of hypoxia.

Linda notes the pulse oximetry values begin to rise. John notes gurgling in the airway and immediately suctions it. Given the potential for vomiting, they choose to intubate Travis to protect his airway. Linda checks the equipment (laryngoscope and endotracheal tube) carefully to assure it operates properly. Linda carefully inserts the endotracheal tube into the trachea, and inflates the cuff. Linda assures the endotracheal tube is properly placed in the trachea by watching the tube go through the vocal folds, noting bilateral breath sounds with ventilation and by the rising pulseoximetry readings. They also attach an endtidal CO_2 monitor and note ventilations are producing CO_2 readings, another sign the endotracheal tube is in the trachea. The depth of tube insertion is noted and it is secured firmly in place. John and Linda will frequently note its position and assess the pulseoximetry and endtidal CO_2 values and breath sounds to assure the endotracheal tube does not displace.

Content Self-Evaluation

Multiple Choice

______ 1. The nasal cavity is responsible for all of the functions listed below EXCEPT
- A. warming the air.
- B. deoxygenating the air.
- C. humidifying the air.
- D. cleansing the air.
- E. the sense of smell.

______ 2. The space located between the tongue and the epiglottis is called the
- A. vallecula.
- B. cricoid.
- C. arytenoid fold.
- D. epiglottic fossa.
- E. glottic opening.

______ 3. The oxygenated circulation that provides perfusion for the lung tissue itself flows through the
- A. pulmonary arteries.
- B. pulmonary veins.
- C. bronchial arteries.
- D. bronchial veins.
- E. none of the above

______ 4. The normal oxygen saturation of hemoglobin in blood as it leaves the lungs is about
- A. 75 percent.
- B. 85 percent.
- C. 90 percent.
- D. 95 percent.
- E. 97 percent.

©2008 Pearson Education, Inc.
Intermediate Emergency Care: 1985, 3rd ed.

______ 5. The majority of the carbon dioxide carried by the blood is
A. carried by the hemoglobin.
B. dissolved in the plasma.
C. transported as calcium.
D. found as free gas in the blood.
E. bicarbonate, carried in the blood.

______ 6. The primary center controlling respiration is located in the
A. medulla.
B. pons.
C. spinal cord.
D. cerebrum.
E. cerebellum.

______ 7. Which of the following would not increase the production of carbon dioxide?
A. fever
B. hyperventilation
C. shivering
D. release of metabolic acids
E. exercise

______ 8. The reflex that responds to the stretch of the lungs by inhibiting respirations is the
A. apneustic reflex.
B. pneumotaxic reflex.
C. Frank-Starling reflex.
D. Hering-Breuer reflex.
E. baroreceptor response.

______ 9. Which of the following is the primary stimulus that causes respiration to occur?
A. increase in pH of the blood
B. decrease in pH of the blood
C. increase in pH of the cerebrospinal fluid
D. decrease in pH of the cerebrospinal fluid
E. reduced oxygen in the blood

______ 10. The amount of air moved with one normal breath is called
A. minute volume.
B. alveolar air.
C. tidal volume.
D. dead air space.
E. vital capacity.

______ 11. Which of the following is the most common cause of upper airway obstruction?
A. the tongue
B. foreign bodies
C. trauma
D. laryngeal swelling
E. aspiration of blood or vomitus

______ 12. The normal respiratory rate for an adult at rest is
A. 8 to 12.
B. 12 to 20.
C. 18 to 24.
D. 24 to 32.
E. 40 to 60.

______ 13. Which of the following is a breathing pattern associated with flail chest?
A. abdominal breathing
B. paradoxical breathing
C. diaphragmatic breathing
D. intercostal retraction
E. A and C

______ 14. It is rare that a patient will have significant hypoxia and not display cyanosis.
A. True
B. False

______ 15. The respiratory pattern that presents with deep and rapid respirations is
A. apneustic respirations.
B. Cheyne-Stokes respirations.
C. Biot's respirations.
D. central neurogenic hyperventilation.
E. agonal respirations.

______ 16. Which modified form of respiration is designed to expand alveoli that may have collapsed during periods of inactivity or rest?
A. coughing
B. sneezing
C. hiccoughing
D. grunting
E. sighing

©2008 Pearson Education, Inc.
Intermediate Emergency Care: 1985, 3rd ed.

_____ 17. Stridor is most commonly associated with
A. laryngeal constriction or edema.
B. the tongue blocking the airway.
C. narrowing of the bronchioles.
D. fluids within the airway.
E. foreign bodies in the lower airway.

_____ 18. The absence of CO_2 in exhaled air, as identified by a capnometer or end-expiratory CO_2 detector, suggests
A. ventilation is not deep enough.
B. ventilations are not occurring fast enough.
C. the endotracheal tube may be in the esophagus.
D. the oxygen percentage of inspired air is insufficient.
E. all of the above

_____ 19. Which of the following devices delivers the highest concentration of oxygen to the patient?
A. nasal cannula
B. simple face mask
C. nonrebreather mask
D. Venturi mask
E. A and D

_____ 20. Which of the devices below delivers the most controlled concentration of oxygen to a patient?
A. nasal cannula
B. simple face mask
C. nonrebreather mask
D. Venturi mask
E. B and C

_____ 21. In the head-tilt/chin-lift maneuver, the fingers under the chin should apply a firm pressure to ensure the jaw remains closed.
A. True
B. False

_____ 22. The intent behind employing Sellick maneuver is to:
A. displace the diaphragm.
B. increase venous return.
C. prevent regurgitation.
D. clear an airway obstruction.
E. increase blood flow to the brain.

_____ 23. The airway adjunct that acts primarily by displacing the tongue forward is the
A. oropharyngeal airway.
B. LMA airway.
C. endotracheal tube.
D. Cobra airway.
E. esophageal gastric tube airway.

_____ 24. Which of the following is an advantage of the nasopharyngeal airway over the oropharyngeal airway?
A. It has a larger diameter.
B. It is easier to insert.
C. It is blocked less frequently by vomitus.
D. It does not stimulate the gag reflex as strongly.
E. It can be used with a BVM.

_____ 25. The bag-valve mask with an oxygen supply attached and oxygen flowing at 15 L per minute delivers what percentage of oxygen to the patient?
A. 21 percent
B. 40 to 60 percent
C. 60 to 80 percent
D. 90 to 95 percent
E. 99.9 percent

_____ 26. One rescuer bag-valve masking is difficult to perform effectively because
A. it is difficult to maintain proper airway positioning.
B. it is difficult to maintain mask seal.
C. it is difficult to squeeze the bag.
D. all of the above
E. none of the above

©2008 Pearson Education, Inc.
Intermediate Emergency Care: 1985, 3rd ed.

______ 27. Hazards of using the demand valve to ventilate a patient include all of the following EXCEPT
A. oxygen toxicity.
B. gastric distention.
C. pulmonary barotrauma.
D. pneumothorax.
E. subcutaneous emphysema.

______ 28. Which of the following is NOT an advantage of automatic ventilators?
A. They free a rescuer when the patient is not breathing.
B. They are convenient and easy to use.
C. They are dependable.
D. They can be used on children younger than age 5.
E. They are lightweight and tolerant to temperature extremes.

______ 29. The light of the laryngoscope should be a bright yellow and flicker slightly when pressure is placed on the blade.
A. True
B. False

______ 30. The tip of the curve of the Macintosh laryngoscope blade is designed to fit into the
A. nasopharynx.
B. glottic opening.
C. vallecula.
D. arytenoid fossa.
E. epiglottis.

______ 31. The purpose of the cuff on the end of the endotracheal tube is to
A. help guide the tube to its proper location.
B. prevent dislodging of the tube after it is correctly placed.
C. seal the airway.
D. center the tube in the trachea.
E. widen the opening of the vocal cords.

______ 32. The major purpose for using a malleable stylet during endotracheal intubation is to
A. maintain a pre-set curve in the tube.
B. keep the tube's lumen open.
C. stiffen the tube so it can be pushed through the glottis.
D. prevent foreign matter from entering the tube.
E. all of the above

______ 33. Which of the following is NOT an indication for endotracheal intubation?
A. respiratory arrest
B. cardiac arrest
C. inability to protect the airway
D. obstruction due to foreign object, swelling, or burns
E. severe epiglottitis

______ 34. When using the laryngoscope to visualize the glottis, it is best to use the teeth as a fulcrum to increase your ability to lift the tissue.
A. True
B. False

______ 35. To reduce the risk of hypoxia, limit attempts at intubation to no more than
A. 15 seconds.
B. 30 seconds.
C. 45 seconds.
D. 60 seconds.
E. 80 seconds.

______ 36. The pilot balloon of the endotracheal tube should be very firm to ensure there is a good seal between the tube and the interior of the trachea.
A. True
B. False

©2008 Pearson Education, Inc.

_____ 37. What volume of air is used to inflate the cuff of an endotracheal tube?
A. 2 to 4 mL
B. 4 to 6 mL
C. 5 to 10 mL
D. 10 to 15 mL
E. 15 to 25 mL

_____ 38. Confirmation of proper endotracheal tube placement is achieved by
A. visualizing the tube passing through the glottis.
B. hearing clear and bilaterally equal breath sounds.
C. noting the absence of gastric sounds with ventilation.
D. observing condensation on the endotracheal tube with exhalation.
E. any three of the above

_____ 39. Which of the following is NOT an indication of esophageal intubation?
A. absence of chest rise with ventilation
B. gurgling sound over the epigastrium
C. a falling pulse oximetry reading
D. skin color turning pink
E. increasing resistance to ventilatory effort

_____ 40. Upon placing the endotracheal tube, you hear very faint breath sounds and some gurgling over the epigastric region. You should next
A. advance the tube slightly.
B. withdraw the tube slightly.
C. inflate the cuff and auscultate again.
D. ventilate more forcibly.
E. remove the tube and re-intubate.

_____ 41. Upon placing the endotracheal tube in a patient, you determine that you can only auscultate breath sounds on the right side. You should next
A. withdraw the tube a few centimeters.
B. withdraw the tube completely.
C. pass the tube a few centimeters further.
D. secure the tube and ventilate more aggressively.
E. check the mask seal.

_____ 42. Which of the following are features of the PTL airway?
A. It can be inserted blindly.
B. It can seal off the nasal and oral cavities.
C. The patient can be ventilated regardless of whether the tube is in the trachea or esophagus.
D. It can be inserted without moving the cervical spine.
E. all of the above

_____ 43. The proper size LMA for the adult patient is which of the following?
A. 1
B. 2
C. 3
D. 4
E. 5

_____ 44. A major disadvantage to the use of the esophageal tracheal CombiTube is that
A. it does not completely isolate the trachea.
B. the tube must be in the trachea.
C. it is associated with gastric distention and vomiting.
D. it cannot be used in the trauma patient.
E. it is somewhat time-consuming to insert.

_____ 45. The major advantage of the King airway over the LMA and Cobra airway is that it stabilizes the tongue.
A. True
B. False

©2008 Pearson Education, Inc.
Intermediate Emergency Care: 1985, 3rd ed.

Label the Diagram

46. Write the names of the components of the upper airway marked A, B, C, D, E, F, G, and H on the figure below.

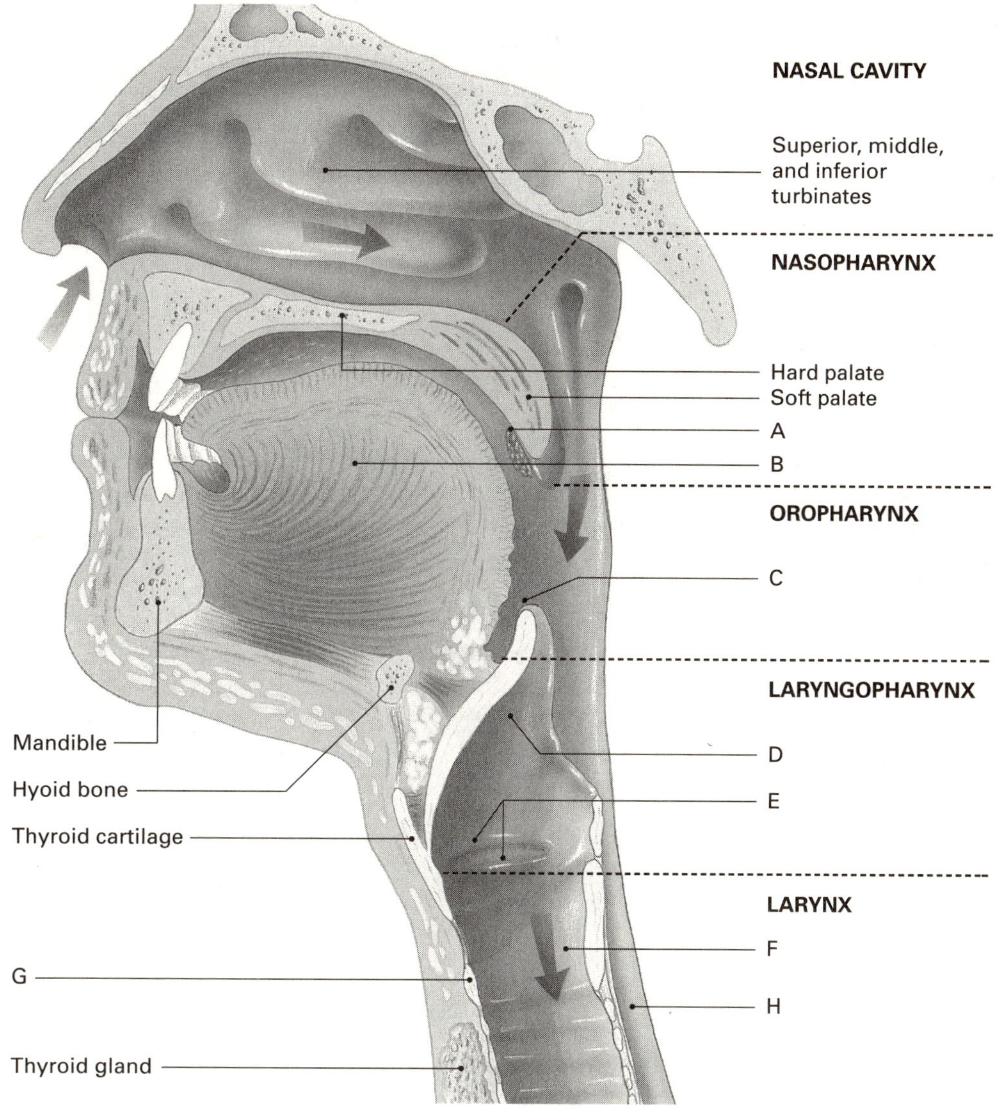

A.

B.

C.

D.

E.

F.

G.

H.

©2008 Pearson Education, Inc.

Special Project

Airway Obstruction

List the five causes of airway obstruction, and identify the mechanism that causes each problem.

1. ______________________________
2. ______________________________
3. ______________________________
4. ______________________________
5. ______________________________

Special Project

Problem Solving—Airway Maintenance

You have been called to a report of a man down and arrive with another EMT and one paramedic. You find bystanders doing CPR on a male in his mid-50s in a parking lot. You take the patient's head and determine the bystanders are doing a fine job of ventilating the patient. You get out your airway bag and prepare to place an endotracheal tube.

What equipment would you prepare?

How would you check your equipment?

©2008 Pearson Education, Inc.
Intermediate Emergency Care: 1985, 3rd ed.

Chapter

10

Fluids and Shock

Review of Chapter Objectives

After reading this chapter, you should be able to do the following:

1. Identify the body's major fluid compartments and the proportion of total body water they contain. **pp. 346–347**

Total body water (TBW)—accounts for 60 percent of the body weight, or about 42 liters in the 70 kg person; divided between two major compartments (intracellular and extracellular)
Intracellular fluid (ICF)—accounts for 75 percent of body fluid
Extracellular fluid (ECF)—accounts for 25 percent of body fluid; subdivided into two compartments (interstitial and intravascular)
Interstitial fluid—accounts for about 17.5 percent of body fluid; remains outside the cells, yet not within the vascular space
Intravascular fluid—accounts for 7.5 percent of body fluid; contained within the circulatory system

2. Identify the abnormal states of hydration, and describe their common causes and effects on the human system. **pp. 347–348**

Dehydration—net loss of body fluid may be caused by vomiting, diarrhea, disorders of absorption, fever states, diaphoresis, seeping wounds, or third space losses; can leave the cardiovascular system without the medium (plasma) to transport essential body materials effectively
Overhydration—net accumulation of fluid caused by the inability of the person to eliminate fluid (as in kidney failure) or an excessive intake of fluids (as in aggressive intravenous fluid administration); excess fluid flows out of the vascular space into the interstitial spaces and lungs causing peripheral edema or pulmonary edema

3. List the major electrolytes, and discuss the role they play in maintaining fluid balance within the human body. **pp. 348–349**

Sodium—chief extracellular cation (positively charged particle); plays a role in regulating the distribution of water
Potassium—chief intracellular cation; plays a major role in the transmission of electrical impulses
Calcium—plays a major role in muscle contraction and nervous impulse transmission
Magnesium—is involved in many biochemical processes
Chloride—body's chief anion (negatively charged particle); plays an important role in kidney function and fluid balance
Bicarbonate—is the principle buffer in the body
Phosphate—is important in body energy stores, renal function and provides some buffer function.

©2008 Pearson Education, Inc.

4. Define diffusion, osmosis, active transport, and facilitated diffusion, and explain the roles they play in human fluid dynamics. **pp. 350–351**

Diffusion—tendency of molecules within a solution to move toward an equilibrium; keeps the fluids within each body compartment consistent in mixture

Osmosis—movement of solvent (body water) from an area of lesser particle concentration to one of greater concentration; causes body water to follow the various electrolytes into the intracellular, intravascular, and interstitial spaces

Active transport—biochemically powered movement of a substance across a cell's membrane, often against an osmotic gradient; essential activity of the cell membrane, which allows the body to control movement of electrolytes and essential molecules; faster than osmosis or diffusion, but it requires cell energy

Facilitated diffusion—assisted transport across the cell membrane; mechanism by which glucose is brought into the body's cells

5. Describe the three mechanisms that help to control pH in the human body. **pp. 352–354**

The three major systems are part of the process to maintain the acid-base balance, since hydrogen ions must be constantly eliminated from the body.

Bicarbonate Buffer System. In a healthy individual, for every molecule of carbonic acid, there are 20 molecules of bicarbonate ion. Any change in this 20:1 ratio is immediately corrected without significant change in the total body pH. An increase in hydrogen ion (acidosis) is corrected as the excess hydrogen ions combine with bicarbonate ions to form carbonic acid. Conversely, when there is a deficit in hydrogen ions (alkalosis), carbonic acid will dissociate into bicarbonate ions and hydrogen ions.

Respiratory Function. An increase in respiration causes increased elimination of CO_2, which results in a decrease in hydrogen ions and an increase in pH. Conversely, decreased respirations cause CO_2 to be retained, causing an increase in hydrogen ions and a decrease in pH.

Kidney Function. The kidneys also regulate the pH by altering the concentration of bicarbonate ions (HCO_3) in the blood. Increased elimination of HCO_3 results in a lowered pH. Conversely, retention of HCO_3 causes an increase in pH.

6. Describe the effects of acidosis and alkalosis. **pp. 354–355**

The total number of hydrogen ions present in the body at any given time is very high. Because of this the pH system is used. The pH scale ranges from 1 to 14. A pH of 1 means that only hydrogen ions are present. A pH of 14 means that virtually no hydrogen ions are present. The pH of the body is normally 7.35 to 7.45. A pH below 7.35 is called acidosis. A pH above 7.45 is called alkalosis.

A variation in humans of only 0.4 of a pH unit in either direction from normal can be fatal. Respiratory acidosis occurs with decreased ventilation and results in a buildup of CO_2. Respiratory alkalosis occurs with an increase in ventilation and a decrease in CO_2.

Metabolic acidosis is an increase in body acidity due to low bicarbonate levels, the kidneys not able to excrete acid, or high body acid production or a combination of these factors.

Metabolic alkalosis is a decrease in body acidity due to decreased kidney activity, excessive vomiting, or ingestion of large amounts of bicarbonate.

7. Explain the factors that maintain and regulate blood pressure. **pp. 355–357**

Blood pressure (BP) is the tension exerted by blood against the arterial walls and is dependent upon both cardiac output and peripheral vascular resistance. Thus the BP equals the cardiac output times the peripheral vascular resistance (PVR). The PVR is the pressure against which the heart must pump. Since the circulatory system is a closed system, increasing either cardiac output or peripheral vascular resistance will increase BP. Likewise, a decrease in cardiac output or a decrease in peripheral vascular resistance will decrease BP.

The body does its best to keep the BP relatively constant by employing compensatory mechanisms and negative feedback loops to regulate the elements of the above formula. As noted earlier, baroreceptors in the carotid sinuses and in the arch of the aorta closely monitor BP. If BP increases,

©2008 Pearson Education, Inc.
Intermediate Emergency Care: 1985, 3rd ed.

the baroreceptors send signals to the brain that cause the BP to return to its normal values. This is accomplished by decreasing the heart rate, decreasing the preload, or decreasing peripheral vascular resistance.

The baroreceptors are also stimulated if the BP falls. The heart rate is increased, as is the strength of the cardiac contractions. There is also arteriolar constriction, venous constriction, and overall increased PVR. Also, the adrenal medulla is stimulated. This results in the secretion of epinephrine and norepinephrine, which further enhance the response.

8. Discuss the pathophysiology of shock. **p. 360**

The cardiovascular system is a closed system of interconnected tubes (blood vessels) that direct blood to the essential organs and tissues of the body. Arteries distribute blood to the various organs and tissues of the body. Arterioles determine the amount of blood perfusing the tissue of an organ and together constrict and increase peripheral vascular resistance or dilate and reduce peripheral vascular resistance. Progressive vasoconstriction can help maintain blood pressure and circulation to the most critical organs as the body loses blood during hemorrhage or fluid during other forms of shock. The venous system collects blood and returns it to the heart. It contains about 60 percent of the total blood volume and, when constricted, can return a relatively great volume (up to 1 liter) to the active circulation.

The cardiovascular system is powered by the central pump, the heart. It circulates the blood and, against the peripheral vascular resistance, drives the blood pressure. Its output is a factor of preload (the blood delivered to it by the venous system), stroke volume (the amount of blood ejected into the aorta with each contraction), rate, and afterload (the peripheral vascular resistance). The heart can help compensate for blood loss by attempting to maintain cardiac output by increasing its stroke volume (which is hard to do in hypovolemic states) or by increasing its rate.

Finally, the cardiovascular system contains the precious fluid, blood. Blood provides oxygen and nutrients to the body cells and removes carbon dioxide and waste products of metabolism. Blood also contains clotting factors that will occlude blood vessels if they are torn or disrupted.

The central nervous system provides control of the cardiovascular system using baroreceptors in the carotid arteries and aortic arch to sense fluctuations in blood pressure. It will maintain blood pressure by increasing heart rate, cardiac preload, and peripheral vascular resistance. Hormones from the kidneys and elsewhere help control blood volume and electrolytes as well as the production of erythrocytes.

9. Describe the body's physiologic response to changes in blood volume, blood pressure, and perfusion. **pp. 355–364**

Increased peripheral resistance is caused by the constriction of the arterioles and provides two mechanisms that combat shock. The arterioles constrict and maintain the blood pressure, and they divert blood to only the critical organs. This reduction in perfusion to the less critical organs results in the increased capillary refill time and the cool, clammy, and ashen skin often associated with shock states. It also results in reduced pulse pressure and weak pulses.

Venous constriction compensates for some blood loss and helps maintain cardiac preload. Since the veins account for about 60 percent of the blood volume, this is reasonably effective in minor to moderate blood loss.

As the cardiac preload drops, the heart rate increases in an attempt to maintain cardiac output and blood pressure. In the presence of significantly reduced preload, this may not be effective.

Peripheral vascular shunting directs the blood away from the skin, conserves body heat, and reduces fluid loss through evaporation. It also redirects blood to more critical areas.

Fluid shifts are the result of drawing fluid from the interstitial and cellular spaces. Fluid moves into the vascular space. While this is a slow mechanism, it can provide the vascular system with several liters of fluid.

10. Describe the effects of decreased perfusion at the capillary level. **pp. 355–364**

Decreased capillary perfusion limits the amount of oxygen and nutrients delivered to the body cells. It usually causes the release of histamine that, in turn, causes precapillary sphincter dilation

©2008 Pearson Education, Inc.

and an increase in perfusion. However, in shock states this is not effective, and the cells must revert to anaerobic metabolism while the byproducts of metabolism accumulate and the available oxygen is exhausted. Carbon dioxide, metabolic acids, and other waste products accumulate while body cells begin to die.

11. Discuss the cellular ischemic, capillary stagnation, and capillary washout phases related to hemorrhagic shock. **pp. 363–364**

Cellular ischemia. As shock ensues, decreased perfusion, first to the non-critical organs, then to all organs, diminishes blood flow through the microcirculation. At the cellular level this diminishes the supply of oxygen and nutrients to the cells and restricts the removal of carbon dioxide and the waste products of metabolism. The cells quickly exhaust their supply of oxygen and begin to use anaerobic metabolism as their sole source of energy to remain alive. This produces an accumulation of pyruvic acid, which in turn, converts to lactic acid and the cells become more acidotic. As cells begin to die, their decomposition releases even more toxins that then begin to affect other cells.

Capillary stagnation. With diminished capillary flow, coupled with the increasingly hypoxic and acidic environment caused by the ischemic cells, the red blood cells become sticky and clump together. They form columns of coagulated erythrocytes called rouleaux that either block the capillary to further flow of blood or will wash out and cause microemboli.

Capillary washout. The toxic environment of the ischemic tissue associated with severe shock finally causes the post-capillary sphincters to dilate and release the hypoxic and acidotic blood as well as the rouleaux into the venous circulation. As this washout becomes extensive, it further reduces the effectiveness of the cardiovascular system and the body moves quickly toward irreversible shock.

12. Identify the need for intervention and transport of the patient with hemorrhage or shock. **pp. 364–371**

Hemorrhage and shock are progressive pathologies that eventually become irreversible. To be effective in care, we must carefully assess our patients for the earliest of signs and intervene with rapid transport to a facility that can rapidly provide surgical intervention (to halt the internal bleeding). We also must immediately halt any external hemorrhage and provide supplemental high-flow oxygen. Intravenous fluids may be run to replace volume, but care must be used to prevent increased internal hemorrhage and hemodilution.

13. Discuss the assessment findings and management of internal and external hemorrhage and shock. **pp. 364–371**

Tachycardia is a compensatory cardiac action to maintain cardiac output when a reduced preload is present. A weak pulse reflects a narrowing pulse pressure and increasing peripheral vascular resistance to maintain systolic blood pressure. Cool, clammy skin is due to the redirection of blood to more critical organs than the skin. Ashen, pale skin may present due to hypoxia and peripheral vasoconstriction. Agitation, restlessness, and reduced level of consciousness occur as the brain receives a reduced flow of oxygenated blood. The hypoxia causes the defense mechanisms of agitation and restlessness, followed by a noticeable reduction in the level of consciousness. Dull, lackluster eyes occur secondary to low perfusion and hypoxic states. Rapid, shallow respiration may occur as shock progresses, the respiratory muscles tire in the hypoxic state, and respiratory effort becomes less efficient. Dropping oxygen saturation may also provide evidence to support developing shock. As the peripheral circulation slows, the readings may drop or become erratic. Falling blood pressure heralds the progression from compensated to decompensated shock. As a late sign, it should not be used to determine the presence of shock.

External hemorrhage must be controlled by direct pressure. If direct pressure alone does not work, use elevation, pressure points or, as a last resort, the tourniquet, to stop the hemorrhage. If all sites of hemorrhage are controlled and you can rule out internal hemorrhage, provide fluid resuscitation to return the blood pressure and vital signs to normal.

©2008 Pearson Education, Inc.
Intermediate Emergency Care: 1985, 3rd ed.

Should the mechanism of injury or any early development of shock signs or symptoms suggest internal hemorrhage, or external hemorrhage cannot be controlled, transport should be expedited and care initiated immediately. Provide high-flow oxygen and ventalitory support as needed and infuse fluids to maintain the blood pressure just below 100 mmHg, ensuring it does not drop below 50 mmHg.

14. Differentiate between the administration rate and volume of IV fluid in patients with controlled versus uncontrolled hemorrhage. **pp. 368–369**

If hemorrhage has been controlled (as with external hemorrhage) then fluid resuscitation can be aimed at returning the blood pressure and other vital signs toward normal. However, if the hemorrhage is internal, and especially if it involves the chest, abdomen, or pelvis, great care must be exercised not to enhance the hemorrhage or excessively dilute the remaining blood. Resuscitation is generally aimed at stabilizing the blood pressure and preventing it from dropping below 50 mmHg. To maintain these parameters, lactated Ringer's solution (preferred) or normal saline should be run rapidly through trauma or blood tubing and large-bore short catheters. Pressure infusers may be necessary as the blood pressure begins to fall below 50 mmHg. Usually prehospital care is limited to between 1 and 3 liters of crystalloid.

15. Define and differentiate between compensated and decompensated hemorrhagic shock. **pp. 361–362**

Compensated shock is a state in which the body is effectively compensating for fluid loss, or other shock-inducing pathology, and is able to maintain blood pressure and critical organ perfusion. If the original problem is not corrected or reversed, compensated shock may progress to decompensated shock.

Decompensated shock is a state in which the cardiovascular system cannot maintain critical circulation and begins to fail. Hypoxia affects the blood vessels and heart so they cannot maintain blood pressure and circulation.

Irreversible shock is a state of shock in which the human system is so damaged that it cannot be resuscitated. Once this stage of shock sets in, the patient will die, even if resuscitation efforts restore a pulse and blood pressure.

16. Discuss the pathophysiological changes, assessment findings, and management associated with compensated and decompensated shock. **pp. 361–371**

As the body experiences a stressor that induces shock, the cardiovascular system is quick to compensate. The venous system constricts to maintain a full vascular system and preload. The heart rate increases to maintain cardiac output, and the arterioles constrict, increasing peripheral vascular resistance to maintain blood pressure (the pressure of perfusion). As these actions become significant, the patient becomes anxious and slightly tachycardic, and the skin becomes cool and pale (circulation is shunted from the skin to more vital organs). With increasing blood loss, the compensation becomes more significant, and thirst, a rapid, weak pulse, and restlessness become apparent. These signs become more apparent as greater compensation is required to maintain the blood pressure. When the body reaches the limits of its compensation and it can no longer maintain the blood pressure, BP drops precipitously, circulation all but stops, and the patient moves very quickly into irreversible shock.

Care for the shock patient includes high-flow oxygen, hemorrhage control, and fluid resuscitation to maintain vital signs when hemorrhage is controlled, with a stable blood pressure just below 100 mmHg (88 mmHg may be optimal with continuing hemorrhage), or use aggressive fluid resuscitation if the blood pressure drops below 50 mmHg.

17. Identify the need for intervention and transport of patients with compensated and decompensated shock. **pp. 361–371**

The body's ability to compensate for shock is limited. While it can maintain blood pressure, the compensation is not without cost. As the arterioles constrict, they deny blood flow to some organs and themselves use energy and tire. The venous vessels tire as they constrict to reduce the volume of the vascular system. If compensation is significant or prolonged, the body may move into

©2008 Pearson Education, Inc.

decompensation, especially if the hemorrhage is not controlled. Most serious internal hemorrhage can only be halted with surgical intervention, most commonly at a trauma center. In the time between our recognition of shock and arrival at the trauma center, we can help the body with its compensation by providing oxygen and fluid resuscitation.

18. Describe the differences in administration of intravenous fluid in normotensive, hypotensive, or profoundly hypotensive patients. pp. 368–369

Administration of intravenous fluids in the normotensive patient without hypovolemia permits the rapid administration of medications and may be indicated when hypovolemia is anticipated (the burn patient). In the patient who is in compensated shock and maintains a relatively normal systolic blood pressure, fluid resuscitation is indicated if hemorrhage is controlled. If the hemorrhage is internal and cannot be controlled in the field, aggressive fluid resuscitation may lead to increased internal hemorrhage and hemodilution making perfusion and clotting less effective. Generally, the administration of intravenous fluids in the normotensive patient is limited.

In the patient who is hypotensive (BP <100 mmHg), intravenous fluids are administered to maintain, not increase, the blood pressure. Here again aggressive fluid resuscitation would dilute the blood and decrease the effectiveness of perfusion and clotting. An increase in blood pressure would also likely break apart clots that are reducing the internal hemorrhage.

In the patient who is profoundly hypotensive (absent pulses and you are unable to determine a blood pressure, or it is <50 mmHg), aggressive fluid resuscitation is indicated. Here the consequences of severe hypoperfusion outweigh the risks of further hemorrhage.

19. Discuss the physiologic changes associated with application and inflation of the pneumatic anti-shock garment (PASG). pp. 369–370

The pneumatic anti-shock garment (PASG) is an air bladder that circumferentially applies pressure to the lower extremities and abdomen. In theory, it compresses the venous blood vessels, returning some blood to the critical circulation, and compresses the arteries, increasing peripheral vascular resistance. These actions increase circulating blood volume and blood pressure, which should help the patient in shock. However, in some cases of shock, this may increase the rate of internal hemorrhage and may disrupt the clotting mechanisms that are restricting blood loss associated with internal injury.

20. Discuss the indications and contraindications for the application and inflation of the PASG. pp. 370

The PASG is indicated for any patient who displays internal or external hemorrhage in the lower abdomen, pelvis, or lower extremities. It is recommended for the stabilization of any pelvic fracture and may be helpful with bilateral femoral fractures with the signs and symptoms of shock.

The PASG should not be used in the patient who is experiencing pulmonary edema or has a head or penetrating chest injury. It should be used with caution on any patient who is experiencing dyspnea as it may increase intra-abdominal pressure and restrict the movement of the diaphragm. The abdominal section should not be employed if the patient is in the third trimester of pregnancy, has an abdominal evisceration, or an impaled object in the abdomen.

Prior to application of the PASG, the patient's blood pressure, pulse rate and strength, and level of consciousness should be assessed and recorded. The abdomen, lower back, and lower extremities should be visualized to ensure that no sharp debris that could harm either the patient or the garment is present.

21. Differentiate between the management of compensated and decompensated shock. pp. 364–371

The management for compensated shock is directed at preventing decompensated shock through patient support. The care involves hemorrhage control, high-flow/high concentrations of oxygen, fluid administration, maintenance of body temperature, body positioning, and general patient support. Once decompensation occurs, as recognized by dropping blood pressure and the lowering of the level of consciousness, aggressive fluid resuscitation and the use of PASG may be indicated. In both cases, however, the patient must be transported immediately to the emergency department.

©2008 Pearson Education, Inc.
Intermediate Emergency Care: 1985, 3rd ed.

Case Study Review

Reread the case study in Chapter 10 and then read the following discussion. This case study presents an example of aggressive and appropriate care for a patient who, by mechanism of injury alone, is suspected of advancing into shock. It highlights both the elements of shock assessment and care.

Arriving on the scene, Dave is presented with a situation that presents with no noticeable hazards and one patient with a mechanism of injury that indicates the potential for serious internal bleeding. The overturned bulldozer trapped the patient's legs and pelvis and may have fractured the pelvis and femurs. These injuries are frequently associated with severe internal blood loss and shock.

Dave suspects, as the vehicle is lifted off Ken, internal bleeding will occur more rapidly. In preparation, he ensures good oxygenation and assesses the visible portion of the patient. He gathers a baseline set of vital signs (all of which indicate that the patient is not yet in decompensated shock), including a pulse oximeter reading. Dave requests air medical service for this patient as it may reduce the patient transport time since there is an expected delay in extrication. He starts two IV lines using normal saline, infusing both at a to-keep-open rate. The PASG is set out on the long spine board so the patient can be moved in one step to the board and immediately have the PASG applied. Dave and his fellow rescuers converse with Ken not only to calm and reassure him, but also to maintain a continuous assessment of Ken's level of consciousness and determine a patient history.

As the bulldozer is removed, Ken is quickly assessed and then moved to the awaiting spine board. The pelvic, femoral, and tibial fractures suggest shock will develop quickly, so the PASG is inflated immediately, not only to stabilize the fractured pelvis and femurs but to tamponade the internal hemorrhage expected with these injuries. As the blood pressure drops to 62/40, both IVs are run wide open to infuse a quick 500 mL of lactated Ringer's solution and the patient is prepared for rapid transport. After the fluid is run, a repeat of the vital signs reflects no change in the blood pressure so another 500 mL of LR is run. As the patient is prepared for flight, his vitals improve and the fluid flow returns to TKO.

Communication with the hospital and the medical direction physician provide the hospital with updated information on the patient's condition so they can be ready with packed red blood cells. The packed red cells are required because the replacement of blood lost through hemorrhage with crystalloid solution dilutes the number of red blood cells and clotting factors available.

If any one of a number of critical steps in the care of this patient had not been completed, this patient probably would not have survived the trip to the hospital. Dave moved quickly and decisively, performing the skills that stabilized his patient, yet omitting care that would have been provided had the patient not been critical. The EMT-I must, through experience, be quickly able to distinguish the patient who needs rapid transport and aggressive care from the patient who will best benefit from meticulous care at the scene and during transport.

Content Self-Evaluation

Multiple Choice

______ **1.** The intravascular fluid accounts for what percentage of the total body water?
- **A.** 7.5%
- **B.** 15%
- **C.** 35.6%
- **D.** 45%
- **E.** 75%

______ **2.** Dehydration classically presents with all of the following signs EXCEPT
- **A.** slow pulse rate.
- **B.** decreased blood pressure.
- **C.** excessive thirst.
- **D.** poor skin turgor.
- **E.** sunken anterior fontanelle (infants).

______ **3.** The most prevalent extracellular cation is
- **A.** potassium.
- **B.** sodium.
- **C.** calcium.
- **D.** chloride.
- **E.** bicarbonate.

©2008 Pearson Education, Inc.

_____ 4. The process by which a solvent (usually water) travels through a semi-permeable membrane from a lesser concentration of solute particles to a greater concentration is called
A. diffusion.
B. active transport.
C. osmosis.
D. facilitated transport.
E. facilitated diffusion.

_____ 5. The process that causes a solute to distribute itself equally throughout a solvent is called
A. osmosis.
B. diffusion.
C. active transport.
D. facilitated transport.
E. permeation.

_____ 6. The higher the pH value, the lower the concentration of hydrogen ions.
A. True
B. False

_____ 7. The normal pH range in the human body is
A. 6.9 to 7.35.
B. 7.35 to 7.45.
C. 7.45 to 7.8.
D. 6.9 to 7.8.
E. none of the above

_____ 8. Which of the following would be considered alkalosis in the human?
A. 6.9 to 7.35
B. 7.35 to 7.45
C. 7.45 to 7.8
D. 6.4 to 6.9
E. none of the above

_____ 9. A decrease in pH of 1 would reflect which change in the concentration of hydrogen ions?
A. 100 times as great
B. 10 times as great
C. 1/10th as great
D. 1/100th as great
E. a doubling

_____ 10. The cellular environment of the human body is slightly acidic.
A. True
B. False

_____ 11. The body system that responds most rapidly to a change in the pH is the
A. respiratory system.
B. cardiovascular system.
C. digestive system.
D. buffer system.
E. genitourinary system.

_____ 12. The addition of hydrogen ions to the bloodstream will result in an increase in carbon dioxide.
A. True
B. False

_____ 13. An inadequate delivery of oxygenated blood to body cells is
A. hypoxia.
B. anoxia.
C. hypoperfusion.
D. ischemia.
E. infarction.

_____ 14. The normal cardiac stroke volume is about
A. 50 mL.
B. 60 mL.
C. 70 mL.
D. 100 mL.
E. 120 mL.

_____ 15. Which of the following affects the cardiac output?
A. preload
B. afterload
C. cardiac contractile force
D. cardiac rate
E. all of the above

©2008 Pearson Education, Inc.
Intermediate Emergency Care: 1985, 3rd ed.

______ 16. The arteriole has the ability to change its internal diameter by as much as
A. twofold.
B. threefold.
C. fourfold.
D. fivefold.
E. sevenfold.

______ 17. Which of the following blood vessel(s) have (has) the greatest effect on blood pressure?
A. aorta
B. the major arteries
C. the veins
D. arterioles
E. venules

______ 18. Which list places the stages of shock in the order of their occurrence?
A. irreversible, decompensated, compensated
B. compensated, decompensated, irreversible
C. compensated, irreversible, decompensated
D. decompensated, irreversible, compensated
E. decompensated, compensated, irreversible

______ 19. Which stage of shock begins with a precipitous drop in blood pressure?
A. compensated
B. decompensated
C. irreversible
D. hypovolemic
E. none of the above

______ 20. Which of the following does NOT occur during the compensated stage of shock?
A. increasing pulse rate
B. decreasing pulse strength
C. decreasing systolic blood pressure
D. skin becomes cool and clammy
E. the patient experiences thirst and weakness

______ 21. Once the patient becomes profoundly unconscious and loses his vital signs, he moves into irreversible shock.
A. True
B. False

______ 22. When using a pulse oximeter, you should use oxygen and ventilation to keep the reading above which oxygen saturation value?
A. 45 percent
B. 80 percent
C. 85 percent
D. 95 percent
E. 99 percent

______ 23. Which of the following is NOT a type of shock category?
A. hypovolemic
B. cardiogenic
C. psychoneurotic
D. obstructive
E. distributive

______ 24. As peripheral vascular resistance rises to maintain systolic blood pressure, what occurs?
A. heart rate increase
B. respirations increase
C. body temperature rises
D. diastolic blood pressure rises
E. all of the above

______ 25. The column of coagulated erythrocytes caused by capillary stagnation is called
A. ischemia.
B. rouleaux.
C. capillary washout.
D. hydrostatic reflux.
E. compensated reflux.

______ 26. Which of the following suggests significant blood loss (shock)?
A. a pulse rate above 120 in the adult
B. a pulse rate above 140 in the school-age child
C. a pulse rate above 160 in the preschooler
D. a pulse rate above 180 in the infant
E. all of the above

©2008 Pearson Education, Inc.

_____ 27. The color, temperature, and general appearance of the skin can indicate shock before there are changes in the blood pressure.
A. True
B. False

_____ 28. Which of the following signs might be suggestive of obstructive shock (as with tension pneumothorax)?
A. dyspnea
B. resonant percussion
C. subcutaneous emphysema
D. distended jugular veins
E. all of the above

_____ 29. During assessment you note that the patient's lower extremities and lower abdomen are warm and pink while the upper extremities, thorax, and upper abdomen are cool and clammy. This presentation is consistent with which type of shock?
A. hypovolemic
B. neurogenic
C. obstructive
D. cardiogenic
E. respiratory

_____ 30. Which of the following may be an indication to employ overdrive respiration?
A. severe rib fractures
B. flail chest
C. diaphragmatic respirations
D. head injury
E. all of the above

_____ 31. Which of these fluid replacement choices would be most desirable for the patient who is losing blood through internal bleeding?
A. packed red blood cells
B. fresh frozen plasma
C. whole blood
D. colloids
E. crystalloids

_____ 32. Most of the solutions used in prehospital care for infusion are
A. hypotonic colloids.
B. isotonic colloids.
C. hypertonic colloids.
D. hypotonic crystalloids.
E. isotonic crystalloids.

_____ 33. Which of the following characteristics of a catheter will ensure that fluids run rapidly through it?
A. short length, small lumen
B. short length, large lumen
C. long length, small lumen
D. long length, large lumen
E. large lumen and either long or short length

_____ 34. In the patient that has internal bleeding and hypovolemia, the objective blood pressure to maintain by PASG and fluid infusions is
A. 120 mmHg.
B. 90 mmHg.
C. 50 mmHg.
D. below 50 mmHg.
E. at a steady level.

_____ 35. The PASG may return what volume of blood to the central circulation?
A. 250 mL
B. 500 mL
C. 750 mL
D. 1,000 mL
E. none at all

©2008 Pearson Education, Inc.
Intermediate Emergency Care: 1985, 3rd ed.

Chapter 11

Intravenous Access and Medication Administration

Review of Chapter Objectives

After reading this chapter, you should be able to do the following:

1. Describe the indications, equipment, techniques, precautions, and general principles of peripheral venous and external jugular cannulation. **pp. 378–400**

Peripheral venous access is the preferable route for medication administration in the emergency prehospital setting. Most emergency drugs are administered this way because it provides a direct route into the venous system, then to the heart, where the drug and blood are further mixed, and then to the body as distributed by the arterial system. Vascular access can be obtained using a steel needle with a beveled sharp edge. Most commonly, an over-the-needle catheter is advanced into the vein, with the needle then withdrawn, leaving the catheter to permit introduction of drugs or fluid or withdrawal of blood for diagnostic testing. The veins of the hands, arms, antecubital fossa, feet, and legs and the external jugular veins are common sites for intravenous cannulation.

The equipment used for intravenous therapy includes a venous constricting band to help engorge the veins; the needle for venipuncture; an antiseptic to cleanse the site; administration tubing to direct and control fluid administration from an IV bag or a syringe to draw up, then administer medication; tape or commercial devices to secure the intravenous catheter; and bacteriostatic ointment to protect the site from infection. An ideal location for venipuncture is free of injury and with relatively prominent veins. The caregiver should take appropriate body substance isolation measures before beginning the procedure. Then the venous constricting band is secured just proximal to the selected site and a vein is chosen. The area is cleansed with an alcohol or betadine swab, using concentric circles moving outward from the selected site. An over-the-needle catheter is selected, with 14- to 18-gauge for blood, thick medications such as glucose, or fluid volume administration or a 20- to 22-gauge catheter for pediatric or geriatric patients or patients who do not need a larger catheter. The catheter is directed, bevel up, through the skin at an angle of 10 to 30 degrees until a "pop" is felt or blood appears in the flash chamber. Once in the vein, the catheter is advanced an additional 0.5 cm and then the catheter is threaded into the vein. The needle is withdrawn, the constricting band is released, and the administration set or saline or heparin lock is attached. A small amount of fluid is run to ensure that the catheter is patent. Watch for edema around the site, which is suggestive of infiltration. Intravenous cannulation and infusion may result in local pain, infiltration, pyrogenic reactions, allergic reactions, catheter shear and embolism, inadvertent arterial puncture, circulatory overload, thrombophlebitis, thrombus formation, air embolism, and necrosis.

Fluid is infused through a venipuncture site to hydrate the patient or to keep the drug route open and quickly available. Most prehospital infusions use isotonic (same osmotic pressure as the plasma) solutions such as normal saline, 5 percent dextrose in water, or lactated Ringer's solution. These solutions flow through the administration set, where their rate of administration is regulated

©2008 Pearson Education, Inc.

by adjusting the drip rate in a chamber. Most commonly 10 (macro) or 60 (micro) drops traveling through a drip chamber equal 1 milliliter. The administration set contains one or more injection ports to accommodate the administration of drugs or additional fluid administration. A special type of administration set is the measured volume administration set, which contains a calibrated chamber that will permit the discrete administration of a volume of fluid.

The external jugular vein is an alternate venous access site located on the lateral anterior neck. It is a large, easily found vein that permits venous access when other veins are collapsed due to hypovolemia or other vascular problems. It is close to the central circulation, so it provides almost immediate absorption of any drugs administered through it. The jugular vein can be engorged by placing digital pressure along the vein just above the clavical. External jugular cannulation is painful and risks damage to the airway or arterial structures in the neck.

2. Describe the indications, equipment, techniques, precautions, and general principles of intraosseous needle placement and infusion. **pp. 400–403**

Intraosseous needle placement is indicated for the critical pediatric patient under 5 when you cannot establish other IV access sites or for the adult patient when you also cannot perform peripheral venous access because of disease or extreme hypovolemia. A special needle is introduced through the compact bone of the tibia and into the medullary space. There fluids or drugs are readily available for absorption and distribution by the venous system.

In the child, the needle is placed at 90 degrees to the tibial plateau, just medial and about two finger widths below the tibial tuberosity (the anterior bump just below the patella). Don gloves and cleanse the site with an antiseptic swab. With a firm twisting motion, introduce the needle into the bone for a few centimeters until you feel a "pop" or reduced resistance. Remove the trocar, attach a syringe, and draw back on the syringe to aspirate bone marrow and blood. Rotate the plastic disk to engage the skin and secure the needle. Connect the IV fluid administration set and secure the needle with bulky dressings and tape. Adult or geriatric IO administration uses the flat tibial plate just two finger widths above the medial malleolus. IO infusion may result in bone fracture, infiltration, growth-plate damage, pulmonary embolism, and the problems associated with venous cannulation.

In the adult, insert the needle into the medullary canal of the sternum, iliac crest, tibia or humerus. The sternum is frequently used because of its convenient location and its thin, uniform overlying bone thickness. Commercially available devices such as the EZ-IO, F.A.S.T., and Bone Injection Gun devices penetrate the thicker adult bone more easily than the standard pediatric devices. The insertion procedure is similar to that used for the pediatric patient, as are the complications.

3. Describe the purpose, equipment, techniques, complications, and general principles for obtaining a blood sample. **pp. 396–399**

Blood composition, the presence of toxins, and blood gas levels are important values to determine for learning what is wrong with a patient. Since emergency care may alter these figures, it is sometimes important to draw blood in the prehospital setting. Blood is withdrawn from a vein through either a needle or catheter and is either directly placed in special containers (blood tubes) or into a syringe for distribution into the blood tubes. A large vein must be used, because the withdrawal of blood may collapse smaller veins. A needled vacutainer is introduced into an engorged vein and blood tubes are introduced, one at a time. The vacuum withdraws blood from the vein and into the tubes, which are then manually agitated to mix the blood with an anticoagulant (all but the red top tube). If a vacutainer is not available, 20 mL of blood may be drawn up in a syringe and distributed among the containers. It is important to fill the containers in order of red, blue, green, purple, and gray (as available), because they contain various anticoagulants and another order may cross-contaminate the blood.

4. Review the specific anatomy and physiology pertinent to medication administration. **pp. 378, 387, 388–389, 394–396, 400, 406, 413–429**

Chapter 2 reviewed human anatomy as it pertains to the absorption, distribution, metabolization, and elimination of the drugs we use to treat disease and trauma. This chapter identifies the anatomy and physiology related to medication administration.

The percutaneous routes of drug administration include transdermal and mucous membrane administration. Transdermal administration permits drug absorption through the skin via

©2008 Pearson Education, Inc.
Intermediate Emergency Care: 1985, 3rd ed.

topical application in which the medication is slowly and steadily absorbed. Mucous membrane administration methods include sublingual, buccal, ocular, nasal, and aural administration, in which a drug is given under the tongue, between the cheek and gum, in the eye, into the nose, or into the ear respectively. Sublingual and buccal routes result in systemic absorption, while the remaining routes result in more local effects.

Pulmonary administration introduces a drug by nebulizer or metered dose inhaler or through an endotracheal tube. All three methods direct the drug to the lung tissue for action; however, endotracheal administration is an emergency route for systemic administration.

Enteral administration delivers a drug to the gastrointestinal tract, where it is absorbed. This is a relatively safe and simple route for drug administration and is the most common route for over-the-counter and prescription drug administration. The disadvantage of this route is that many factors can affect absorption including stress, diet, and metabolic rate. Liver function metabolizes some drugs, and a dysfunctional liver may alter the medication's metabolization or distribution. The enteral methods of administration include oral, gastric tube, and rectal administration. (Rectal administration is not subject to hepatic [liver] alteration.)

With parenteral administration, a drug is injected into the dermis (intradermal), the subcutaneous layer (subcutaneous), muscle (intramuscular), or veins (intravenous). The intradermal route provides little or no systemic absorption and is used for diagnostic testing and for the administration of local anesthetic. Subcutaneous injection promotes slow, sustained systemic absorption of a drug, while intramuscular injection permits systemic drug absorption at a moderate rate. Because intravenous drug administration injects the drug directly into the bloodstream, where it is directed to the heart, mixed with the returning venous blood, and then distributed systemically, it is the fastest parenteral administration route.

Anatomically, subcutaneous injections may be made into the skin regions over the deltoid muscle, the thighs, and, in some cases, the upper abdomen. Intramuscular injections may be given into the deltoid muscle, 2 inches below the acromial process; into the gluteal muscle, in the upper outer quadrant of the buttocks; into the anterolateral aspect of the thigh muscle (vastus lateralis); and into the central and lateral segment of the mid-thigh (rectus femoris).

5. Discuss legal aspects affecting medication administration, including the "six rights" of drug administration. **pp. 403–404**

The administration of the wrong medication or withholding the right medication or providing it in the wrong dose or by the wrong route can have catastrophic consequences. Hence, medication administration is an area of EMT-I practice where the EMT-I is exposed to legal liability. You must ensure that you receive informed and expressed consent from the patient (when possible), provide medications in strict compliance with system protocols and the direction of on-line medical direction, and follow proper administration techniques. Once a medication is administered, it is essential that you document the indication for the drug, any online authorization for the administration, the name of the person who delivered the drug, the drug name, dose, route and rate of delivery, and the resulting patient response, whether positive or negative. These actions will go a long way to limiting your liability in drug administration.

There are basically six rights of drug administration. They are the right patient, the right drug, the right dose, the right time, the right route, and the right documentation.

The right patient. Ensure that the patient is the right person and properly matched to the medication. This is an infrequent problem in prehospital care, but as EMS moves to the out-of-hospital environment, we may be treating some patients on a routine basis. Ensure the medication order is for the patient you are attending.

The right drug. Ensure the drug is what is intended for the patient. Review your standing orders or, if the order is received from medical direction, repeat ("echo") the order back to the physician so you are both clear on the drug, dose, route, and timing of the order. Also examine the drug packaging to ensure that it contains the medication you wish to administer and that the medication is still sterile, has not expired, and is not contaminated or discolored.

The right dose. Carefully calculate the exact dose (usually weight dependent) for the patient before you draw up the medication and again just before you administer it. If the drug

©2008 Pearson Education, Inc.

package you select has significantly more or less of the drug than you intend to use, recheck the packaging to ensure it is the right drug and right concentration, and recheck your calculations to ensure the right dosage. Never overdose or underdose your patient.

The right time. Usually prehospital medications are given rather rapidly and not on a schedule. Check the packaging and your protocols for administration rates and ensure that you follow the sequencing, time intervals between, and drip rates for emergency drugs.

The right route. Specific drugs require specific routes of administration. While most emergency drugs are administered by the IV route, be aware of alternate drug administration routes, the drugs that can be administered by those routes, and the circumstances requiring the use of those routes. With each medication administration, ensure you are using the right route.

The right documentation. Documentation of drug administration is of paramount importance. You must carefully record the patient's condition (the circumstances that require the drug's administration), the drug name, dose, and route of administration, and who administered the drug and at what time. It is also essential that you record the patient's response to the drug, whether good or bad.

6. Discuss medical asepsis and the differences between clean and sterile techniques, and uses of antiseptics and disinfectants. pp. 404–405

Medical asepsis describes a medical environment free of pathogens. The most aseptic environment is a sterile one, one free of all living organisms. However, in prehospital care we frequently cannot attain such a state. We utilize equipment and supplies that are sterile when packaged and then use medically clean techniques to reduce the risk of spreading infection. These techniques include the use of disinfectants to kill microorganisms on equipment and in the ambulance and of antiseptics to reduce the bacterial load on the patient's skin when we utilize procedures like venipuncture.

Antiseptics are agents that are designed for topical use to destroy or inhibit pathogenic microorganisms already on living tissue. They are used to cleanse the skin before parenteral drug administration to prevent infection secondary to the needle stick.

Disinfectants are powerful agents that are toxic to living tissue. They are not designed for topical administration but for the direct cleaning of durable patient care equipment.

7. Describe how standard precautions relate to medication administration. p. 380

Any time there is the possibility of contact with body substances or patient wounds, you must use body substance isolation measures. Gloves, at a minimum, provide barrier protection to the caregiver from possibly infectious material at the scene and to the patient from the caregiver. Goggles and a mask also provide protection, as does hand washing after contact with a patient or possibly infected material.

8. Describe the equipment, techniques, complications, and general principles for the preparation and administration of parenteral medication. pp. 406–407, 413–429

Parenteral administration includes the routes utilizing needles to administer drugs into the tissues or vascular system—intradermal, subcutaneous, intramuscular, intravenous, and intraosseous routes. Begin the parenteral administration process by cleansing the patient's skin at the injection site with an antiseptic such as alcohol or a betadine solution. The medication for injection is in solution and drawn up in a syringe, then injected with a needle (bevel up). For subcutaneous and intramuscular injection, consider injecting a 0.1-mL air bubble after the medication to limit leakage, and then massage the region to enhance absorption. Most emergency medications are injected via the intravenous route because of its rapid distribution throughout the body.

Intradermal drug administration calls for insertion of a 25- to 27-gauge needle at a 10- to 15-degree angle just into a segment of skin that is pulled taut. Slow injection of up to 1 mL of solution will create a small wheal of medication. Then remove the needle. Intradermal injection results in a very slow absorption rate greatly affected by local perfusion rates and is used for diagnostic testing and the administration of local anesthetics.

For subcutaneous administration, place a 24- to 26-gauge needle into a 1-inch "pinch" of the patient's skin at a 45-degree angle and inject no more than 1 ml of medication. The skin must be

©2008 Pearson Education, Inc.
Intermediate Emergency Care: 1985, 3rd ed.

free of scarring, superficial nerves, blood vessels and tendons, tattoos, and bruising. Pulling the plunger back ensures that the needle is not in a blood vessel (aspiration of blood indicates a blood vessel entry). Subcutaneous injection may be given at many locations around the body, including the tissue under the tongue.

For intramuscular injections, use a 21- to 23-gauge needle inserted at a 90-degree angle into the deltoid (up to 2 mL), dorsal gluteal (up to 5 mL), vastus lateralis (up to 5 mL), or rectus femoris (up to 5 mL) muscle. Again, pulling back on the plunger ensures that the needle is not in a blood vessel. Intramuscular injection provides a predictable systemic absorption and is used for several prehospital drugs including glucagon and morphine. Careful placement of parenteral needles is important because of potential damage to nerves and arteries. Needles for intradermal, subcutaneous, and intramuscular injection are 3/8 to 1 inch in length.

9. Describe proper disposal of contaminated items and sharps. **p. 405**

Sharps and contaminated materials pose a risk for the spread of infection. Do not recap needles unless absolutely necessary and, in such instance, do so using only one hand. Used needles represent a real risk for introducing pathogens from the patient's blood into someone stuck with the needle. Dispose of all needles in a puncture-proof biohazard container. Ensure all medical waste is placed in a biohazardous waste bag and is not left at the scene. Follow your service's biohazard exposure plan should you receive a needlestick.

10. Synthesize a pharmacologic management plan including medication administration. **pp. 403–429**

As you care for patients with serious medical and trauma emergencies, you will often need to administer medications to them via the sublingual, oral, pulmonary, subcutaneous, intramuscular, intravenous, and intraosseous routes. The procedures described in this chapter must become an integral part of your patient management skills.

11. Integrate pathophysiological principles of medication administration with patient management. **pp. 403–429**

Drug administration is a fundamental skill used in the treatment of the sick and injured. For medications to be effective, they must be safely delivered to the body by the appropriate route. Many different routes for drug delivery are available to the EMT-I; however, specific drugs require specific routes for administration. It is the responsibility of the EMT-I to know the best medication to give by the best route in the appropriate dose at the appropriate time to manage his patient's condition according to the treatment protocols and local medical direction. You have learned in this chapter, for example, that certain medications do not work well when administered orally to a patient in shock or by IM to a patient with poor distal perfusion. By integrating the pathophysiologic principles of medication administration with and understanding of your assessment of the patient's medical condition, you will be able to better manage the patient's needs.

12. Describe the indications, equipment, techniques, precautions, and general principles of administering medications by inhalation routes. **pp. 426–429**

Pulmonary medications are administered via nebulizer, metered dose inhaler, and endotracheal tube. Drugs indicated for inhalation include those that cause bronchodilation, mucolytics, antibiotics, and topical steroids for respiratory emergencies, congestion, infection, and inflammation respectively.

A nebulizer aerosolizes a small volume of liquid (or dissolves) medication using oxygen, which is then inhaled into the lungs and absorbed quickly. The device is assembled (mouth piece, medication reservoir, oxygen port, relief valve, and oxygen tubing and source), and 3 to 5 ml of solution (or a medication dissolved in 3 to 5 ml of sterile water) is placed in the medication reservoir. Oxygen is set to run at 5 to 8 liters per minute (without a humidifier), and the mouthpiece is placed in the patient's mouth. The patient should hold the nebulizer and inhale slowly and deeply with each breath, then hold the breath for 1 to 2 seconds before exhaling. The patient should continue doing this until the medication is gone (about 3 to 5 minutes). For nebulized medications to be effective, the patient must have an adequate tidal volume and respiratory rate, although nebulizers can be connected to an endotracheal tube during positive pressure ventilation.

©2008 Pearson Education, Inc.

Metered dose inhalers are frequently used in patients with COPD and asthma to deliver agents to induce bronchodilation. The device consists of a pressurized medication canister, plastic shell and mouthpiece, and possibly a spacer. The patient self-administers the drug by assembling the inhaler, shaking it for 2 to 5 seconds, inverting it, placing the mouthpiece in the mouth, and sealing the lips against the mouthpiece. Then, during the beginning of a deep inhalation, the patient presses the canister downward to release a dose of medication. A second dose may be necessary. Nebulizers are preferable to metered dose inhalers in acute respiratory emergencies because they administer the drug over more time and are less dependent on a single deep inspiration.

Endotracheal administration of a drug involves expressing the drug down the endotracheal tube (in a volume of 10 mL and from 2 to 2.5 times the normal intravenous dose). Narcan, atropine, lidocaine, and epinephrine can be administered this way in an emergency when IV access is not otherwise available. Once the drug is injected down the endotracheal tube, the ventilator provides several deep ventilations to deliver the drug to the pulmonary tissue.

Case Study Review

Reread the case study in Chapter 11 and then read the following discussion.

You and Jay are requested to respond to a full arrest but 3 minutes away. On arrival, you spot CPR in progress. These events suggest a better than average chance to successfully resuscitate your patient. The use of the AED and the officers doing good compressions and ventilations add to this prognosis. However, the rhythm of asystole (no electrical activity) suggests otherwise. While you and Jay care for the airway and circulation, your student prepares for the IV and fluid and medication administration.

Darren readies a 1,000 mL bag of normal saline and checks its clarity and expiration date. He spikes the bag with a macrodrip set, assures it remains medically clean and also tears tape to secure the line. Once that is prepared, Darren swabs the intended site and initiates a large-bore IV (14 gauge). It is clear he has practiced this procedure many times so that it is performed smoothly and efficiently. He uses the blood on the catheter for a glucose analysis, then disposes of the sharps appropriately. He then covers the intravenous site with a tagaderm dressing and uses the two tape strips to secure the IV tubing in a loop so a pull on the tube won't dislodge the catheter.

Darren adjusts the flow rate by turning the wheel and watches the drip chamber. The steady flow of fluid identifies that the IV is running wide open. This rapidly pushes any medications administered, like the epinephrine, quickly into the venous circulation, taking it quickly to the heart where it mixes with other returning blood, circulates through the lungs, travels back through the heart, and then out to the rest of the body. The whole procedure happens in but seconds.

Notice that simultaneously Darren exercises due caution. He wears gloves and goggles, announces that a sharps is located where others might come in contact with it, and carefully places all needles in the sharps container and contaminated materials in a biohazard bay where they are no longer a danger to rescuers or bystanders.

Content Self-Evaluation

Multiple Choice

_____ 1. Which of the following is an indication for intravenous administration?
- A. fluid replacement
- B. blood replacement
- C. drug administration
- D. need of blood for analysis
- E. all of the above

_____ 2. Both central venous and peripheral venous cannulation are common in prehospital care.
- A. True
- B. False

©2008 Pearson Education, Inc.
Intermediate Emergency Care: 1985, 3rd ed.

______ 3. Which of the following is a likely site for intravenous cannulation?
A. the hands
B. the arms
C. the legs
D. the neck
E. all of the above

______ 4. The solution that contains large proteins is a(n)
A. colloid.
B. crystalloid.
C. isotonic.
D. hypotonic.
E. hypertonic.

______ 5. The solution that contains an electrolyte concentration close to that of plasma is a(n)
A. colloid.
B. crystalloid.
C. isotonic.
D. hypotonic.
E. hypertonic.

______ 6. The solution that contains an electrolyte concentration greater than that of plasma is a(n)
A. colloid.
B. crystalloid.
C. isotonic.
D. hypotonic.
E. hypertonic.

______ 7. One example of a hypotonic solution is
A. normal saline.
B. lactated Ringer's solution.
C. plasmanate.
D. 5 percent dextrose in water.
E. dextran.

______ 8. The most desirable replacement for blood lost during trauma is
A. normal saline.
B. lactated Ringer's solution.
C. plasmanate.
D. 5 percent dextrose in water.
E. none of the above

______ 9. Which intravenous fluid bag would you discard?
A. one that is cloudy
B. one that is discolored
C. one that is leaking
D. one that is expired
E. all of the above

______ 10. For optimal fluid delivery, the drip chamber should be how full?
A. 1/4
B. 1/3
C. 1/2
D. 2/3
E. none of the above

______ 11. The administration set most appropriate for administration of intravenous solutions for fluid replacement is the
A. macrodrip administration set.
B. microdrip administration set.
C. measured volume administration set.
D. blood tubing set.
E. none of the above

______ 12. The most common microdrip setting equaling 1 mL is
A. 10 gtts.
B. 20 gtts.
C. 45 gtts.
D. 60 gtts.
E. none of the above

______ 13. The administration set most appropriate for administration of a very specific volume of intravenous solution or drug is the
A. macrodrip administration set.
B. microdrip administration set.
C. measured volume administration set.
D. blood tubing set.
E. none of the above

©2008 Pearson Education, Inc.

_____ 14. The major difference between blood tubing and a standard intravenous administration set is that blood tubing has a filter to remove clots and particulate matter.
A. True
B. False

_____ 15. Blood is not administered with fluids like lactated Ringer's solution because such solutions increase blood's potential for coagulation.
A. True
B. False

_____ 16. The most common intravenous cannula used in the prehospital setting is the
A. over-the-needle.
B. through-the-needle.
C. hollow needle.
D. angiocatheter.
E. A and D

_____ 17. A needle gauge of 18 is smaller than a needle gauge of 22.
A. True
B. False

_____ 18. A venous constricting band should be left in place no longer than
A. 1 minute.
B. 2 minutes.
C. 3 minutes.
D. 5 minutes.
E. 10 minutes.

_____ 19. Leaving the constricting band on for too long is likely to cause
A. collapse of the vein.
B. damage to the distal blood vessels.
C. damage to the vessels under the band.
D. changes in the distal venous blood.
E. all of the above

_____ 20. When cleansing the site for intravenous cannulation, you should make one swipe over the intended site with a betadine or alcohol swab.
A. True
B. False

_____ 21. The angle of insertion for intravenous cannulation is
A. 10 degrees.
B. 10 to 30 degrees.
C. 45 degrees.
D. 60 degrees.
E. 60 to 90 degrees.

_____ 22. After you feel the "pop" associated with intravenous cannulation, you should
A. advance the catheter.
B. advance the needle 0.5 centimeter, then advance the catheter.
C. advance the needle 1 centimeter, then advance the catheter.
D. advance the needle 2 centimeters, then advance the catheter.
E. withdraw the needle, then advance the catheter.

_____ 23. You should consider using the external jugular vein as an IV access site only after you have exhausted other means of peripheral access or when the patient needs immediate fluid administration.
A. True
B. False

_____ 24. During external jugular vein cannulation, the patient's head should be
A. moved to the sniffing position.
B. turned toward the side of access.
C. turned away from the side of access.
D. hyperextended.
E. hyperflexed.

©2008 Pearson Education, Inc.
Intermediate Emergency Care: 1985, 3rd ed.

_____ 25. To fill the jugular access site and make the vessel easier to both locate and cannulate, you should
A. apply a venous constricting band, tightly.
B. apply a venous constricting band, loosely.
C. occlude the vein gently with a finger.
D. perform the procedure without occluding the vein.
E. have the patient take a deep breath and hold it.

_____ 26. When establishing an IV with blood tubing, you must be careful to
A. fill the drip chamber 1/3 full.
B. completely cover the blood filter with blood.
C. fill the set with normal saline first.
D. fill the drip chamber 3/4 full.
E. A and B

_____ 27. Which of the following is a factor that may affect intravenous flow rates?
A. failure to remove a venous constricting band
B. edema at the access site
C. the cannula tip up against a vein valve
D. a clogged catheter
E. all of the above

_____ 28. The complication of peripheral venous access in which a plastic embolus can form is
A. pyrogenic reaction.
B. pain.
C. thrombophlebitis.
D. catheter shear.
E. all of the above

_____ 29. The most common cause of catheter shear is
A. cannulating thick veins.
B. cannulating underneath the constricting band.
C. withdrawing the needle from within the catheter.
D. withdrawing the catheter from the needle.
E. faulty catheter construction.

_____ 30. If a blood clot appears to stop or slow intravenous fluid flow, forcefully inject a small amount of heparin into the catheter and continue the infusion.
A. True
B. False

_____ 31. The reason venous blood sampling is important in the prehospital setting is that our interventions may alter the blood's composition or erase important information about it.
A. True
B. False

_____ 32. Drawing blood and injecting it into the blood tubes in the wrong order may result in
A. leaving the wrong volume of blood in a tube.
B. cross-contamination of the blood with anticoagulants.
C. depletion of the vacuum in the tubes at too early a stage.
D. coagulation in the last tubes to be filled.
E. all but C

_____ 33. Do not use a blood tube after its expiration date because the anticoagulant and vacuum may have become ineffective.
A. True
B. False

_____ 34. The device that accepts the blood tube to permit its filling is
A. the leur lock.
B. the Huber needle.
C. the vacutainer.
D. the leur-sampling needle.
E. A or C

©2008 Pearson Education, Inc.

______ 35. You should fill the blood tube to between a third and a half of its volume because the anticoagulant is measured for this amount of blood.
A. True
B. False

______ 36. When using a syringe to fill your blood tubes, you should draw a volume of blood of about
A. 5 mL.
B. 10 mL.
C. 20 mL.
D. 35 mL.
E. 50 mL.

______ 37. The complication from drawing blood in which red blood cells are destroyed is
A. hematocrit.
B. hemoconcentration.
C. hemolysis.
D. hemotypsis.
E. hematuria.

______ 38. Hemoconcentration occurs during drawing blood
A. when the constricting band is left in place too long.
B. when blood is drawn back through a needle that is too small.
C. with premature mixing of the anticoagulant.
D. with too vigorous a mixing of the blood and anticoagulant.
E. with too forceful an aspiration of blood into the syringe.

______ 39. When an IV catheter is withdrawn, place pressure on the venipuncture site with a sterile gauze pad for about 5 minutes.
A. True
B. False

______ 40. Any solution or drug that can be administered via the intravenous route may also be administered by the intraosseous route.
A. True
B. False

______ 41. Acceptable intraosseous infusion sites for the adult include all of the following EXCEPT
A. sternum.
B. tibia.
C. pelvis.
D. humerus.
E. all of the above

______ 42. Confirmation that you are in the medullary space is achieved by
A. feeling the bone "pop."
B. pushing the needle 2 to 4 mm.
C. aspirating bone marrow and blood.
D. feeling resistance to the twisting of insertion.
E. none of the above

______ 43. Complications of intraosseous cannulation include all of the following EXCEPT
A. pulmonary embolism.
B. fracture.
C. growth plate damage.
D. aspiration of bone marrow.
E. complete insertion.

______ 44. Medication administration is an important part of the medical care provided by EMT-Is.
A. True
B. False

______ 45. Which of the following is NOT one of the six rights of drug administration?
A. the right dosage
B. the right indication
C. the right time
D. the right documentation
E. the right patient

©2008 Pearson Education, Inc.
Intermediate Emergency Care: 1985, 3rd ed.

______ **46.** The process you use to ensure you hear and correctly understand the medical direction physician's order to administer a medication is
A. protocol compliance.
B. order confirmation with your partner.
C. redundant physician orders.
D. echoing the order back to the physician.
E. asking the physician to repeat the order.

______ **47.** Which of the following must you know about the drugs you are authorized to administer?
A. their usual dosages
B. their contraindications
C. their common side effects
D. their routes of administration
E. all of the above

______ **48.** When you administer drugs, which of the following standard precautions should you always employ?
A. gloves
B. a mask
C. goggles
D. a gown
E. A and D

______ **49.** The condition in which a medical environment is free of all pathogens is described as
A. asepsis.
B. uncontaminated.
C. medically clean.
D. disinfection.
E. none of the above

______ **50.** The environment that EMT-Is should strive to maintain while delivering prehospital emergency care is
A. aseptic.
B. sterile.
C. medically clean.
D. disinfected.
E. none of the above

______ **51.** To cleanse the site of a parenteral injection, you would use a(n)
A. aseptic.
B. disinfectant.
C. detergent.
D. antiseptic.
E. dilutant.

______ **52.** When possible, you should recap needles
A. as a last resort.
B. in a moving ambulance only.
C. except in a moving ambulance.
D. only when they have not been used on a patient.
E. when directed by a physician.

______ **53.** Documentation regarding the administration of a drug should include all of the following EXCEPT the
A. time of administration.
B. route of administration.
C. class of drug administered.
D. positive patient responses.
E. negative patient responses.

______ **54.** A syringe should be chosen for drug administration that is slightly smaller than the volume of drug to be administered.
A. True
B. False

______ **55.** The smaller the gauge of a hypodermic needle, the smaller the diameter of its lumen.
A. True
B. False

©2008 Pearson Education, Inc.

______ 56. What is the total dose of a drug contained in an ampule with 5 mL of a drug in a 0.3 mg/mL concentration?
A. 0.3 mg
B. 1.5 mg
C. 5 mg
D. 15 mg
E. none of the above

______ 57. Which of the following drug containers may contain multiple doses of a drug?
A. vial
B. ampule
C. Mix-o-Vial
D. preloaded syringe
E. medicated solutions

______ 58. Prior to drawing medication from a vial, you must first inject an equal volume of air into the vial.
A. True
B. False

______ 59. Which of the following must be cleansed with an alcohol swab before the drug is withdrawn?
A. vial
B. ampule
C. Mix-O-Vial
D. preloaded syringe
E. A and C

______ 60. Which of the following is a common emergency drug administered sublingually?
A. sodium bicarbonate
B. epinephrine
C. nitroglycerin
D. aspirin
E. magnesium

______ 61. The drug route that calls for insertion of the needle at 10 to 15 degrees is
A. intradermal.
B. subcutaneous.
C. intramuscular.
D. intraosseous.
E. none of the above

______ 62. Which of the following is most likely to be an acceptable site for subcutaneous injection?
A. forearms
B. calves
C. abdomen
D. buttocks
E. all of the above

______ 63. Through which of the following routes should you inject no more than 1 mL of a drug?
A. intradermal
B. subcutaneous
C. intramuscular
D. A and B
E. all of the above

______ 64. For intradermal and subcutaneous injections, the needle is inserted with the bevel down.
A. True
B. False

______ 65. At which of the following intramuscular injection sites should you administer a maximum of 2 mL of a drug?
A. deltoid
B. gluteal
C. vastus lateralis
D. rectus femoris
E. B and C

______ 66. When you pull back on the syringe plunger during subcutaneous or intramuscular injection and blood appears, you should
A. inject the drug.
B. inject the drug followed by a small bubble of air.
C. insert the needle 1 cm further.
D. attempt the injection at another site.
E. consider the appearance of blood insignificant.

©2008 Pearson Education, Inc.
Intermediate Emergency Care: 1985, 3rd ed.

______ 67. The drug route that calls for use of a 21- to 23-gauge needle is
A. intradermal.
B. subcutaneous.
C. intramuscular.
D. intraosseous.
E. none of the above

______ 68. The drug route that calls for use of a needle 3/8 to 1 inch long is
A. intradermal.
B. subcutaneous.
C. intramuscular.
D. all of the above
E. none of the above

______ 69. The recommended angle of insertion for the needle when administering an intramuscular injection is
A. 10 degrees.
B. 15 degrees.
C. 45 degrees.
D. 90 degrees.
E. between 10 and 15 degrees.

______ 70. After injecting an intramuscular drug, massaging the site is contraindicated because it will slow absorption.
A. True
B. False

______ 71. Never administer an intravenous drug infusion as the primary IV line.
A. True
B. False

______ 72. Which of the following information would you expect to find on the label of a premixed intravenous solution bag?
A. name of the medication
B. total dosage of the drug
C. concentration of the drug
D. expiration date
E. all of the above

______ 73. The volume of heparin needed to fill the standard heparin lock is
A. 1 to 2 mL.
B. 3 to 5 mL.
C. 7 to 15 mL.
D. 10 to 20 mL.
E. none of the above

______ 74. Once a drug is administered through a heparin lock, you should infuse what volume of saline?
A. 1 to 2 mL
B. 3 to 5 mL
C. 7 to 15 mL
D. 10 to 20 mL
E. none of the above

______ 75. The small volume nebulizer often used in prehospital emergency medical service administers what volume of medication?
A. 1 to 2 mL
B. 3 to 5 mL
C. 5 to 10 mL
D. 10 to 15 mL
E. 15 to 20 mL

______ 76. The small volume nebulizer's major advantage over the metered dose inhaler is that the patient does not need an adequate tidal volume for effective medication delivery.
A. True
B. False

______ 77. The metered dose inhaler is activated to release its medication
A. just before the patient seals his lips to the mouthpiece.
B. as the patient exhales.
C. as the patient inhales.
D. during both inhalation and exhalation.
E. between inhalation and exhalation.

©2008 Pearson Education, Inc.

______ 78. Nebulizers and metered dose inhalers are advantageous in respiratory emergencies because they deliver their medication to the exact site of action.
A. True
B. False

______ 79. Endotracheal medication administration calls for drugs to be diluted to what volume?
A. 1 mL
B. 2 mL
C. 3 mL
D. 5 mL
E. 10 mL

______ 80. Which of the following drugs is NOT administered via the endotracheal route?
A. meperidine
B. naloxone
C. atropine
D. lidocaine
E. epinephrine

©2008 Pearson Education, Inc.
Intermediate Emergency Care: 1985, 3rd ed.

Chapter 12

Pharmacology

Review of Chapter Objectives

After reading this chapter, you should be able to do the following:

1. List the four main sources of drug products. **p. 434**

There are four main sources of drugs. They are plants, animals, minerals, and synthetic substances (laboratory).

2. List the components of a drug profile. **pp. 437–438**

Names: The generic, trade, and sometimes the chemical names
Classification: The broad group to which the drug belongs
Mechanism of action: The way the drug causes its desired effects (its pharmacodynamics)
Indications: The conditions appropriate for the drug's administration
Pharmacokinetics: How the drug is absorbed, distributed, and eliminated, including its onset and duration of action
Side effects/adverse reactions: The drug's untoward or undesired effects
Routes of administration: How the drug is given
Contraindications: Conditions that make it inappropriate to administer a drug (including conditions in which administration is likely to cause a harmful outcome)
Dosage: The amount of drug that should be given
How supplied: The typical concentrations and preparations of the drug
Special considerations: How the drug may affect pregnant, pediatric, and geriatric patients

3. Differentiate among the chemical, generic (nonproprietary), and trade (proprietary) names of a drug. **p. 434**

The chemical name of a drug represents its chemical composition and molecular structure. An example is 7-chloro-1, 3-dihydro-1-methyl-5-phenyl-2H-1, 4-benzodiazepine-2-one.

The generic name of a drug is suggested by the original manufacturer and confirmed by the United States Adopted Name Council. An example, for which the chemical name is given above, is diazepam.

The brand, trade, or proprietary name of a drug is the name given the drug by a specific manufacturer. This name is a proper name and should be capitalized and may be followed by a trademark insignia. An example is Valium®, a brand name for diazepam.

4. List and differentiate the phases of drug activity, including the pharmaceutical, pharmacokinetic, and pharmacodynamic phases. **pp. 438–442**

The pharmaceutical phase of drug activity addresses the drug's intrinsic characteristics such as how the drug dissolves or disintegrates once injected or ingested. Pharmacokinetics refers to the processes by which a drug is absorbed, distributed, biotransformed, and eliminated by the body.

©2008 Pearson Education, Inc.

Pharmacodynamics is the mechanism (or mechanisms) by which a drug interacts with the body to accomplish its action.

5. Describe the processes called pharmacokinetics and pharmacodynamics, including theories of drug action, drug-response relationship, factors altering drug responses, predictable drug responses, and unpredictable adverse drug responses. pp. 438–442

There are two important elements of pharmacology: how drugs are transported into or out of the body (pharmacokinetics) and how drugs interact with the body to cause their effects (pharmacodynamics).

Pharmacokinetics examines the absorption, distribution, biotransformation, and elimination of drugs.

For a drug to perform its action, it must first reach its site of action, a process referred to as **absorption**. While some drugs affect target tissue directly (like antacids in the stomach), most must first find their way to the bloodstream. Drugs administered directly into a venous or arterial vessel are quickly transported to the heart, mixed with the blood, and distributed throughout the body. A drug injected into the muscle tissue and, to a somewhat lesser degree, into the subcutaneous tissue, is transported quickly to the bloodstream because of the more than adequate circulation in these tissues. However, shock and hypothermia may slow the process, while fever and hyperthermia may speed it. Oral medications must survive the gastric acidity and be somewhat lipid soluble to be transported across the intestinal membrane. The differing acid content of the digestive tract also impacts the dissociation of the drug into ions that are more difficult to move into the circulation. And finally, the drug's concentration affects its uptake by the bloodstream and, ultimately, its distribution. The end result of the absorption process is the concentration of the drug in the bloodstream and its availability for activation of the target tissue, called its bioavailability.

Once a drug enters the bloodstream, it must be carried throughout the body and to its site of action. The term for this process is **distribution**. Many factors affect the release and uptake of a drug by the body's cells. Some drugs bind to the plasma proteins of the blood and are released over a prolonged period of time. An increase in the blood's pH may increase the rate of release of the drug, or competition from other drugs for binding sites may cause more of a drug to become available. Distribution of some drugs is dependent upon their ability to cross the blood-brain or placental barriers. Other drugs are easily deposited in fatty tissue, bones, and teeth.

Once in the body, drugs are broken down into metabolites in a process called **biotransformation**. This process makes the drug more or less active and can make the drug more water soluble and easier to eliminate. Some drugs are totally metabolized, some are partially metabolized, while still others are not metabolized at all. The liver is responsible for most biotransformation, while the lungs, kidneys, and GI tract do some limited biotransformation.

Elimination is the excretion of the drug in urine, expired air, or in feces. Renal excretion is the major mechanism for eliminating drugs from the body. Drugs are eliminated as the blood pressure pushes and filters blood through kidney structures. This effect is enhanced by special cells that "pump" (active transport) some metabolites into the tubules. Kidney reabsorption also plays a part in drug excretion. Protein-soluble molecules and electrolytes are easily absorbed, but the uptake may be affected by the blood's pH.

A drug's effects on the body are referred to as **pharmacodynamics**. Drugs may cause their effects by binding on a receptor site, by changing physical properties, by chemically combining with other substances, or by altering a normal metabolic pathway.

Most drugs effect their actions by binding to receptor sites, especially those of the autonomic nervous system. The drug either inhibits or stimulates the cells or tissue. The force of attraction of a drug is referred to as its **affinity**. Affinity becomes important when different drugs compete for a site. The drug's **efficacy** is its ability to cause the expected response. Binding to a receptor site causes a change within the cell and induces the drug's effect. However, some drugs may establish a chain-reaction effect whereby other drugs are released and cause the desired effect. The number of receptor sites may change as the drug becomes available and uses them, thereby reducing the drug's continuing effect. Chemicals that bind to the receptor and cause the expected response are termed **agonists**. **Antagonists** bind to the site and do not cause the expected response. Some drugs

©2008 Pearson Education, Inc.
Intermediate Emergency Care: 1985, 3rd ed.

have both properties. Drugs may also act by modifying the physical properties of a part of the body. For example, the drug mannitol changes the blood's osmolarity and increases urine output.

Some drugs chemically combine with other substances to cause their desired effect. For example, antacids interact with the hydrochloric acid in the stomach to reduce the pH.

Other drugs act by altering normal biologic processes and the metabolic pathways. Such drugs are used to treat cancers and viral infections.

The **drug-response relationship** is the relationship between a drug's pharmaceutical, pharmacokinetic, and pharmacodynamic properties. It most commonly relates to the blood plasma level of the drug. Other important factors include the speed of onset, duration of action, minimum effective concentration, and biologic half-life. Another very important factor in the drug-response relationship is the **therapeutic index**, or the ratio between the drug's lethal and effective doses.

Factors altering drug response include the patient's age, body mass, sex, pathologic state, genetic factors, and psychological factors as well as environmental considerations and the time of administration. These factors may increase or decrease the drug's ability to generate its desired affect.

Responses to drug administration may include unintended responses, or **side effects**. These are care-provider induced (iatrogenic) and include allergic reactions, idiosyncratic (unique to an individual) reactions, tolerance, cross-tolerance, tachyphylaxis, cumulative effects, dependency, drug interactions, drug antagonisms, summation, synergistic reactions (a result greater than the expected additive result of two drugs administered together), potentiation, and interference. Some of these effects may be predictable and desired and some may be unexpected.

6. List and describe general properties of drugs. pp. 437–438

- An **agonist** is a drug that causes the expected effect when bound to the receptor site.
- An **antagonist** is a drug that does not cause the expected effect when bound to the receptor site.
- An **agonist-antagonist** is a drug that binds to a receptor site, causing some expected effects and blocking others.

7. Describe mechanisms of drug action. pp. 440–441

How a drug interacts with the body to cause its effects is referred to as pharmacodynamics. Drugs induce their effects by binding to a receptor site, changing the physical properties of the body, chemically combining with other substances, or altering a normal metabolic pathway.

8. Discuss considerations for storing and securing drugs. pp. 435–437

Federal laws require certain drugs be stored, secured, and accounted for. Because of the complexity of the issue, the large variability in the drugs used by EMS systems, and how states, EMS systems, and ambulance services meet these requirements, it is important that you consult with your service operations officer, your system protocols and guidelines, and your system medical director to identify the proper criteria for storing and securing drugs.

9. Review mathematical principles, equivalents, and conversions. pp. 445–448

The metric system's three fundamental units are grams, meters, and liters. If you know the prefixes and their numeric equivalents, you can easily convert measurements to smaller or larger units. To convert to a smaller unit multiply the original measurement by the numerical equivalent of the smaller measurement's prefix. To convert a measurement to a larger unit, divide the original measurement by the numerical equivalent of the smaller measurement's prefix.

The metric system has replaced the traditional apothecary and household systems of measure although there are still some occasional holdovers that you may run into. The international thermometric scale measures temperature in degrees Celsius. The centigrade is slightly different from Celsius, yet based on a similar system of 100 equal parts. The more popular Fahrenheit measurement is still used but not the basis for medicine. Thus the EMT-I should learn to convert from Fahrenheit to Celsius and back again.

©2008 Pearson Education, Inc.

10. Calculate oral and parenteral drug dosages for all emergency medications administered to adults, infants, and children. **pp. 448–451**

To calculate basic drug dosage, either oral or parenteral, you need to know the desired dose, the dose on hand, and the volume on hand. The desired dose is the specific quantity of medication needed. Dosages may be standard or calculated according to body weight or age. Concentration refers to weight per volume. A liquid medication's concentration is the drug's weight per volume of liquid in which it is dissolved. From the concentration, you can determine the dosage on hand and the volume on hand. Because you cannot see the desired dose dissolved in liquid, you must convert its weight to volume using the formula:

$$\text{Volume to be administered} = \frac{\text{Volume on hand (desired dose)}}{\text{Dosage on hand}}$$

Remember to express all weight and volume measurements with the same metric prefix.

11. Calculate intravenous infusion rates for adults, infants, and children. **pp. 451–452**

To deliver fluid or medication through an IV infusion, you must calculate the correct infusion rate in drops per minute. To calculate the correct IV infusion rate you must first know the administration tubing's drip chamber factor, as well as the volume on hand, desired dose, and dosage on hand. The correct formula to use is as follows:

$$\text{Drops/minute} = \frac{\text{Volume on hand} \times \text{drop} \times \text{drip factor} \times \text{desired dose}}{\text{Dosage on hand}}$$

Fluids being administered, either with or without medication, require a specific period of time to infuse. To calculate the time to infuse, the following formula is used:

$$\text{Drops/minute} = \frac{\text{Volume to be administered (drip factor)}}{\text{Time in minutes}}$$

Remember that the dosages in infants and children are weight dependent and your calculation of their weight should be accurate.

12. List and describe the drugs that an EMT-Intermediate may administer in a pharmacological management plan. **pp. 452–461**

At the end of this workbook is a series of drug cards. Cut them out and review them to assure you can list and describe the drugs used in your system.

Case Study Review

Reread the case study in Chapter 12 and then read the following discussion. This case study exemplifies the importance of knowing the effects of the drugs we administer and their potential impact on patients with preexisting medical problems. The study further examines the importance of a thorough patient history and how the information revealed by it can impact the administration of emergency drugs.

The crew of Unit 151 is presented with a 68-year-old female patient with a history of asthma and complaining of dyspnea. She has a moderately rapid respiratory rate and only slightly labored breathing. The crew reports diffuse wheezes, confirming a probable asthma event. Her heart rate is only slightly elevated, her blood pressure normal, and her oxygen saturation is 95%, reason only for slight concern. They administer oxygen by nonrebreather at 15 lpm and watch the saturation rise to 100%.

The history from this patient is quite revealing. The report of her inhaler running out last evening and her need for 3 to 5 doses per day explain her dyspnea and wheezing. However, the careful investigation into her past medical history identifies the past myocardial infarctions and the use of nitroglycerin and propranolol, a potent beta blocker. This information is very important, as propranolol is

©2008 Pearson Education, Inc.
Intermediate Emergency Care: 1985, 3rd ed.

prescribed to slow the heart rate while the common drugs administered for asthma are likely to increase its rate. This coupled with her age (which probably limits her ability to metabolize the drugs) will cause these care providers to be very careful in the administration of albuterol and her past history of cardiac problems contraindicates the use of epinephrine. Following the nebulized albuterol, they are also very watchful of the patient to assure the drugs they do administer do not have adverse effects. They are especially watchful for the signs of an MI, including chest pain, nausea, or dizziness. Without the attention to detail this crew observed, the care they would have given this patient might very well have caused more problems than it would have corrected.

Content Self-Evaluation

Multiple Choice

______ 1. The study of drugs and their interactions with the body is
A. pharmaceutics.
B. pharmacokinetics.
C. pharmacodynamics.
D. pharmacology.
E. pharmacopedia.

______ 2. Which of the following types of drug names is 7-chloro-1, 3-dihydro-1-methyl-5-phenyl-2H-1, 4-benzodiazepine-2-one?
A. chemical name
B. generic name
C. official name
D. brand name
E. common name

______ 3. Which of the following types of drug names is diazepam?
A. chemical name
B. generic name
C. official name
D. brand name
E. common name

______ 4. Digitalis is an example of a drug derived from
A. a plant.
B. an animal.
C. a mineral.
D. synthetic production.
E. a lipid base.

______ 5. Bovine insulin is an example of a drug derived from
A. a plant.
B. an animal.
C. a mineral.
D. synthetic production.
E. a lipid base.

______ 6. The drug reference that presents manufacturer-provided drug information and some photos of drugs is the
A. *EMS Guide to Drugs.*
B. *Physician's Desk Reference.*
C. *AMA Drug Evaluations.*
D. *Monthly Prescribing Reference.*
E. all of the above

______ 7. The broad group to which a drug belongs is its
A. indication.
B. pharmacokinetics.
C. classification.
D. mechanism of action.
E. none of the above

______ 8. Conditions in which it is inappropriate to give a drug are referred to as its
A. mechanisms of action.
B. indications.
C. contraindications.
D. side effects.
E. special considerations.

©2008 Pearson Education, Inc.

______ 9. Drugs do not confer any new properties on cells or tissues; they only modify or exploit existing functions.
A. True
B. False

______ 10. Which of the following is NOT one of the four basic processes of pharmacokinetics?
A. absorption
B. distribution
C. receptor binding
D. biotransformation
E. elimination

______ 11. Which of the following represents an energy-consuming movement of ions against the concentration gradient?
A. diffusion
B. active transport
C. osmosis
D. filtration
E. facilitated transport

______ 12. Which of the following represents movement of molecules across a membrane from an area of higher pressure to an area of lower pressure?
A. diffusion
B. active transport
C. osmosis
D. filtration
E. facilitated transport

______ 13. The measure of the amount of a drug that is still active after it reaches the target organ is its
A. bioavailability.
B. biotransformativity.
C. metabolism.
D. pro-drug effect.
E. active distribution.

______ 14. Which of the following is a significant medium for elimination of drugs from the body?
A. urine
B. respiratory air
C. saliva
D. sweat
E. all are significant

______ 15. Pharmacodynamics are best described as
A. interactions between drugs.
B. the processes by which drugs are eliminated from the body.
C. the effects of a drug on the body.
D. the processes by which drugs bind to receptor sites.
E. the process by which a drug is administered.

______ 16. The location where a drug combines with a protein, resulting in a biochemical effect, is a(n)
A. second messenger.
B. antagonist.
C. receptor.
D. agonist.
E. protein block.

______ 17. A drug's ability to cause the receptor to initiate its expected response is referred to as its
A. affinity.
B. efficacy.
C. agonist.
D. antagonist.
E. equilibrium.

______ 18. A chemical that binds to a receptor site but does not cause the expected effect is a(n)
A. partial-antagonist.
B. competitive antagonist.
C. agonist.
D. antagonist.
E. noncompetitive antagonist.

______ 19. A drug reaction that is unique to an individual is referred to as
A. idiosyncrasy.
B. tachyphylaxis.
C. antagonism.
D. synergism.
E. potentiation.

©2008 Pearson Education, Inc.
Intermediate Emergency Care: 1985, 3rd ed.

______ 20. A drug reaction that is greater than expected from the administration of two drugs that have the same effect at the same time is referred to as

A. idiosyncrasy.
B. tachyphylaxis.
C. antagonism.
D. synergism.
E. potentiation.

______ 21. Which of the following is NOT a division of the nervous system?

A. central nervous system
B. peripheral nervous system
C. autonomic nervous system
D. sympathetic nervous system
E. antagonistic nervous system

______ 22. Which nervous system controls motor functions?

A. somatic
B. autonomic
C. sympathetic
D. parasympathetic
E. antagonistic

______ 23. Which nervous system is responsible for the "feed-or-breed" response?

A. somatic
B. autonomic
C. sympathetic
D. parasympathetic
E. antagonistic

______ 24. Which nervous system works in opposition to the parasympathetic nervous system?

A. central
B. sympathetic
C. autonomic
D. somatic
E. antagonistic

______ 25. The agents that transport impulses through the synapse between neurons and between nerve cells and the target organs are called

A. neuroeffectors.
B. neurotransmitters.
C. intrasynaptic agents.
D. neuroleptic ions.
E. transport cells.

______ 26. The cholinergic neurotransmitter is

A. acetylcholine.
B. epinephrine.
C. norepinephrine.
D. muscarinic antagonist.
E. muscarinic agonist.

______ 27. Which neurotransmitter serves both the sympathetic and parasympathetic nervous systems?

A. acetylcholine
B. epinephrine
C. norepinephrine
D. dopamine
E. none of the above

______ 28. A drug that stimulates the parasympathetic nervous system is called a(n)

A. sympatholytic.
B. sympathomimetic.
C. parasympatholytic.
D. parasympathomimetic.
E. antiemetic.

______ 29. Which of the following is a fundamental unit of the metric system?

A. liter
B. gram
C. meter
D. pound
E. all except D

______ 30. Which of the prefixes below represents 1/1,000?

A. deci
B. kilo
C. micro
D. centi
E. milli

©2008 Pearson Education, Inc.

Special Project

Pharmacology (Drip and Drug) Math

Guide to Easier Drug Calculations

While there might be more rapid systems to calculate drip rates and concentrations, the following stepwise approach is designed to help you understand the math so you are able to solve almost any problem. While math is an essential skill for the EMT-I, most drip calculations are simple, standard, and easy to perform once you become familiar with the drugs and drip rates used in your system.

Step I: Identify all known elements.

Elements for most drug dose calculations:

C = Concentration (g, mg, or μg per ml)
Dd = Desired dose
Va = Volume to be administered
Dh = Weight (Dose on hand) (g, mg, or μg)
Vh = Volume on hand (convert to mL)

Elements for most drip calculations:

R = Rate (either in drops/min, drops/mcg, or mL/min)
V = Volume (convert to mL)
T = Time (convert to minutes)
D = Drip conversion (drops per mL)

Step II: Select the proper formula.

The element that you don't know (and need to find) should be equal to the remainder of the formula.

Concentration = Dose on hand/Volume on hand $\quad C = Dh/Vh$

Dose on hand = Volume on hand × Concentration $\quad Dh = Vh \times C$

Volume on hand = Dose on hand/Concentration $\quad Vh = Dh/C$

$$\text{Volume to be administered} = \frac{\text{Volume on hand} \times \text{Desired dose}}{\text{Dosage on hand}} \qquad Va = \frac{Vh \times Dd}{Dh}$$

$$\text{Dose on hand} = \frac{\text{Volume on hand} \times \text{Desired dose}}{\text{Volume to be administered}} \qquad Dh = \frac{Vh \times Dd}{Va}$$

$$\text{Desired dose} = \frac{\text{Volume to be administered} \times \text{Dosage on hand}}{\text{Volume on hand}} \qquad Dd = \frac{Va \times Dh}{Vh}$$

$$\text{Volume on hand} = \frac{\text{Volume to be administered} \times \text{Dosage on hand}}{\text{Desired dose}} \qquad Vh = \frac{Va \times Dh}{Dd}$$

Rate = Volume/Time($R = V/T$)

Volume = Rate × Time($V = R \times T$)

Time = Volume/Rate($T = V/R$)

©2008 Pearson Education, Inc.
Intermediate Emergency Care: 1985, 3rd ed.

Step III: Convert all variables into common terms.

Use the drip conversion figure or other conversion formula to convert all values to metric and standard values.

Rate—into milliliters or milligrams/minute
Volume—into milliliters
Concentration—into milligrams/milliliter
Time—into minutes
Weight—into milligrams

Step IV: Plug in the known values.

Complete the formula, inserting the values identified in Step I.

Step V: Cancel out labels.

Cross-multiply labels to cancel them out. The result should leave you with the label in terms of the unknown value.

$$\text{Volume} = \frac{\text{Rate} \times \text{Time}}{\text{min}} = \frac{\text{X ml} \times \text{Y}\cancel{\text{min}}}{\cancel{\text{min}}} = \text{X ml} \times \text{Y} = \text{X} \times \text{Y ml}$$

Step VI: Do the mathematical operations.

Multiply, divide, add, or subtract as necessary.

$3 \times 7 = 21 \quad 3/7 = 0.43 \quad 7 + 3 = 10 \quad 7 - 3 = 4$

Step VII: Apply any needed conversions.

Use the mathematical conversions needed, such as the drip conversion, to determine the final answer. Ensure that your answer is provided in the form and label the question asks for.

$$\frac{\text{X ml/min}}{\text{min}} \text{ using a } \frac{\text{Y gtts/ml}}{\text{ml}} = \text{X ml} \times \text{gtts} = \frac{\text{X} \times \text{Y gtts}}{\text{min}} = \text{X} \times \text{Y gtts/min}$$

There are two particular types of math used in prehospital care. One deals with continuous intravenous infusions (drip math) and the other deals with parenteral bolus or enteral administration (drug math). Included within this workbook are exercises for drip and drug math.

Drip Math Worksheet 1

Formulas

Rate = Volume/Time mL/min = drops per min/drops per mL

Volume = Rate × Time drops/min = mL per min × drops per mL

Time = Volume/Rate mL = drops/drops per mL

Please complete the following drip math problems.

1. You are running a D_5W drip (60 drops/ml) into a patient at 15 drops/min. During a 25-minute trip to the hospital, how much fluid would you infuse?
2. Medical direction requests that you infuse 250 mL of a solution during a 1 hour transport. What rate do you need to set:

   A. for a 60 drops/mL infusion set?

   B. for a 10 drops/mL infusion set?

©2008 Pearson Education, Inc.

3. If a 50 mL bag of normal saline is hung and running through a 45 drops/mL administration set at 32 drops per minute, how long will the fluid last?
4. If you are running a macro drip (10 drops/mL) at 4 drops per second, how much fluid could you infuse in 45 minutes?
5. Medical direction orders you to infuse 1.5 mL of a solution every minute. What drip rate would you set:
   A. with a 60 drops/mL set?
   B. with a 45 drops/mL set?
   C. with a 10 drops/mL set?

Drug Math Worksheet 1

Formulas

$$\text{Concentration} = \text{Dose on hand/Volume on hand} \quad C = Dh/Vh$$

$$\text{Dose on hand} = \text{Volume on hand} \times \text{Concentration} \quad Dh = Vh \times C$$

$$\text{Volume on hand} = \text{Dose on hand/Concentration} \quad Vh = Dh/C$$

$$\text{Volume to be administered} = \frac{\text{Volume on hand} \times \text{Desired dose}}{\text{Dose on hand}} \quad Va = \frac{Vh \times Dd}{Dh}$$

$$\text{Dose on hand} = \frac{\text{Volume on hand} \times \text{Desired dose}}{\text{Volume to be administered}} \quad Dh = \frac{Vh \times Dd}{Va}$$

$$\text{Desired dose} = \frac{\text{Volume to be administered} \times \text{Dose on hand}}{\text{Volume on hand}} \quad Dd = \frac{Va \times Dh}{Vh}$$

$$\text{Volume on hand} = \frac{\text{Volume to be administered} \times \text{Dose on hand}}{\text{Desired dose}} \quad Vh = \frac{Va \times Dh}{Dd}$$

$$1\text{ kg} = 2.2\text{ lb} \quad 1\text{ g} = 1{,}000\text{ mg} \quad 1\text{ mg} = 1{,}000\ \mu\text{g}$$

Please complete the following drug math problems.

1. What volume of atropine, provided as 1 mg in 5 mL, would you administer to provide 0.5 mg of drug to the patient?
2. The medical direction physician asks you to administer 40 mg of furosemide to a patient. It comes in an ampule with 80 mg in 4 mL. What volume will you administer?
3. What volume of epinephrine would you administer to provide a patient with 1 mg of the drug:
   A. if provided as a 1:1,000 solution? (1 g/1,000 mL)
   B. if provided as a 1:10,000 solution? (1 g/10,000 mL)
4. Protocol calls for the administration of 0.2 mg/kg of adenosine for a pediatric patient. Your patient weighs 6 kilograms, and the drug is supplied in a vial with 6 mg in 2 mL. What volume would you administer to your patient?

©2008 Pearson Education, Inc.
Intermediate Emergency Care: 1985, 3rd ed.

Chapter

13 Cardiac Emergencies

Review of Chapter Objectives

After reading this chapter, you should be able to do the following:

1. Describe the incidence, morbidity, and mortality of cardiovascular disease. **pp. 468–469**

Cardiovascular disease (CVD) is serious and extremely common, with more than 60 million Americans affected. Morbidity is considerable: An American has a nonfatal heart attack (myocardial infarction, MI) roughly every 29 seconds. Coronary heart disease (CHD), one type of CVD, is the single largest killer of Americans and Canadians. Roughly 466,000 Americans die annually from CHD, half of them before reaching a hospital. Many deaths from CHD are sudden and involve lethal cardiac dysrhythmias. Many deaths from MI occur within the first 24 hours, frequently within the first hour.

2. Review cardiovascular anatomy and physiology. **pp. 469–472**

Cardiac anatomy and physiology were discussed in detail in Chapter 2. The adult heart is the size of a clenched fist and lies in the center of the mediastinum posterior to the sternum and anterior to the spine. It is a muscular organ, with three tissue layers: endocardium, or innermost layer that lines the chambers; the myocardium, or middle layer with its unique ability to generate and conduct electrical impulses causing the heart to contract; and the pericardium, which is a protective sac surrounding the heart. Normally, about 25 mL of pericardial fluid is contained between the two layers of pericardium, and the heart can move freely within the pericardial sac.

The heart contains four chambers, two superior, the atria, and two inferior, the ventricles. Valves control the flow of blood through the heart. The mitral valve is between the left atrium and ventricle; the tricuspid valve is between the left ventricle and aorta and the pulmonary valve between the right ventricle and the pulmonary artery.

The right atrium receives deoxygenated blood from the body via the superior and inferior venae cava. The right ventricle sends the deoxygenated blood to the lungs via the pulmonary artery. Oxygenated blood is returned from the lungs to the left atrium via the pulmonary veins. The left ventricle pumps the oxygenated blood to the body via the aorta. Oxygenated blood is pumped from the heart to the tissues via the arteries, and deoxygenated blood is transported from the tissues back to the heart via the veins. The capillaries connect arteries and veins. The exchange of oxygen and carbon dioxide with the body tissues takes place through the very thin capillary walls.

The heart receives its nutrients from the coronary arteries that originate in the aorta and spread over the heart. The left coronary artery supplies the left ventricles, interventricular septum, part of the right ventricle, and the conduction system. Its two main branches are the anterior descending artery and circumflex artery. The right coronary artery supplies a portion of the right atrium and right ventricle and part of the conduction system. Its two major branches are the posterior descending artery and marginal artery.

The cardiac cycle consists of diastole, the relaxation phase that takes place at the end of a cardiac contraction, and systole, the contraction phase. Normally when the heart contracts, each ventricle ejects about two thirds of its blood, which is about 70 mL. This volume is known as the ejection fraction or the stroke volume and it depends on three factors: preload, cardiac contractility, and afterload. Preload is the end-diastolic volume and influences the force of the next contraction because of the stretch it exerts. Frank Starling's law of the heart states that the more myocardial muscle is stretched, the greater its force of contraction will be. Afterload is the resistance against which the heart muscle must pump. An increase in peripheral vascular resistance will decrease stroke volume.

Cardiac output is calculated as stroke volume times the heart rate. Since the normal heart rate is 60–100 beats per minute and the average stroke volume is 70 mL, the average cardiac output is about 5 liters per minute (70 mL × 70 bpm = 4,900 mL/min).

The heart function is regulated by the sympathetic and parasympathetic nervous components of the autonomic nervous system, working in opposition to one another to maintain a balance. During stress, the sympathetic system dominates to raise the heart rate and increase contractile force. During sleep, the parasympathetic system dominates to decrease heart rate and contractile force. The autonomic control of the heart is defined by three terms: chronotropy or rate, inotropy or contractile strength, and dromotropy or rate of impulse conduction. Lastly, the cardiac function depends heavily on electrolyte balances. Electrolytes that affect cardiac function include sodium, potassium, chloride, and magnesium.

3. Discuss prevention strategies that may reduce the morbidity and mortality of cardiovascular disease. p. 469

There are two public health prevention strategies. The first is to educate people about the risk factors for CVD and encourage lifestyle modifications to minimize the potential impact of risk factors. The second strategy is to teach signs and symptoms of a heart attack so patients can receive medical intervention as soon as possible. As you will see, the likelihood of success with fibrinolytic therapy for a heart attack in evolution (treatment with a clot-buster drug to dissolve the clot causing myocardial ischemia/hypoxia) is highest when care is instituted very early in the course of the attack.

4. Identify the risk factors most predisposing to coronary artery disease. p. 477

Factors proven to increase the risk of CVD include (1) smoking, (2) older age, (3) family history of cardiac disease, (4) hypertension, (5) hypercholesterolemia, (6) diabetes mellitus, (7) cocaine use, and (8) male gender. Factors that are thought to increase risk include (1) diet, (2) obesity, (3) oral contraceptives, (4) sedentary lifestyle, (5) Type A personality (competitive and aggressive), and (6) psychosocial tension (stress).

5. Identify and describe the components of assessment as it relates to the patient with cardiovascular compromise. pp. 472–480

The focused history for cardiac situations uses the SAMPLE format: Symptoms, Allergies, Medications, Past medical history, Last oral intake, and Events preceding the incident.

- **Signs/Symptoms.** The most common symptoms of cardiac disease/compromise include chest pain or discomfort, dyspnea, cough, syncope, and palpitations.

  Use the OPQRST format (also something you encountered with pulmonology) to assess chest pain or discomfort: Onset of pain, Provocation/Palliation of pain, Quality of pain, Region where felt/Radiation, Severity, and Timing (duration). Questions concerning dyspnea are similar: You want to know how long it has lasted and whether it is continuous or intermittent. Was onset rapid or gradual? Does anything specific either worsen or palliate the dyspnea, and is it exertional or not? Last, be sure to see if orthopnea exists: Does sitting upright give any relief? Questions about cough center on whether it is chronic or acute and whether it suggests congestive heart failure (dry or productive, presence of any wheezing with cough, etc.).

  In addition, observe and question for these possible signs/symptoms: level of consciousness, diaphoresis, restlessness/anxiety, feeling of impending doom, nausea/vomiting, fatigue, palpitations,

©2008 Pearson Education, Inc.
Intermidiate Emergency Care: 1985, 3rd ed.

edema of extremities or positional (sacral), syncope, behavioral change, facial expression, limitation of activity, signs of recent trauma. Many signs/symptoms of cardiovascular disease and compromise can be subtle or change (either rapidly or gradually) over time.

- **Allergies.** Check for allergies to medication (prescription and over-the-counter). Try to distinguish between details suggestive of side effect (such as GI upset) and those of allergy (rash, hives, anaphylactic shock).
- **Medications.** Check both for current medications (again, prescription and over-the-counter) and recent medication changes. If there has been a recent change, ask why. Look for use of cardiovascular drugs such as nitroglycerin, propranolol or other beta blockers, digitalis (digoxin, Lanoxin), diuretics (Lasix, Dyazide), antihypertensives (Capoten, Prinivil, Vasotec), antidysrhythmics (Quinaglute, Mexitil, Tambocor), lipid-lowering agents (Mevacor, Lopid), and erectile dysfunction medications (Viagra, Levitra, Cialis). If possible, check directly (by inspecting med tray, if there is one) or indirectly (by history) about drug compliance and bring containers to the hospital with you.
- **Past medical history.** Ask directed questions about history of heart disease, MI, stroke, high blood pressure, as well as why suggestive drugs are taken. Specific problems you should inquire about include history of rheumatic heart disease (valvular problems), previous cardiac surgery, congenital cardiac anomalies, pericarditis or other inflammatory cardiac disease, or congestive heart failure (CHF). Relevant problems of other organ systems include pulmonary disease/COPD, diabetes mellitus, renal disease, hypertension, atherosclerosis. Also ask whether there is any family history of illness/death (particularly early deaths before age 50) from cardiovascular disease or other relevant disorders. Last, be sure to ask whether patient smokes or smoked tobacco and whether he/she knows his/her cholesterol level.
- **Last oral intake.** Valuable as a screening question for anyone with a possible surgical condition, this also gives you the chance to ask about most recent caffeine or tobacco use, as well as whether there was a recent fatty meal. (For some patients, this may help steer you to gallbladder disorders.)
- **Events preceding incident.** Ask what the patient was doing just before onset of symptoms. Was there emotional stress or physical exertion? Was there sexual activity? If the patient is male, does he take Viagra? It is often uncomfortable to take a sexual history, but sometimes the information gained is lifesaving, and you can explain to the patient the possible importance of the answer.

6. Explain the purpose of ECG monitoring and its limitations. p. 480

The electrocardiogram (*electro* = electrical, *cardio* = heart, *gram* = record) visualizes the heart's electrical activity as recorded from skin-surface electrodes. The heart is the largest generator of electrical energy in the body, and this is conducted through the body to the skin. An ECG machine records changes in current as a positive impulse (shown on the machine or on a paper printout as an upward deflection), a negative impulse (shown as a downward deflection), or no change (a flat, isoelectric line). The pattern shown over time is a chronological record of the heart's electrical activity, and it is called a rhythm strip.

The ECG in no way assesses the contractility of the myocardium or the pumping ability of the left ventricle, only the electrical activity in the different regions of the heart. There are other limitations of ECG monitoring. Artifacts may occur on the tracing, deflections that do NOT reflect the electrical activity of the heart. Artifacts may be due to a variety of causes, including muscle tremor, shivering movements by the patient, loose electrodes, interference at the 60-hertz range, and machine malfunction. It is important that you be able to recognize artifacts and try to eliminate them from the tracing.

7. Describe how ECG wave forms are produced and correlate the electrophysiological and hemodynamic events occurring throughout the entire cardiac cycle with the various ECG wave forms, segments, and intervals. pp. 482–488

The components of an ECG tracing reflect the electrical changes in the heart with each impulse conducted through the heart:

- **P wave.** This first component of the ECG reflects atrial depolarization. On Lead II, it appears as a positive, rounded wave that comes before the QRS complex. Normally, this correlates hemodynamically with the opening of the AV valves and atrial contraction, which completes the filling of the ventricles with blood.
- **QRS complex.** This second component of the ECG reflects ventricular depolarization. The Q wave is the initial negative deflection after the P wave; the R wave is the first positive deflection after the P wave; and the S wave is the first negative deflection after the R wave. You should note that not all three waves need be present, and the shape of the QRS complex can vary among individuals. Normally, this correlates hemodynamically with the opening of the semilunar valves and ventricular contraction, pumping blood into the pulmonary arteries and aorta.
- **T wave.** The T wave, which follows the QRS complex, reflects repolarization of the ventricles. It is normally positive in Lead II, rounded, and moves in the same direction as the QRS complex. This is the correlate of ventricular relaxation after contraction.
- **U wave.** A U wave is an occasional finding; when it occurs, it follows the T wave and is usually positive in deflection. U waves are normal in some individuals. You should note that it reflects electrolyte abnormalities in other patients.

In addition, three time intervals and a segment of the ECG reading also have clinical significance:

- **P-R interval (called PRI or P-Q interval, PQI).** The P-R interval is the distance from the beginning of the P wave (the beginning of atrial depolarization) to the beginning of the QRS complex (the beginning of ventricular depolarization). It represents the time taken to send the impulse from the atria to the ventricles (the delay at the AV junction and node). The R wave is absent in some individuals, and in these patients you will see a P-Q interval instead. The terms PRI and PQI are used interchangeably.
- **QRS interval.** The QRS interval is the distance from the first deflection of the QRS complex to the last, and it represents the time necessary for ventricular depolarization and onset of ventricular contraction.
- **Q-T interval.** This is the distance from the beginning of the Q wave to the beginning of the T wave, and it represents the total duration of ventricular depolarization. The duration of the Q-T interval normally has an inverse relationship with heart rate. At increased heart rates (tachycardia), the Q-T interval is generally shortened. With bradycardia, Q-T interval is generally lengthened.
- **S-T segment.** This is the distance from the S wave to the beginning of the T wave, and generally it is isoelectric. In some states such as myocardial ischemia, this segment may be either elevated or depressed.

8. Identify how heart rates may be determined from ECG recordings. pp. 488–489

ECG graph paper is standardized such that paper always moves across the recording stylus at 22 mm/sec. (Each small box represents 0.04 second, and each large box is equivalent to five small boxes, or 0.20 second.) ECG paper also has time interval markings at the top of the paper, with marks placed at 3-second intervals (or 15 large boxes, $15 \times 0.20 = 3.0$ seconds).

Three methods exist for quickly establishing heart rate. First, if a patient has a regular rhythm, you can take the number of heartbeats in 6 seconds, multiply by 10, and get rate in beats per minute (bpm). Second, you can measure the R-R interval (also in a patient with a regular rhythm) in seconds, divide into 60, and you have heart rate per minute. If the R-R interval is 0.65 second, $60 \div 0.65 = 92$ bpm. (Other methods using the R-R interval are described on text page 488.) The triplicate method, also useful only in the case of a regular rhythm, requires you to find an R wave that falls on a dark line bordering a large box. You can then assign numbers corresponding to heart rate to the next six dark lines to the right: This equates to 300, 150, 100, 75, 60, and 50 bpm. The number corresponding to the dark line closest to the peak of the next R wave is a rough estimate of heart rate. Last, you can use a commercial heart rate calculator ruler. If you prefer this method, make sure you are comfortable with at least one alternative method that does not require a physical aid.

©2008 Pearson Education, Inc.
Intermidiate Emergency Care: 1985, 3rd ed.

9. Describe a systematic approach to the analysis and interpretation of cardiac dysrhythmias. **pp. 488–489**

The following characterize normal sinus rhythm: (1) heart rate between 60 and 100 bpm; (2) regular rhythm, with constant P-P and R-R intervals; (3) P waves that are normal in shape, upright, and appear only before each QRS complex; (4) P-R interval that is constant and lasting 0.12–0.20 second; and (5) QRS complex with normal shape and duration less than 0.12 second. Any deviation from the normal electrical rhythm constitutes a dysrhythmia. The term arrhythmia is properly reserved for states in which there is no cardiac electrical activity.

10. Identify the specific mechanical, pharmacological, and electrical therapeutic interventions for patients with dysrhythmias causing compromise. **pp. 490–500**

- **Sinus bradycardia.** The overall goal of treatment is satisfactory heart rate, with subsequently adequate cardiac output and blood pressure and decreased risk of more dangerous dysrhythmias. Thus, treatment is based on symptoms, and no treatment may be needed unless hypotension or ventricular irritability is present. If treatment is needed, give a 0.5 mg bolus atropine sulfate, and repeat every 3–5 minutes until rate is satisfactory or you have given 3.0 mg atropine. If atropine fails, consider transcutaneous cardiac pacing (TCP), if available.
- **Sinus tachycardia.** Treatment is directed at the underlying cause. Hypovolemia, fever, anemia, or other cause should be corrected. The overall goal is to reduce heart rate to a level compatible with adequate ventricular filling time, with supports in place to maintain an adequate stroke volume.
- **Premature ventricular contractions (PVCs).** Treatment is indicated for patients with a prior history of heart disease or symptoms or if the PVCs are malignant. Administer oxygen and establish IV access. If the patient is symptomatic, give lidocaine at a dose of 1.0–1.5 mg/kg body weight. Give an additional bolus of 0.5–0.75 mg/kg every 5–10 minutes as needed until a total of 3.0 mg/kg has been reached. If PVCs are effectively suppressed, start a lidocaine drip at a rate of 2–4 mg/minute. Reduce dose in appropriate patients. As an alternative to lidocaine, consider amiodarone. Overall goal is adequate ventricular filling and cardiac output and prevention of ventricular tachycardia or ventricular fibrillation.
- **Ventricular tachycardia (VT).** If there is a pulse (perfusing VT), give oxygen and place an IV line. Give amiodarone, 150 mg in 20 ml of D5W over 10 minutes. If conversion is successful, administer a 1mg/min. drip to a total dose of 360 mg. Alternately, give lidocaine IV at 1.0–1.5 mg/kg and additional doses of 0.5–0.75 mg/kg up to a total of 3.0 mg/kg. If there is no pulse (nonperfusing VT), treat as for ventricular fibrillation. Treatment goals are to maintain adequacy of cardiac output and coronary artery perfusion and to prevent ventricular fibrillation.
- **Ventricular fibrillation.** Treatment of ventricular fibrillation and nonperfusing VT is the same: Initiate CPR for 2 minutes and follow with defibrillation at 360 joules (or biphasic equivalent). Continue CPR (without pulse check), control airway, and establish IV access. Administer epinephrine 1:10,000 or vasopressin as the drug of first choice; give epinephrine every 3–5 minutes as needed. If unsuccessful, consider second-line agents such as lidocaine or amiodarone.
- **Asystole** (or *cardiac standstill*). Treatment is CPR, airway management, oxygenation, and medication (epinephrine and atropine). If there is any doubt of an underlying rhythm, attempt defibrillation.

11. Describe the indications for and process of defibrillation. **pp. 500–507**

Defibrillation is indicated for the patient who is in ventricular fibrillation or pulseless ventricular tachycardia. On arrival, question bystanders about the circumstances of the patient collapse and verify that the patient is unconscious, pulseless, and apneic. Provide 2 minutes of CPR while setting up the AED. Assure the patient is in a safe defibrillation environment dry and away from metal objects. Turn the power on and apply the defibrillation pads to the patient's chest. Clear personnel from the patient and allow the AED to analyze the rhythm. If advised, deliver the shock. Continue CPR without taking the pulse for two minutes before checking pulse and administering additional shocks. For manual defibrillator, follow the same procedure but administer the shock at 360 joules or the machine's biphasic equivalent.

©2008 Pearson Education, Inc.

12. Define angina pectoris and myocardial infarction (MI). **pp. 508–511, 512**

Angina pectoris, or pain in the chest, occurs when the myocardial demand for oxygen exceeds the available supply through the coronary arteries. Myocardial ischemia causes the chest pain. Usually, reduced blood flow through the coronary arteries is correlated with permanent partial obstruction by atherosclerotic lesions.

Each year about 466,000 Americans die from coronary heart disease (CHD) and myocardial infarction (MI) is the usual direct cause of death. In addition, an American suffers a nonfatal MI every 29 seconds. Myocardial infarction, the death of myocardial tissue, is the result of prolonged oxygen deprivation or when myocardial oxygen demand exceeds oxygen supply for an extended period. MI is most often associated with atherosclerotic heart disease (ASHD, which is the same as atherosclerotic coronary heart disease). The precipitating event is often development of a thrombus in a partially occluded artery, with the thrombus completely occluding the vessel. Other pathophysiologic bases for MI include coronary artery spasm, microemboli as can be seen with cocaine use, acute volume overload, hypotension (causing myocardial hypoperfusion), or acute respiratory failure (leading to acute hypoxia). Trauma can also cause MI, often by loosening atherosclerotic plaque in the coronary artery, blocking it.

The region of the heart affected and the size of the eventual infarcted area depend on the coronary artery involved and the specific site of the obstruction. Most infarctions involve the left ventricle. Obstruction of the left coronary artery or its branches may result in infarction of the anterior or lateral ventricle or the interventricular septum. Right coronary artery occlusions tend to result in infarction of the inferior or posterior wall of the left ventricle or infarction of the right ventricle.

The pathophysiologic progression of events starts with ischemia, followed by cell death. The infarcted tissue becomes necrotic and eventually forms scar tissue, if the affected individual survives. Ischemic tissue at the periphery of the infarct will survive but may become the origin of dysrhythmias. Dysrhythmias are the most common complication of MI and the most common cause of death from an MI.

Infarction of myocardium can cause congestive heart failure. Heart failure implies that the heart is working poorly but adequately. If the heart cannot meet body oxygen demand, cardiogenic shock results. Last, if the damaged portion of the ventricular wall is too weakened, it may form a ventricular aneurysm and rupture, causing death.

Based on pathophysiology, the basic strategies of intervention are pain relief and reperfusion. For reperfusion to be effective, rapid, safe transport is essential.

13. List other clinical conditions that may mimic signs and symptoms of angina pectoris and myocardial infarction. **pp. 473–474, 508–511, 512**

Causes of chest pain fall into four categories: cardiovascular, respiratory, gastrointestinal, and musculoskeletal. You'll note that the causes range from the troublesome but benign (dyspepsia, or heartburn) to the life threatening (aortic dissection). Cardiovascular causes include coronary artery disease and angina, but also pericarditis and dissection of the thoracic aorta. Respiratory causes include pulmonary embolism, pneumothorax, pneumonia, and pleurisy (pleural inflammation). GI causes are diverse: cholecystitis (gallbladder origin), pancreatitis, hiatal hernia, esophageal disease, gastroesophageal reflux (GERD), peptic ulcer disease, and dyspepsia. Musculoskeletal causes include chest wall syndrome, costochondritis, acromioclavicular disease, herpes zoster (shingles), chest wall trauma, and chest wall tumors. You should always be prepared to treat patients with chest pain as if they may have cardiac ischemia or another major disease process. Only after you have excluded these possibilities should you consider the less critical causes.

14. List the mechanisms by which an MI may be produced by traumatic and non-traumatic events. **p. 509**

See Objectives 3 and 4 above.

©2008 Pearson Education, Inc.
Intermidiate Emergency Care: 1985, 3rd ed.

15. List and describe the assessment parameters to be evaluated in a patient with chest pain. **pp. 472–480, 508, 510–511, 512**

Initial size-up, inspection, and vital signs may reveal a lot. Is breathing labored? Is the patient diaphoretic and pale? Are there other signs of shock? Remember that blood pressure usually elevates during an episode of ischemia and then returns to normal. Hypotension more likely suggests cardiac compromise and possible shock. Peripheral pulses should be regular and equal. Irregularities may suggest dysrhythmia. (Assess the OPQRST of the chief complaint.)

16. List and describe the initial assessment parameters to be evaluated in—and the anticipated presentation of—a patient with chest pain that may be myocardial in origin. **p. 510**

See Objective 15. In addition, as you move through the OPQRST mnemonic, look for these signs of MI: sudden onset chest pain that proves to be severe, constant, and unrelenting over a period longer than 30 minutes. Pain may radiate to the arms (usually the left), neck, back, or into the epigastrium. Myocardial ischemia can easily produce pain in the 8–10 range and the pain may be associated with nausea and vomiting. Unlike the situation with angina, neither rest nor nitroglycerin will palliate MI pain. Remember that patients with diabetes mellitus may NOT have this picture even when an MI is in evolution. These patients may minimize the severity of their discomfort or simply complain of feeling unwell. Typically, these patients do not have nausea and vomiting. MIs typically evolve over 48–72 hours, and so the pain seen at 24–48 hours may be very different than if you had seen the patient in the first 12–24 hours after onset of discomfort.

Emotion may suggest MI. Patients with severe chest pain often are very frightened and complain of a sense of doom or fear of death. Denial of emotional upset or severity of pain does not mean a benign episode. Denial may hide severe fear or pain.

Other physical findings typical of MI include pallor and diaphoresis, coldness in the extremities, and possible change in body temperature. Heart rate and rhythm may be irregular or not. Blood pressure may be baseline, high, or low. The ECG should be checked first for underlying rhythm and any sign of dysrhythmia.

Next, assess whether the patient is a likely candidate for rapid transport and reperfusion therapy with fibrinolytic agents. Consult medical direction. Note that some patients will have contraindications to fibrinolytic therapy, including bleeding or clotting disorders, possible blood in the stool, uncontrolled hypertension, recent trauma, recent hemorrhagic stroke, or recent surgery. If you are uncertain whether the patient meets criteria for reperfusion therapy, assume that he/she does.

17. Describe the pharmacological agents available to the EMT-Intermediate for use in the management of dysrhythmias and cardiovascular emergencies. **pp. 490–500, 508–519, 522–523**

The classes of drugs you are most likely to use in the setting of an MI are antidysrhythmics, sympathomimetics, and other drugs used in cardiovascular emergencies. Please refer to the drug card in the back of this workbook for the specific indications, contraindications, and dosages.

Antidysrhythmics

Antidysrhythmics control or suppress dysrhythmias. Among the most commonly used are atropine, lidocaine, procainamide, adenosine, and amiodarone.

- Atropine sulfate.
- Lidocaine.
- Adenosine.
- Amiodarone.

Sympathomimetics

Sympathomimetic agents are similar to the naturally occurring hormones epinephrine and norepinephrine, and they mimic sympathetic nervous system stimulation on either alpha or beta adrenergic receptors. Alpha receptor stimulation causes peripheral vasoconstriction and beta receptor stimulation increases heart rate and cardiac contractility, causes bronchodilation and peripheral

©2008 Pearson Education, Inc.

vasodilation. Stimulation of dopaminergic receptors in the renal and mesenteric vascular beds causes dilation. Commonly used sympathomimetic agents include epinephrine, vasopressin, and dopamine.

- Epinephrine.
- Vasopressin.
- Dopamine.

Other drugs used for cardiovascular emergencies

Other drugs used to treat cardiovascular emergencies include oxygen, nitroglycerin, morphine, aspirin, and furosemide.

18. Develop, execute, and evaluate a treatment plan based on the field impression for the patient with chest pain that may be indicative of angina or myocardial infarction. pp. 508–511, 512

Act expediently and calmly and keep the patient in as much physical and emotional rest as possible. Provide supplemental oxygen to decrease myocardial oxygen demand and increase available oxygen. Always have good IV access (possibly more than one IV line). Be sure to ask about medication allergies (especially to any that may have been used previously in a cardiac setting) before the patient or family may become unable to give you this information. Transport as rapidly as possible with no lights or sirens if possible. Delay in transport, however, is preferable to a patient's refusal to leave the scene.

Management includes placing the patient at physical and emotional rest to decrease myocardial oxygen demand: Give oxygen, generally at high-flow rate. Establish IV access on scene or en route to the hospital. Conduct the ECG; do not, however, delay transport to perform it. You can give nitroglycerin sublingually as a tablet or spray. If symptoms persist after 1–2 doses, raise your suspicion for a more serious condition such as acute MI. Morphine may be used for nonresponsive chest pain.

Patients with an initial episode of angina or an episode that does not respond to medication are usually admitted for observation. Immediate transport is indicated if relief does not come after oxygen and nitrates. The absence of relief may signal the beginning of infarction, and in this case reperfusion is crucial. Hypotension may occur, especially if nitroglycerin has been given. It indicates transport as well because it can lead to or worsen hypoperfusion of myocardial tissue. Transport should be WITHOUT lights or siren, if possible, in order to minimize patient anxiety.

If the patient refuses transport, be sure you clearly explain that immediate evaluation is vital because of the potential for problems such as MI. If you can't reverse the patient's decision, be sure the patient reads and signs the refusal and understands the potential risks. Ask that he contact his cardiologist or other physician for follow-up as soon as possible.

19. Define the terms "congestive heart failure" and "pulmonary edema" and the cardiac and non-cardiac causes and terminology associated with them. pp. 513–515

Congestive heart failure (CHF) is a general term for ventricular failure (left, right, or both) that causes excess fluid to accumulate in body tissues (hence, congestion). The excess fluid is manifest as edema, which may be pulmonary, peripheral, sacral, or within the abdomen as ascites. You may find it in the acute setting of MI, pulmonary edema, or pulmonary hypertension. In the chronic setting, it can reflect cardiac enlargement.

Manage a patient with severe CHF by assessing in an ongoing manner for life-threatening symptoms and intervene promptly while readying the patient for rapid transport. Do not allow the patient to exert in any way, including standing up. Positioning in a seated position with feet dangling promotes venous pooling and, consequently, reduced preload. Administer high-flow oxygen. If necessary, provide positive-pressure ventilations with either a demand valve or a bag-valve-mask device. Establish an IV line at a keep-vein-open rate or place a saline or heparin lock. Place ECG electrodes. If the patient is extremely diaphoretic, apply tincture of benzoin first so electrodes will adhere tightly to skin. Record a baseline ECG and continue monitoring.

©2008 Pearson Education, Inc.
Intermidiate Emergency Care: 1985, 3rd ed.

Medication use will be according to your local protocols or the order of medical direction. Always remember to ask about drug allergies or reactions to any medication. Common medications used in the care of congestive heart failure include: morphine sulfate, nitroglycerin, furosemide, and dopamine

Transport as a nonemergency unless clinical conditions say otherwise. Indications for emergency transport include hypertension or hypotension, severe respiratory distress or pending respiratory failure, or life-threatening dysrhythmias. If you feel nonemergency transport will compromise the patient's condition, use lights and siren.

As the left ventricle's pumping ability falls, it cannot pump out all of the blood delivered to it from the lungs. Consequently, left atrial pressure rises and is transmitted to the pulmonary veins and the pulmonary capillary beds. When pulmonary capillary pressure increases sufficiently, blood plasma is forced into the alveoli and interstitial spaces; this is pulmonary edema. Progressive fluid accumulation in the alveoli decreases the lungs' oxygenation capacity and can cause hypoxia that can be fatal.

For left ventricular failure, the cardinal symptom is dyspnea due to pulmonary edema. Signs include cyanosis, tachycardia, noisy, labored breathing, rales, cough, blood-tinged, frothy sputum, and a gallop rhythm of the heart. The major signs of right ventricular failure: neck veins engorged and pulsating, edema of body and extremities, engorged liver and spleen, abdominal distention with ascites (fluid), as well as tachycardia.

20. Describe the early and late signs and symptoms of pulmonary edema. **p. 514**

Pulmonary edema reflects backup of fluid into the pulmonary alveoli and interstitium, but it does not necessarily imply etiology. Left ventricular failure, however, is probably the best known and most common cause, and you should look for other signs of congestive heart failure in a patient who presents with signs of pulmonary edema. If pulmonary edema seems to be very acute in onset, look for precipitating causes, such as cardiac dysrhythmia or acute MI. Dependent edema represents edema in the gravity-dependent portions of the body. For a bedridden patient, this often manifests as sacral edema. Sometimes edema will be so severe it will eliminate your ability to find a pulse in the affected area (such as a pedal pulse). If edema is severe enough it may become pitting edema (a situation in which you press firmly into the affected tissue, lift the finger, and find that the depression caused by your finger persists).

21. Explain the clinical significance of paroxysmal nocturnal dyspnea. **p. 514**

Paroxysmal nocturnal dyspnea (PND) is an episode of waking during the night due to shortness of breath, and it reflects the presence of pulmonary edema. If these episodes become more frequent (more nights or more times/night), it suggests worsening of the underlying pathophysiologic process.

22. Define the term "hypertensive emergency." **p. 522**

A hypertensive emergency is a life-threatening elevation in blood pressure. It occurs in 1% or less of patients with hypertension, usually when the hypertension is poorly controlled or left untreated. It is characterized by a rapid increase in diastolic pressure, usually to above 100 mmHg, and/or a systolic blood pressure above 160 mmHg. The patient may experience restlessness, confusion, blurred vision, nausea, and vomiting. It often occurs with hypertensive encephalopathy.

23. Describe the clinical features of the patient in a hypertensive emergency. **p. 522**

Clinically, the emergency is usually characterized by a rapid increase in diastolic pressure generally, to greater than 100 mmHg and a systolic blood pressure above 160 mmHg. It is often accompanied by restlessness and confusion, blurred vision, and nausea and vomiting. It often occurs with hypertensive encephalopathy, a consequence of severe hypertension marked by severe headache, vomiting, visual changes including transient blindness, paralysis, seizures, and stupor or coma. With modern medications, hypertensive encephalopathy has become rare, although it is still seen in the hospital setting. Both ischemic and hemorrhagic strokes are more common results

©2008 Pearson Education, Inc.

of severe hypertension and can have devastating consequences. Hypertensive emergency can also cause left ventricular failure and pulmonary edema.

The major causes of hypertensive emergency include noncompliance with antihypertensive drugs or other prescribed medications and lack of treatment for hypertension. Risk factors include age (older age) and race (hypertension is more common in African Americans, and morbidity and mortality appear to be higher, too). Among pregnant women, one cause of hypertension is preeclampsia (also called toxemia of pregnancy), which can appear at any point after the 20th week of pregnancy.

Assessment findings on physical exam of a patient with hypertensive emergency commonly include a chief complaint of headache accompanied by any of the following: nausea, vomiting, blurred vision, shortness of breath, epistaxis, and dizziness (vertigo). The patient may be semi-conscious or unconscious and seizing. In toxemia of pregnancy, the woman usually has edema of hands or face. Photosensitivity and headache are common complaints in this group. Determine whether there is a documented history of hypertension and to what degree prescribed medications have been taken. Find out whether the patient may have borrowed someone else's medications or taken herbal or over-the-counter drugs. Skin may be pale or flushed, normal, cool, or warm. Look for edema. The patient may confirm PND, orthopnea, vertigo, epistaxis, tinnitus, or visual acuities. Look for possible motor or sensory deficits in parts of the body or on one side. ECG findings are generally inconclusive unless there is an underlying cardiac condition such as angina or MI. If left ventricular failure is present, pulmonary edema may be present. Otherwise, lungs are generally clear. The pulse is strong and may feel bounding.

24. List the interventions prescribed for the patient with a hypertensive emergency. p. 523

Management centers on positioning for comfort and watching for possible airway compromise if vomiting or stroke occurs. Give oxygen and decide upon transport based on clinical presentation. Attempt supportive IV therapy on-scene or en route. Place pregnant patients on their left sides and transport as smoothly and quietly as possible.

Medications that may be used in the prehospital setting have notably changed recently; know your local protocol. Medications often used include morphine, furosemide, and nitroglycerin.

25. Define the term "cardiogenic shock." p. 515

Cardiogenic shock is the extreme state of heart failure: Cardiac output is so low it cannot sustain minimal physiologic activity. Clinically, you will see it after existing dysrhythmias, hypovolemia, or altered vascular tone have been corrected, leaving only the possibility of endogenous pump failure. This failure of the heart and overwhelming of any compensatory mechanisms usually happens after an extensive MI, often involving more than 40% of the left ventricle, or with diffuse ischemia. Note that cardiogenic shock can occur at any age, but it is most often seen as an end-stage event in geriatric patients with underlying disease. Mortality rate is high for elderly patients following massive MI or septic shock because end-organ damage is so severe that life cannot be sustained.

26. Identify the clinical criteria for cardiogenic shock. pp. 515–516

Numerous mechanisms can lead to cardiogenic shock, and onset may be gradual or acute. Among mechanical causes are tension pneumothorax and cardiac tamponade. Interference with ventricular emptying or afterload (such as pulmonary embolism and prosthetic or natural valve dysfunction) can also cause shock. Impairment in cardiac contractility is also a general cause: examples include MI, myocarditis, and recreational drug use. Trauma is another general cause, either primarily through cardiac damage or secondarily through hypovolemia. Finally, shock can develop secondarily to underlying conditions such as neurologic, GI, renal, or metabolic disorders.

Assessment findings depend on whether the patient is in an early phase of shock or a most advanced state. Look for evidence of a possible contributing cause such as hypovolemia, sepsis, or trauma. Among direct cardiac causes, you will most often see cardiogenic shock in the setting of MI. Information about the patient's medications may give clues about preexisting pump compromise. Inquire about the degree of compliance with medication regimens and ask about borrowed or over-the-counter drugs, which might have unpredictable interaction effects.

©2008 Pearson Education, Inc.
Intermidiate Emergency Care: 1985, 3rd ed.

The altered mental status associated with advancing shock may begin as restlessness and progress through confusion to loss of consciousness. Airway findings include dyspnea, productive cough, or labored breathing. Tachypnea is often present due to pulmonary edema. Also common is a history of paroxysmal nocturnal dyspnea. Typical ECG findings include tachycardia and ectopy (PVCs) is also common.

MI often precedes cardiogenic shock; symptoms will be compatible with those expected with MI. Expect hypotension to develop as shock progresses. Systolic pressure will often fall to less than 80 mmHg. Try to correct any discovered dysrhythmias.

Management of cardiogenic shock begins by placing the patient in a position of comfort. With pulmonary edema, this may be sitting upright. Treatment consists mostly of caring for underlying conditions (such as MI or CHF) and supportive care. Remember to treat heart rate and rhythm and transport rapidly. Medications that may be used in this setting include the vasopressor dopamine. Other medications include morphine, nitroglycerin, and furosemide.

27. Define the term "cardiac arrest." **p. 518**

Cardiac arrest and sudden death account for 60% of all deaths from coronary heart disease. Cardiac arrest is defined as the absence of ventricular contractions that immediately results in systemic circulatory failure. Sudden death is any death that occurs within one hour of the onset of symptoms. At autopsy, signs of MI are not present, and authorities generally believe lethal dysrhythmia secondary to severe atherosclerosis is the most common cause of death. The risk factors for sudden death are similar to those for ASHD and CHD. Other causes of sudden death include drowning, acid-base imbalance, electrocution, drug intoxication, electrolyte imbalance, hypoxia, hypothermia, pulmonary embolism, stroke, hyperkalemia, trauma, and end-stage renal disease.

28. Define the term "resuscitation." **p. 518**

Resuscitation and management start with simultaneous efforts on the ABCs. Ventilate with a bag-valve mask using 100% oxygen. Intubate or insert an airway as quickly as possible. If ECG changes indicate defibrillation, perform it in conjunction with CPR, stopping CPR only long enough to apply the pads or paddles and deliver the shock.

After starting CPR and advanced airway management, get IV access with a venous site as close to the heart as possible (for instance, the antecubital area in the arm or the external jugular vein). Follow IV medications with a 30–45 second flush to ensure complete delivery. After each flush, set the line to a keep-vein-open rate. Agents used with cardiac arrest include atropine, lidocaine, procainamide, epinephrine, norepinephrine, isoproterenol, dopamine, and dobutamine.

If blood pressure and pulse return, be aware that the blood pressure itself may be low, normal, or high because of the drugs administered. Pulse may return with a bradycardic, normal, or tachycardic rate. Ventricular ectopy is the most serious concern. If the patient presented in ventricular tachycardia or ventricular fibrillation or if ectopy is seen postarrest, use an antidysrhythmic such as lidocaine and amiodarone.

Transport should be done as safely and smoothly as possible and with lights and siren.

29. Identify local protocol dictating circumstances and situations where resuscitation efforts would not be initiated or would be discontinued. **pp. 519, 520–521**

In some situations, the patient will not survive despite resuscitation efforts, and in these cases resuscitation is contraindicated and should not be begun: these settings are rigor mortis, fixed dependent lividity (pooling of blood in gravity-dependent fashion), decapitation, and incineration. Less obvious but equally important settings include those where there is an advance directive to withhold resuscitation. Some considerations regarding the decision to initiate or discontinue include those circumstances in support of the resuscitation decision: younger than 18 years, a cause that could benefit from in-hospital resuscitation (hypothermia), persistent ventricular fibrillation/tachycardia, transient return of a pulse, EMS witnessed arrest, family opposed to termination. Conditions supporting termination: traumatic asystolic arrest, resuscitation for more than 25 minutes or four rounds of ACLS drugs.

©2008 Pearson Education, Inc.

30. Identify the critical actions necessary in caring for the patient in cardiac arrest. pp. 518–519

Assessment for cardiac arrest shows an unresponsive, apneic, pulseless individual. After initiating CPR, place ECG leads and initiate monitoring. Dysrhythmias you may find include ventricular tachycardia or fibrillation, asystole, or PEA. If you find asystole, confirm it in two or more leads. Question bystanders with the goal of finding some specific, prognostic information: Did anyone witness the arrest? If CPR was begun before you arrived, try to learn as precisely as possible the length of time between arrest and initiation of effective CPR. Often, the emergency room physician will also want to know total down time from the beginning of the arrest until arrival at the emergency department. Also, try to get a list of the patient's medications as well as a past history.

31. Synthesize patient history and assessment findings to form a field impression for the patient with chest pain and cardiac dysrhythmias that may be indicative of a cardiac emergency. pp. 472–480

- **Cardiovascular disease.** Assessment findings are specific to the region of the vascular system affected by occlusion. Central findings such as tachypnea and change in heart rate or rhythm suggest pulmonary embolism or aortic aneurysm. Care is largely supportive unless a life-threatening problem (such as hypotension or dysrhythmia) develops.
- **Chest pain.** Chest pain can have a cardiac (pericarditis, angina, or MI) or vascular (aortic aneurysm) origin, or it can reflect problems of the respiratory system, GI tract, or musculoskeletal system. Look for pain on exertion that is relieved by rest and/or nitroglycerin as a sign of possible angina and pain that is unremitting for an MI. With both you may well see sinus tachycardia or other dysrhythmias.
- **Angina pectoris.** The typical presentation for angina is pain lasting from 3–5 minutes, or perhaps as long as 15 minutes, that is relieved by rest and/or nitroglycerin. Relief of pain is generally associated with resolution of ECG disturbances.
- **A suspected myocardial infarction.** The patient with an acute MI has chest pain that is severe, constant, and lasts longer than 30 minutes. Neither rest nor nitroglycerin relieves the pain, and the patient may be fearful or feel a sense of doom. Dysrhythmias can appear without warning.
- **Heart failure.** Heart failure, inadequacy of pumping ability to meet the body's oxygen demand, can be left-sided, right-sided, or both. Left-sided ventricular failure typically presents with dyspnea and the following additional signs: cyanosis, tachycardia, noisy, labored breathing, rales, cough, blood-tinged, often frothy sputum, and galloping heart sounds. Decreased lung sounds on exam reflect pulmonary edema. Right-sided ventricular failure typically presents with tachycardia, jugular venous distention, edema of body and extremities, engorged (palpable) liver and spleen, and abdominal distention due to ascites fluid. History will usually reflect past cardiac disease or pulmonary disease (COPD). Paroxysmal nocturnal dyspnea suggests left heart failure.
- **A hypertensive emergency.** The patient with a hypertensive emergency will have extreme hypertension (diastolic greater than 100 mmHg or systolic blood pressure above 160) and usually will show some signs of hypertensive encephalopathy such as headache, visual change, nausea and vomiting, restlessness, or seizures or coma.
- **Cardiogenic shock.** Cardiogenic shock represents shock of cardiac origin. Exam will show characteristic signs of shock (hyperperfusion to extremities, hypotension, tachycardia) but history and exam will rule out extracardiac causes such as hypovolemia or sepsis. ECG may reveal an underlying acute event such as MI.
- **Cardiac arrest.** Patients in cardiac arrest are unresponsive, apneic, and pulseless. ECG may show asystole, PEA, or ventricular tachycardia or ventricular fibrillation. Confirm arrest in two or more ECG leads before beginning management.

32. Given several preprogrammed patients with cardiac complaints, provide the appropriate assessment, treatment, and transport. pp. 472–524

You will see patients who have the problems or conditions discussed in this chapter because cardiovascular disease is so common and so serious. It accounts for considerable morbidity and mortality. Review the objectives above to familiarize yourself with care in the setting of chest pain, angina, and MI, as well as care of heart failure and other acute cardiovascular emergencies.

©2008 Pearson Education, Inc.
Intermidiate Emergency Care: 1985, 3rd ed.

Case Study Review

Reread the case study in Chapter 13 and then read the following discussion. This case study demonstrates how EMT-Is react to a typical medical emergency involving chest pain. In addition to observing how the team conducts the patient's initial assessment, note how they respond as the situation quickly changes into a more complex and urgent one.

David and Sam are called to a home to evaluate a man with "chest pain." You aren't told if they are given any additional information or if any sense of urgency is conveyed, but a call for chest pain in an adult should always bring several differential diagnoses to mind. Cardiac conditions, including angina and acute MI, should be at the top of that list.

They find a 66-year-old man who reports palpitations, shortness of breath, and dizziness. While David's initial impression of the patient suggests he is stable, the very recent history is suggestive of a cardiac problem. The past history of an MI, 3 years ago, and the calcium channel blocker support that suspicion. They complete a full set of vital signs noting they are within normal limits and the oxygen saturation is 99% on room air. To David's questioning, the patient explains that the "palpitations" have passed and that he is not currently experiencing any chest pain but that he did have some during the episode. While their patient tries to dismiss the episode, David and Sam persuade him to take a trip to the hospital.

It is fortunate David was able to convince the patient of the need to be seen at the hospital. The episode repeats. However, David and Sam have prepared for just such a situation. They have oxygen flowing, a saline lock in place for the administration of medications, if and as needed, a baseline ECG (normal sinus rhythm), and SpO_2 monitoring in place. As the patient reports the episode of palpitations, David quickly checks the monitor and the patient's problem is revealed. Ventricular tachycardia at a rate of 225 displays on the monitor and the blood pressure is now 72/P. This episode of dysrhythmia-induced hypotension clearly explains why the patient experienced the dizziness.

David follows the system protocols by administering amiodarone over 10 minutes and the episode resolves. The amiodarone drip follows and a reassessment of the vital signs reflects a return to normal values. It becomes very clear that David and Sam served this patient well by talking him into the trip to the hospital and preparing for any future events during the transport.

Content Self-Evaluation

MULTIPLE CHOICE

______ 1. Coronary heart disease accounts for about what number of deaths in the United States, annually?
A. 100,000
B. 200,000
C. 500,000
D. 1,000,000
E. 5,000,000

______ 2. From innermost to outermost, the three tissue layers of the heart are
A. the endocardium, the pericardium, and the myocardium.
B. the endocardium, the myocardium, and the syncytium.
C. the endocardium, the myocardium, and the pericardium.
D. the myocardium, the epicardium, and the pericardium.
E. the epicardium, the myocardium, and the endocardium.

______ 3. The blood supply to the left ventricle, interventricular septum, part of the right ventricle, and the heart's conduction system comes from which artery?
A. left coronary artery
B. the right coronary
C. the anterior descending artery
D. the circumflex artery
E. the posterior descending artery

©2008 Pearson Education, Inc.

______ 4. The normal cardiac output over one minute is about
A. 70 mL.
B. 1 liter.
C. 2 liters.
D. 3 liters.
E. 5 liters.

______ 5. The term that describes heart rate is
A. inotropy.
B. chronotropy.
C. dromotropy.
D. atrophy.
E. none of the above

______ 6. The cardiac conductive cells have which of the following properties?
A. excitability
B. conductivity
C. automaticity
D. contractility
E. all of the above

______ 7. Chest pain is the most common chief complaint among patients with cardiac disease, but not all patients with cardiac disease will have chest pain.
A. True
B. False

______ 8. Which of the following is a cause of chest discomfort?
A. pneumothorax
B. esophageal disease
C. herpes zoster
D. pneumonia
E. all of the above

______ 9. Dyspnea may be the only complaint from the patient experiencing an MI.
A. True
B. False

______ 10. The feeling of impending doom, frequently associated with the MI, is due to
A. massive stimulation of the sympathetic nervous system.
B. the fight or flight response.
C. the release of epinephrine.
D. all of the above
E. none of the above

______ 11. Which of the following drugs may cause a myocardial infarction in the absence of coronary artery disease?
A. Cialis
B. cocaine
C. Inderal
D. Nitrostat
E. all of the above

______ 12. Which patient position is necessary to determine abnormal jugular vein distention?
A. the patient seated bolt upright
B. the patient seated at a 45 degree angle
C. the patient lying supine
D. the patient lying with the head down
E. none of the above

______ 13. At least what percent of MI patients will display chest wall tenderness?
A. 15%
B. 25%
C. 35%
D. 45%
E. 60%

______ 14. All of the following can cause an artifact on ECG EXCEPT
A. patient movement.
B. an enlarged heart.
C. movement by the patient.
D. shivering by the patient.
E. loose electrodes.

______ 15. The most common lead used to monitor the heart in the prehospital setting is
A. Lead I.
B. Lead II.
C. Lead III.
D. MCL_1.
E. none of the above

©2008 Pearson Education, Inc.
Intermidiate Emergency Care: 1985, 3rd ed.

______ 16. The ECG cannot provide which of the following?
A. the heart rate
B. the regularity of the heart
C. the timing of electrical conduction
D. the presence of pumping action
E. the presence of electrical disturbances

______ 17. A QRS interval of 0.38 seconds is considered normal.
A. True
B. False

______ 18. The P wave of the normal lead II ECG should be which of the following?
A. upright
B. regular in shape
C. precede each QRS complex
D. all look alike
E. all of the above

______ 19. Common causes of dysrhythmias include all of the following EXCEPT
A. myocardial ischemia or infarction.
B. electrolyte and pH disturbances.
C. CNS or autonomic nervous system damage.
D. drug effects.
E. eupnea.

______ 20. In the bradycardia algorithm, the first drug in the intervention sequence is
A. procainamide.
B. epinephrine.
C. atropine.
D. isoproterenol.
E. dopamine.

______ 21. Criteria that identify malignant PVCs include all EXCEPT
A. R on T phenomenon.
B. couplets or longer runs of ventricular tachycardia.
C. one or two PVCs per minute.
D. multifocal origin within the ventricles.
E. accompanying chest discomfort.

______ 22. The treatment of choice for stable ventricular tachycardia is oxygen and
A. nitroglycerin.
B. lidocaine.
C. atropine.
D. amiodarone.
E. either B or D

______ 23. Nonperfusing ventricular tachycardia and ventricular fibrillation are treated identically, including initiation of CPR followed by
A. epinephrine 1:10,000 IV bolus.
B. adenosine IV bolus.
C. transcutaneous cardiac pacing (TCP).
D. defibrillation at 360 joules.
E. atropine IV bolus.

______ 24. Causes of PEA include all of the following EXCEPT
A. hypovolemia.
B. cardiac tamponade.
C. hypothermia.
D. acidosis.
E. massive pulmonary embolism.

______ 25. The benefit of using biphasic wave form defibrillation is the reduction in myocardial damage and increased battery life.
A. True
B. False

______ 26. Previous countershocks decrease transthoracic resistance, thereby allowing the defibrillator to deliver more energy to the heart.
A. True
B. False

©2008 Pearson Education, Inc.

______ 27. Current resuscitation guidelines for cardiac arrest recommend what before the first defibrillation?
A. no CPR
B. 1 minute of CPR
C. 2 minutes of CPR
D. one dose of amiodarone
E. intubation

______ 28. Which of the following is not true regarding stable angina pectoris?
A. It means chest pain.
B. It is related to stress.
C. It responds quickly to treatment.
D. It continues after rest.
E. They are brief.

______ 29. The most common complication of the MI is
A. dysrhythmia.
B. dizziness.
C. congestive heart failure.
D. hypotension.
E. none of the above

______ 30. Cardiac dysrhythmias are the greatest threat to the MI patient before he or she arrives at the emergency department.
A. True
B. False

______ 31. Medications that might be used by the EMT-I in the treatment of myocardial infarction include oxygen and
A. aspirin.
B. nitroglycerin.
C. oxygen.
D. morphine sulfate.
E. all of the above

______ 32. A significant pulmonary embolism is likely to cause which of the following?
A. left heart failure
B. myocardial infarction
C. angina pain
D. right heart failure
E. dysrhythmias

______ 33. A patient presents coughing up large volumes of a frothy pink sputum. This is most likely due to
A. chest trauma.
B. congestive heart failure.
C. PEA.
D. pericardial tamponade.
E. pulmonary embolism.

______ 34. Causes of cardiogenic shock include all of the following EXCEPT
A. drug toxicity.
B. tension pneumothorax.
C. pulmonary embolism.
D. diffuse myocardial hypoxia.
E. prosthetic valve malfunction.

______ 35. Which of the following is not a common management in treating the cardiogenic shock patient?
A. morphine sulfate
B. nitroglycerin
C. vasopressors such as dopamine
D. supine patient positioning
E. Lasix

______ 36. Which of the following is a frequent cause of sudden death?
A. drug intoxication
B. trauma
C. pulmonary embolism
D. stroke
E. all of the above

______ 37. Return of spontaneous circulation occurs when resuscitation results in resumption of a pulse; spontaneous breathing may or may not return.
A. True
B. False

©2008 Pearson Education, Inc.
Intermidiate Emergency Care: 1985, 3rd ed.

_____ 38. Which of the following is a possible criterion for termination of resuscitation efforts?
   A. persistent ventricular fibrillation of tachycardia
   B. patient is under 18 years of age
   C. transient return of a pulse
   D. systolic arrest is associated with blunt trauma
   E. arrest witnessed by EMS personnel

_____ 39. Characteristics of a hypertensive emergency include which of the following?
   A. rapid increase in blood pressure
   B. systolic blood pressure above 160 mmHg
   C. evidence of end organ dysfunction
   D. diastolic blood pressure above 100 mmHg
   E. all of the above

_____ 40. The use of Lasix and nitroglycerin in a hypertensive emergency is now being questioned as the drop in blood pressure may be harmful.
   A. True
   B. False

MATCHING

Write the letter of the definition or description regarding cardiac function in the space provided next to the term to which it applies. The same description or definition may be used more than once or not at all.

_____ 41. cardiac cycle

_____ 42. diastole

_____ 43. systole

_____ 44. ejection fraction

_____ 45. preload

_____ 46. afterload

_____ 47. cardiac output

_____ 48. stroke volume

A. the ratio of blood pumped from the ventricle compared with the amount contained at the end of diastole

B. the series of events between the end of a cardiac contraction to the end of the next

C. the resistance against which the heart must pump

D. the phase of the cardiac cycle during which the heart contracts

E. the amount of blood pumped by the ventricle during one cardiac contraction

F. the amount of blood pumped by the ventricle during one minute

G. the phase of the cardiac cycle during which the heart muscle is relaxed

H. the end-diastolic volume in the ventricle

I. the phase of the cardiac cycle during which blood enters the coronary arteries

Write the letter of innate rate of impulse discharge in beats per minute (bpm) in the space provided next to the part of the cardiac conduction system to which it applies.

_____ 49. Purkinje system

_____ 50. AV node

_____ 51. SA node

A. 60–100 bpm

B. 15–40 bpm

C. 40–60 bpm

©2008 Pearson Education, Inc.

Label the Diagrams

Supply the missing labels for the drawing showing the chambers of the heart by writing the appropriate letters in the spaces provided for Figure 1.

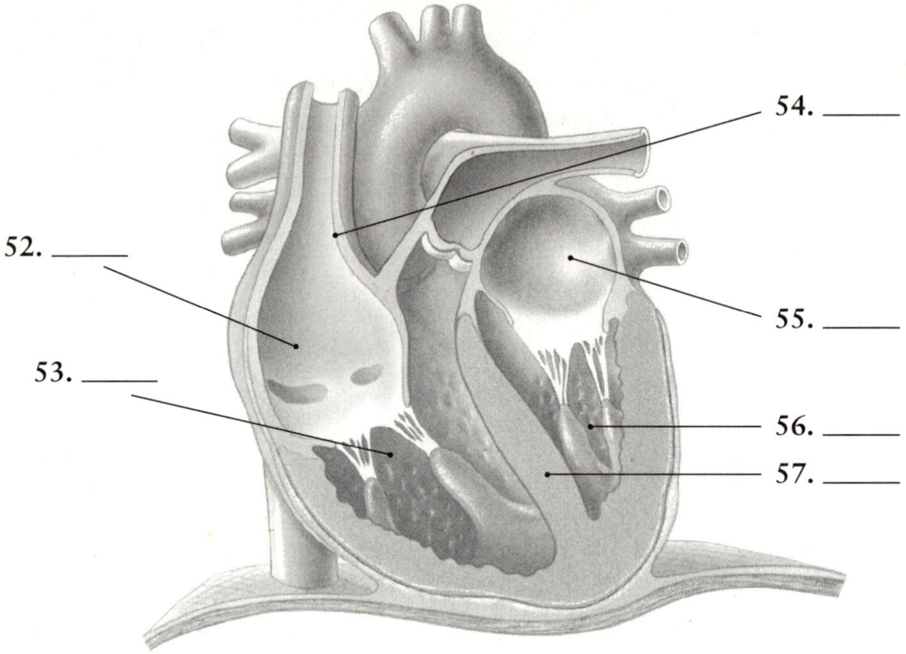

A. right ventricle

B. interatrial septum

C. left atrium

D. right atrium

E. interventricular septum

F. left ventricle

Supply the missing labels for the drawing showing the cardiac conductive system by writing the appropriate letters in the spaces provided for Figure 2.

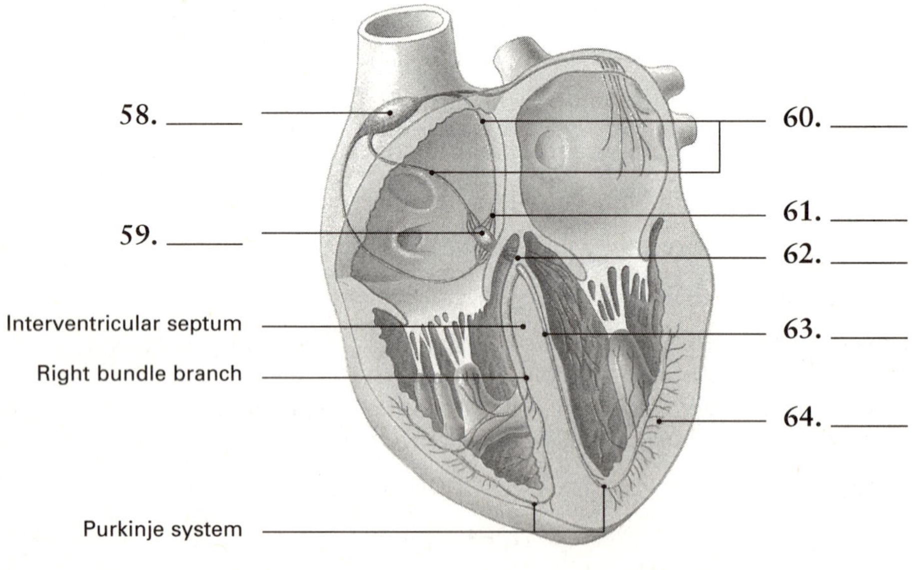

A. Purkinje fibers

B. left bundle branch

C. SA node

D. AV node

E. bundle of His

F. internodal atrial pathway

G. AV junction

©2008 Pearson Education, Inc.
Intermidiate Emergency Care: 1985, 3rd ed.

Use the terms below to fill in the missing labels for Figure 3 in the spaces provided.

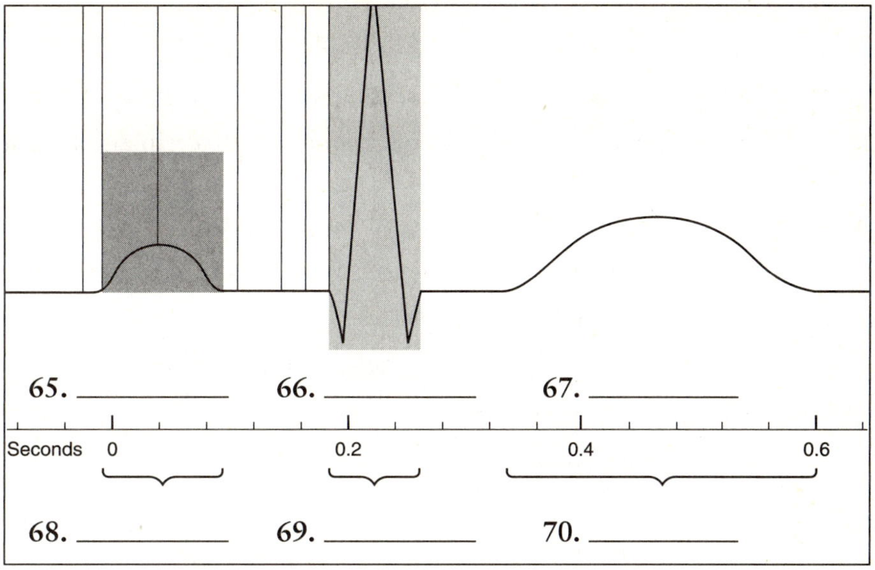

Figure 3

A. QRS complex

B. Ventricular depolarization

C. Atrial depolarization

D. T wave

E. Ventricular repolarization

F. P wave

MATCHING

A letter response may be used more than once or not at all.

A. cardiogenic shock
B. heart failure
C. acute MI
D. left ventricular failure
E. right ventricular failure
F. cardiac arrest
G. stable angina
H. hypertensive encephalopathy

_____ **71.** constant chest pain that is not relieved by rest or nitroglycerin and lasts longer than 30 minutes

_____ **72.** dyspnea, tachycardia, noisy, labored breathing, gallop heart rhythm

_____ **73.** syndrome in which the heart's pumping ability does not meet body needs

_____ **74.** unresponsiveness with apnea and pulselessness

_____ **75.** jugular venous distention, engorged liver, edema, tachycardia

_____ **76.** reproducible chest pain with stress

_____ **77.** hypotension and symptoms of MI

_____ **78.** severe headache, visual disturbance, seizures, stupor, diagnostic vital signs

Special Project

ECG Interpretation

The chapter introduces a five-step procedure for analyzing ECG strips: (1) regularity; (2) rate; and your interpretation. (3) P waves; (4) PRI (analysis of P-R interval); and (5) QRS (analysis of QRS complexes).

Look at each of the three ECG tracings shown and complete the information grid asked for below each tracing.

Rhythm 1

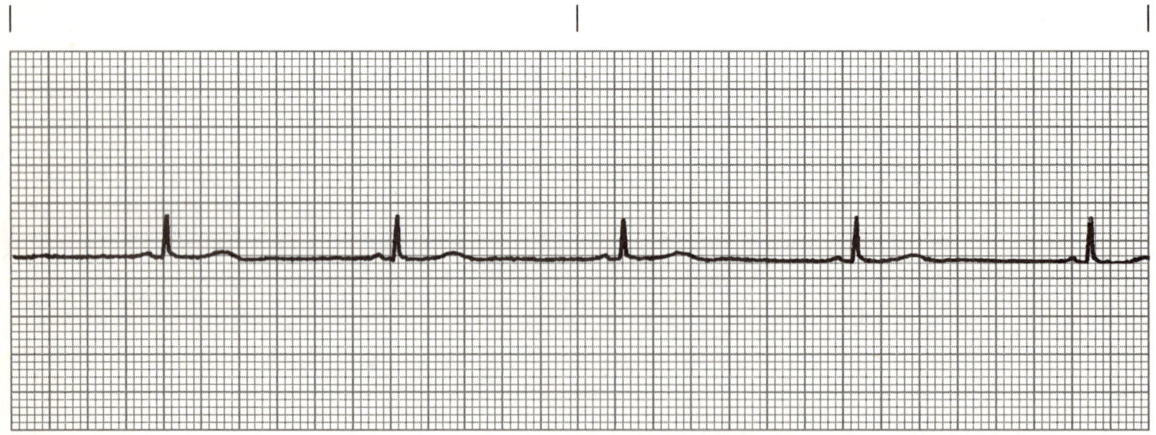

Regularity: ____________ Rate: ____________ P-Waves: ____________

PRI: ____________ QRS: ____________ Interp: ____________

©2008 Pearson Education, Inc.
Intermidiate Emergency Care: 1985, 3rd ed.

Rhythm 2

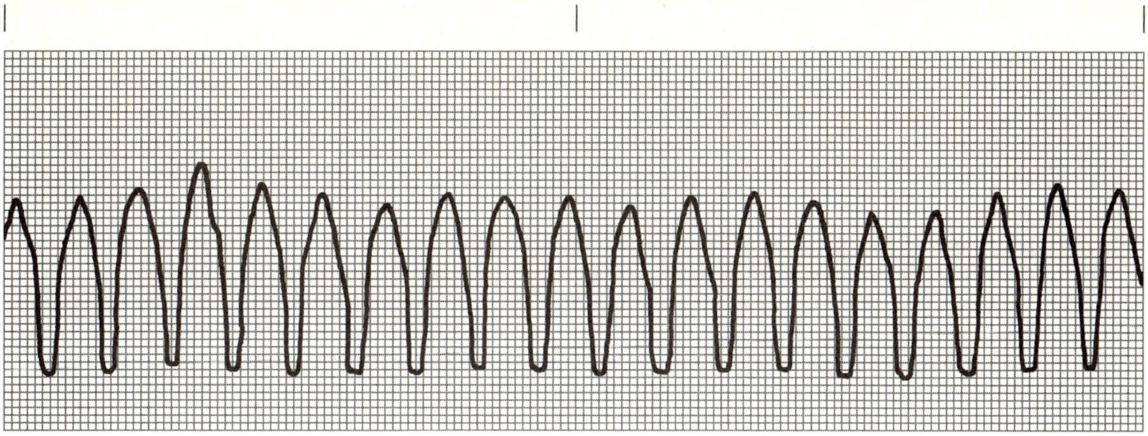

Regularity: ____________________ Rate: ____________________ P-Waves: ____________________

PRI: ____________________ QRS: ____________________ Interp: ____________________

Rhythm 3

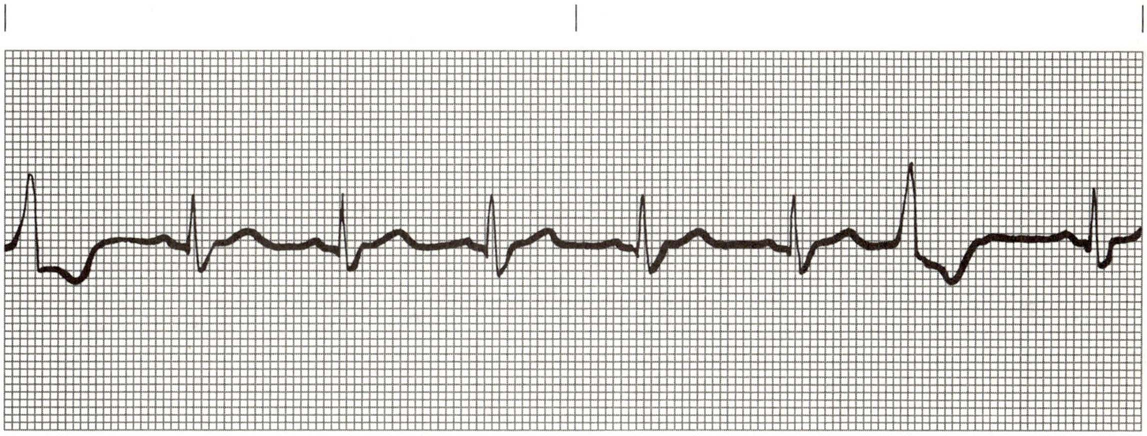

Regularity: ____________________ Rate: ____________________ P-Waves: ____________________

PRI: ____________________ QRS: ____________________ Interp: ____________________

©2008 Pearson Education, Inc.

Rhythm 4

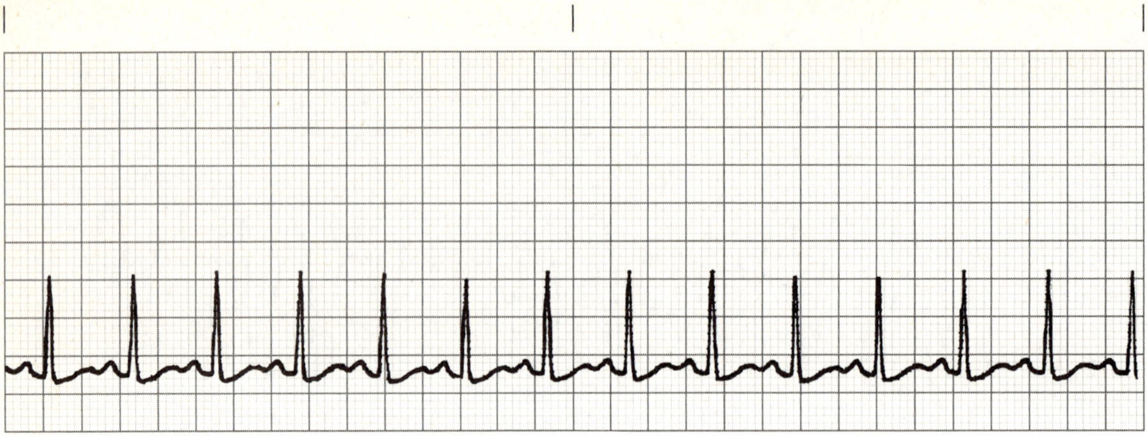

Regularity: ____________________ Rate: ____________________ P-Waves: ____________________

PRI: ____________________ QRS: ____________________ Interp: ____________________

Rhythm 5

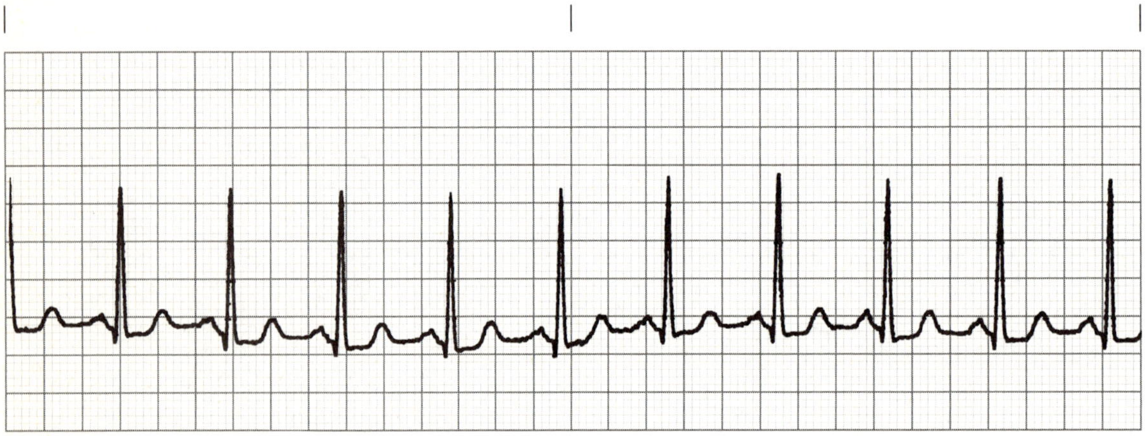

Regularity: ____________________ Rate: ____________________ P-Waves: ____________________

PRI: ____________________ QRS: ____________________ Interp: ____________________

©2008 Pearson Education, Inc.
Intermidiate Emergency Care: 1985, 3rd ed.

Rhythm 6

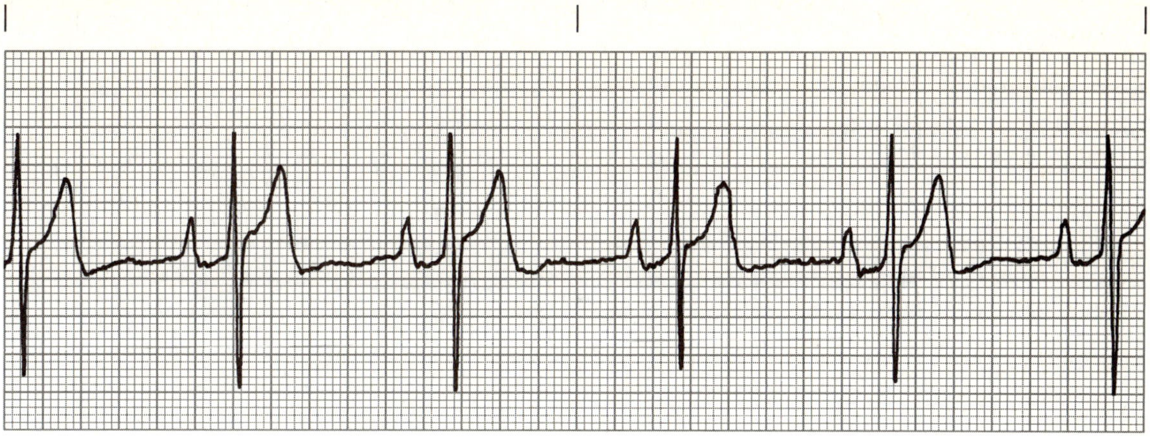

Regularity: ____________________ Rate: ____________________ P-Waves: ____________________

PRI: ____________________ QRS: ____________________ Interp: ____________________

Rhythm 7

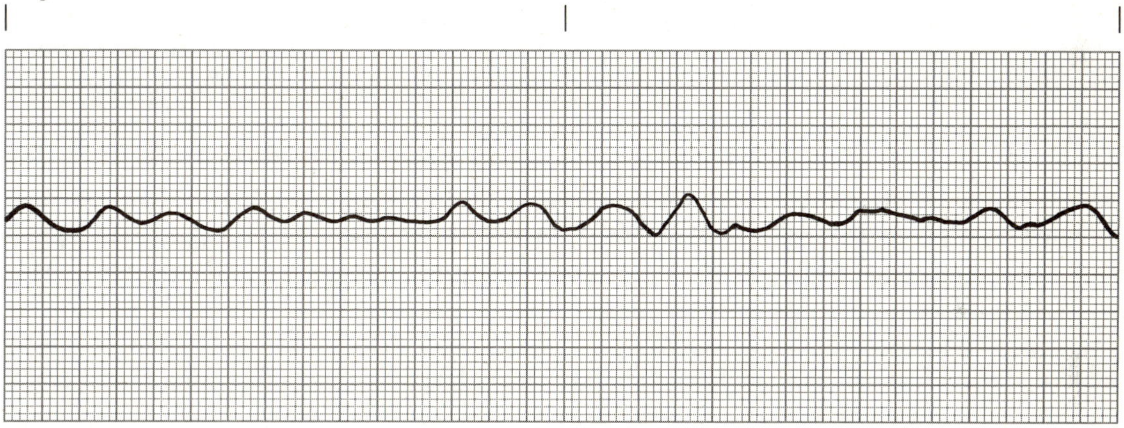

Regularity: ____________________ Rate: ____________________ P-Waves: ____________________

PRI: ____________________ QRS: ____________________ Interp: ____________________

©2008 Pearson Education, Inc.

Rhythm 8

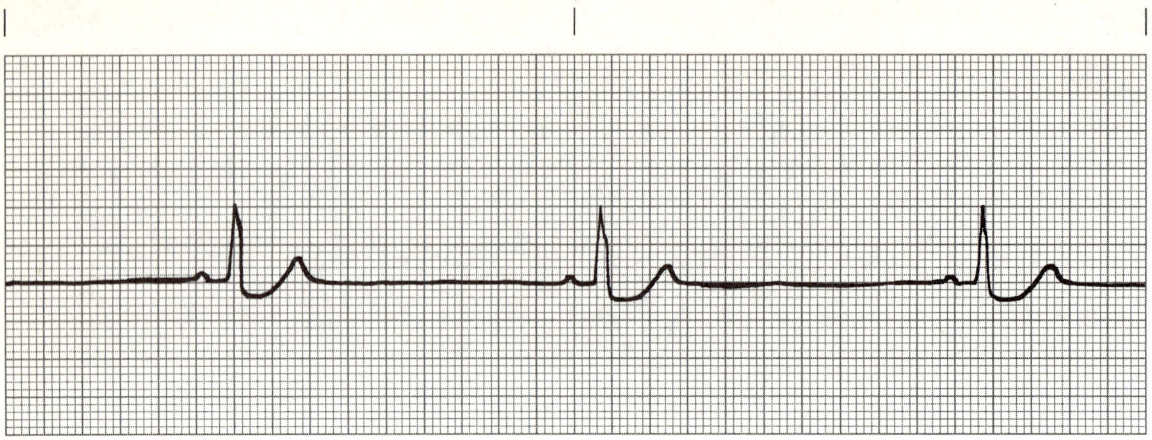

Regularity: ____________ Rate: ____________ P-Waves: ____________

PRI: ____________ QRS: ____________ Interp: ____________

Rhythm 9

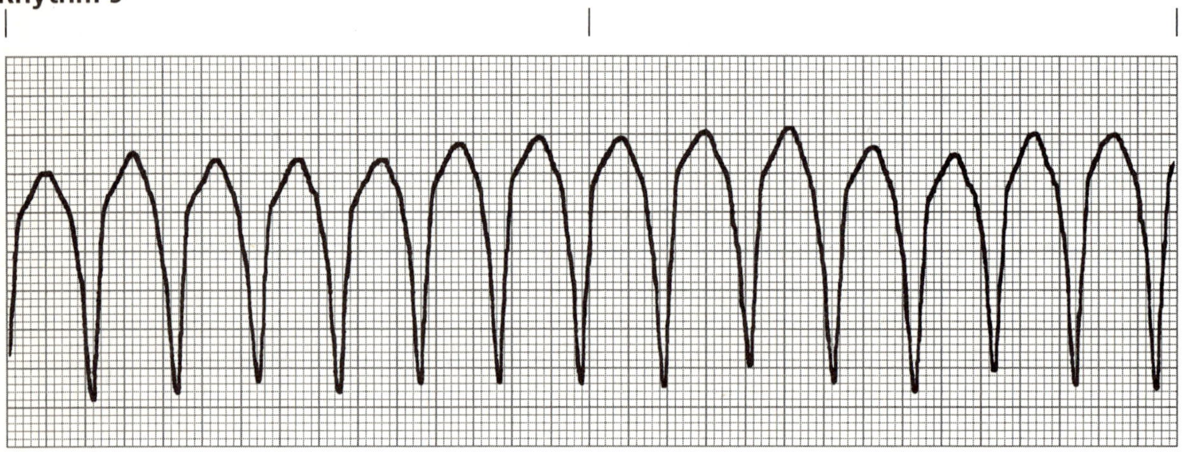

Regularity: ____________ Rate: ____________ P-Waves: ____________

PRI: ____________ QRS: ____________ Interp: ____________

©2008 Pearson Education, Inc.
Intermidiate Emergency Care: 1985, 3rd ed.

Chapter

14 Respiratory Emergencies

Review of Chapter Objectives

After reading this chapter, you should be able to do the following:

1. Describe the general management principles for a patient with acute respiratory insufficiency. **pp. 531–532**

Airway problems always demand the first priority after you assure your own safety. In trauma, protect the spine while positioning the airway and use mechanical airways to maintain the airway as needed. Provide high flow/high concentration oxygen (including the COPD patient). Also provide IPPV with 100% oxygen if the patient's breathing is inadequate or absent.

2. Identify the epidemiology, pathophysiology, assessment findings, and management for the following respiratory diseases and conditions:

a. Upper airway obstruction **p. 532**

The most common cause of upper airway obstruction is the relaxed tongue. However, foreign objects, facial trauma, inflammation, burns, and trauma also cause this threat to the airway. In the supine and unconscious patient the tongue drops back in the airway, obstructing it. Foreign objects can simply lodge in the airway at any point and prevent the passage of air. Swelling, due either to airway thermal or chemical burns or infection, can reduce the internal lumen of the airway and restrict or occlude the passageway. Trauma can disrupt the structures that hold the airway open such as the facial bones, mandible, larynx or tracheal rings.

You may recognize an obstructed airway by the actions of the patient, facial expression and coloring, panic, inability to speak. You may also hear abnormal respiratory sound such as stridor or snoring. In the unconscious patient you may discover airway obstruction as you attempt to ventilate the patient.

Actions in response to upper airway obstruction include asking the patient if he can speak, and if he does not respond or cannot speak, employ 5 abdominal thrusts. In the unconscious patient properly position the head and neck, attempt ventilation. Then if an obstruction is apparent, try to visualize and remove it, try abdominal thrusts. If the obstruction is due to swelling, attempt to position the head and neck for optimum ventilation, try and ventilate past the obstruction and consider epinephrine and diphenhydramine (Benadryl).

b. Emphysema **pp. 534–537**

Emphysema is classified as a chronic obstructive pulmonary disease (COPD). Alveolar walls are destroyed by exposure to noxious substances such as cigarette smoke or other environmental toxins. The disease also causes destruction of the walls of the small bronchioles, which contributes to a trapping of air in the lungs. The result is a decrease in both ventilation and diffusion. Patients tend to breathe through pursed lips, creating a positive pressure that helps to prevent alveolar collapse. A developing decrease in PaO_2 leads to a compensatory increase in red blood cell production (polycythemia). Emphysema patients are more susceptible to acute respiratory infections and cardiac dysrhythmias. They become dependent on bronchodilators

©2008 Pearson Education, Inc.

and corticosteroids and, in the final stages, supplemental oxygen. In contrast to chronic bronchitis sufferers, emphysema patients often lose weight and seldom have a cough except early in the morning. Because of the habit of breathing through pursed lips and the color produced by polycythemia, they are sometimes called "pink puffers." Clubbed fingers are common. Auscultation may reveal diminished breath sounds and, at times, wheezes and rhonchi. There may also be signs of right-sided heart disease. As a result of severe respiratory impairment, COPD patients may exhibit confusion, agitation, somnolence, 1-to-2-word dyspnea, and use of accessory muscles to assist respiration.

c. Chronic bronchitis **pp. 534, 537–539**

Chronic bronchitis is classified, along with emphysema, as a chronic obstructive pulmonary disease (COPD). COPD affects 25 percent of adults, with chronic bronchitis affecting one in five adult males. Chronic bronchitis reduces ventilation as a result of increased mucus production that blocks airway passages. It is often caused by cigarette smoking but also occurs in nonsmokers. There may be a history of frequent respiratory infections. Chronic bronchitis is usually associated with a productive cough and copious sputum. Patients tend to be overweight and often become cyanotic, so they are sometimes called "blue bloaters." Auscultation of the airway often reveals rhonchi due to mucus occlusion.

The goals of treatment are relief of hypoxia and reversal of bronchoconstriction. Because these patients may be dependent on a hypoxic respiratory drive (low oxygen levels stimulate respiration), respiratory effort may become depressed when oxygen is administered. Needed oxygen should not be withheld, but the patient's respirations must be carefully monitored. IV fluids may help loosen mucous congestion. Medical direction may also order administration of a bronchodilator, such as albuterol, metaproterenol, or ipratropium bromide, and may also recommend corticosteroid administration.

d. Asthma **pp. 539–541**

Asthma is an obstructive lung disease that causes abnormal ventilation. While deaths from other respiratory diseases are decreasing, deaths from asthma have been on the increase, with 50 percent of those deaths occurring before the patient reaches the hospital. Asthma is thought to be caused by a combination of genetic predisposition and environmental triggers that differ from individual to individual. These include allergens, cold air, exercise, stress, and certain medications. Exposure to a trigger causes release of histamine which, in turn, causes both bronchial constriction and capillary leakage that leads to bronchial edema. The result is a significant decrease in expiratory airflow, which is the essence of an "asthma attack." In the early phase of an attack, inhaled bronchodilator medications such as albuterol will help. In the late phase, inflammation sets in and anti-inflammatory drugs are required to alleviate the condition.

Assessment must focus first on evaluation and support of the airway and breathing. Most patients will report a history of asthma. The physical exam should focus on the chest and neck to assess breathing effort. The respiratory rate is the most critical of the vital signs. EMS systems should also be able to measure the peak expiratory flow rate. Treatment is aimed at correction of hypoxia (oxygen administration) and relief of bronchospasm and inflammation. A special case is status asthmaticus—a severe, prolonged attack that does not respond to bronchodilators. It is a serious emergency requiring prompt recognition, treatment, and transport. Another special case is asthma in children, which is treated much as for adults but with altered medication dosages and some special medications.

e. Toxic inhalation **pp. 541–542**

Toxic inhalation may cause pain and inflammation, destroy pulmonary tissues, and affect the ability of the alveoli to exchange oxygen. Such injury may be caused by the products of combustion and chemical irritants. Exposure may cause a progressive swelling of the airways and limit the patient's ability to exchange air. History will be the best indicator of possible exposure and you should try to identify the agent and nature of exposure. The patient will likely complain of a painful throat and you will recognize abnormal airway sounds. Care for patients with suspected toxic inhalation first assures that you, other rescuers, bystanders, and the patient are protected from further exposure. Generally, injury is progressive so concentrate on providing humidified oxygen and rapid transport. Also start an IV for rapid venous access.

©2008 Pearson Education, Inc.
Intermediate Emergency Care: 1985, 3rd ed.

f. Carbon monoxide **p. 542**

Carbon monoxide is a tasteless, odorless, colorless gas resulting from incomplete combustion. It replaces oxygen in hemoglobin and thereby reduces the body's ability to transport oxygen to the cells. Be suspicious of the environment when multiple people have symptoms. Those symptoms include ringing in the ears, headache, nausea, vomiting, agitation, confusion, loss of coordination, chest pain, loss of consciousness, seizures, and possibly skin discoloration (ashen or cherry red). Care involves removing all from the environment, providing high flow oxygen and rapid transport. If the patient is not breathing, provide IPPV with 100% oxygen.

g. Pulmonary embolism **pp. 542–543**

A pulmonary embolism is a blood clot (thrombus) that lodges in an artery in the lungs. One in five cases of sudden death is caused by pulmonary thromboembolism. It is a life-threatening condition because it can significantly reduce pulmonary blood flow (perfusion), causing hypoxemia (lack of oxygen in the blood). Immobilization, such as recent surgery, a long bone fracture, or being bedridden, increases the risk of developing an embolism. Other risk factors for clot formation include pregnancy, oral birth control medications, cancer, and sickle cell anemia.

The classic symptom of pulmonary embolism is a sudden onset of severe dyspnea, which may or may not be accompanied by pleuritic pain. The physical exam may reveal other signs including labored breathing, tachypnea, and tachycardia. In severe cases, there may be signs of right-sided heart failure, including jugular vein distention and possibly falling blood pressure. Auscultation may reveal no significant findings. In 50 percent of cases, examination of the extremities will reveal signs suggesting deep venous thrombosis (warm, swollen extremity with thick cord palpated along the medial thigh and pain on palpation or when extending the calf). Because a large embolism may cause cardiac arrest, be prepared to perform resuscitation. Primary care is aimed at support of the airway, breathing, and circulation. As necessary, assist ventilations and provide supplemental oxygen. Endotracheal intubation may be required. Establish IV access, monitor vital signs and cardiac rhythms, and transport expeditiously to a facility that can care for the patient's critical needs.

h. Spontaneous pneumothorax **pp. 543–544**

Spontaneous pneumothorax, which occurs in the absence of trauma, is a relatively common condition, occurring in roughly 18 persons per 100,000 population. It is relatively likely to recur as well (with 50% recurrence rate at two years). Significant risk factors include male gender, age 20 to 40 years, tall, thin stature, and history of cigarette smoking. Presentation is marked by sudden onset pleuritic chest or shoulder pain, often precipitated by a bout of coughing or by heavy lifting. The loss of negative pressure in the affected hemithorax prevents proper chest expansion, and the patient may report dyspnea. In individuals who do NOT have significant underlying pulmonary disease, a pneumothorax of up to 15 to 20% of the chest cavity can be tolerated fairly well. Monitor symptoms and pulse oximetry readings during transport. Be especially attentive in your ongoing assessment of patients who require positive-pressure ventilation. These patients are at higher risk for development of tension pneumothorax, which is marked by increasing resistance to ventilation, along with hypoxia, cyanosis, and possible hypotension. Examination will reveal tracheal deviation away from the affected side of the chest and distention of the jugular vein. Needle decompression of a tension pneumothorax may be required.

i. Hyperventilation syndrome **pp. 544–545**

Hyperventilation, with rapid breathing, chest pain, and numbness in the extremities, is often associated with anxiety, and it is called hyperventilation syndrome in this setting. However, you should remember that a number of significant and common medical conditions can cause hyperventilation, including cardiovascular and pulmonary conditions such as acute myocardial infarction and pulmonary thromboembolism, sepsis, pregnancy, liver failure, and several metabolic and neurologic disorders. Be conservative and consider hyperventilation to be a sign of a serious medical problem until proven otherwise. Management centers on reassurance and assisting the patient to consciously decrease the rate and depth of breathing (maneuvers that will increase PCO_2).

©2008 Pearson Education, Inc.

3. Given several preprogrammed patients with nontraumatic pulmonary problems, provide the appropriate assessment, prehospital care, and transport. **pp. 531–545**

You will see patients who have the problems or conditions discussed in this chapter because pulmonary disease is common and serious. It accounts for considerable morbidity and mortality, second only to cancer and cardiac problems. Review the objectives above to familiarize yourself with care in the setting of common pulmonary emergencies.

Case Study Review

Reread the case study in Chapter 14 and then read the following discussion. This case study demonstrates how EMT-Is can reach a field diagnosis and choose appropriate emergency treatment in a respiratory emergency. On this call, Bob and Linda gather critical information from the patient history.

Bob and Linda prepare for their "difficulty breathing" patient by noting the hot and humid day and, no doubt, recognizing that this alone would increase the likelihood that they will respond to a respiratory related illness today. As they approach the scene they do their survey and note the patient sitting upright in the chair, tripoding (supporting the chest with the arms, allowing gravity to help with the breathing effort) and two empty inhalers sitting on the table. The patient's presentation with his panicked expression and words spoken one at a time (one word dyspnea) also support the diagnosis of a serious breathing problem.

As Linda assesses breath sounds she hears no sounds in the distal reaches of the lungs. This suggests the bronchoconstriction is so severe that the patient cannot move air into the far reaches of the pulmonary tissue. The patient's diaphoresis and cool pale skin suggest shock is imminent. Despite his presentation, the vital signs are rather normal for his level of anxiety and the oxygen saturation is good considering his difficulty breathing. Given that he has taken quite a bit of his own medication (and her knowledge that albuterol works best when given early), Linda anticipates the albuterol will do little to resolve the problem. She quickly plans to transport the patient gently, but quickly, to the hospital. The administration of fluid by IV will help loosen any thick mucus that might be contributing to the dyspnea and also administers some epinephrine SQ to further promote bronchodilation.

Content Self-Evaluation

MULTIPLE CHOICE

_____ 1. Which of the following is considered an intrinsic risk factor for respiratory disease?
A. smokestack pollutants
B. polluted water
C. genetic predisposition
D. cigarette smoking
E. stress

_____ 2. Factors that commonly cause acute aggravation of symptoms due to chronic obstructive pulmonary disease (COPD) include all of the following EXCEPT
A. progression of lung cancer.
B. exertion, including heavy lifting and exercise.
C. allergens such as foods and dust.
D. tobacco smoke.
E. occupational airborne pollutants such as chemical fumes.

_____ 3. Common physical attributes of a person with emphysema include all of the following EXCEPT
A. chronic cough.
B. barrel chest.
C. clubbing of the fingers.
D. pinkish tone to skin.
E. thin build.

©2008 Pearson Education, Inc.
Intermediate Emergency Care: 1985, 3rd ed.

______ 4. Common physical attributes of a person with chronic bronchitis include all of the following EXCEPT
A. chronic cough.
B. thin build.
C. bluish, cyanotic tone to skin.
D. cough producing large amounts of sputum.
E. ankle edema.

______ 5. Two conditions in which respiration is frequently dependent on hypoxic respiratory drive, and use of supplemental oxygen may induce respiratory depression are
A. asthma and pneumonia.
B. spontaneous pneumothorax and pneumonia.
C. asthma and emphysema.
D. asthma and adult respiratory distress syndrome.
E. chronic bronchitis and emphysema.

______ 6. The epidemiology of asthma includes all of the following EXCEPT
A. an increase in mortality rate over the past decade.
B. a death rate in whites that is roughly twice that in blacks.
C. it is a common disorder in both males and females.
D. mortality change seen mostly in persons over age 45 years.
E. the fact that half of asthma deaths occur in the prehospital setting.

______ 7. Medications commonly used by persons with asthma include all of the following EXCEPT
A. beta agonists administered via inhaler.
B. oral doses of aspirin.
C. anticholinergics administered via inhaler.
D. oral doses of corticosteroid.
E. cromolyn sodium administered via inhaler.

______ 8. The chief management goals for an acute asthma attack involve improvement in
A. blood pH (acidosis), hypoxia, and wheezing.
B. hypoxia, bronchospasm, and wheezing.
C. blood pH (acidosis), hypoxia, and local inflammation.
D. hypoxia, bronchospasm, and local inflammation.
E. hypoxia, wheezing, and local inflammation.

______ 9. Be prepared for which of the following when caring for a patient with status asthmaticus?
A. acidosis with dehydration
B. dehydration with early signs of renal failure
C. respiratory depression when administered supplemental oxygen
D. respiratory arrest requiring endotracheal intubation
E. tracheal inflammation causing airway obstruction

______ 10. The mechanism by which toxic inhalation threatens life is
A. edema
B. laryngospasm
C. pulmonary edema
D. all of the above
E. none of the above

______ 11. Intubation attempts in the toxic inhalation patient may result in laryngospasm.
A. True
B. False

______ 12. Carbon monoxide exposure is potentially life threatening because carbon monoxide displaces oxygen from hemoglobin in red blood cells.
A. True
B. False

©2008 Pearson Education, Inc.

______ 13. Which of the following signs of carbon monoxide poisoning is not found during the early stages of the problem?
A. confusion
B. headache
C. chest pain
D. cherry red skin
E. agitation

______ 14. Roughly one in ten cases of pulmonary emboli result in death.
A. True
B. False

______ 15. Risk factors for pulmonary emboli include all of the following EXCEPT
A. obesity
B. pregnancy.
C. prolonged immobilization.
D. thrombophlebitis.
E. use of oral contraceptives, especially in smokers.

______ 16. The ventilation-perfusion mismatch characteristic of pulmonary embolism is due to loss of blood flow to a ventilated segment of lung tissue.
A. True
B. False

______ 17. The processes of ventilation, diffusion, and perfusion allow gas exchange to occur efficiently in the lungs and other body tissues. The derangement in pulmonary embolism is principally of
A. ventilation.
B. diffusion.
C. perfusion.
D. a combination of ventilation and diffusion.
E. a combination of diffusion and perfusion.

______ 18. Common physical findings in pulmonary embolism include all of the following EXCEPT
A. evidence suggestive of deep venous thrombosis.
B. labored, painful breathing.
C. tachypnea and tachycardia.
D. left heart failure.
E. normal chest auscultation.

______ 19. Which of the following statements about spontaneous pneumothorax is FALSE?
A. Most patients have acute onset pain in the chest or shoulder region.
B. Onset of pain often follows coughing or heavy lifting.
C. Spontaneous pneumothorax is much more common in women than in men.
D. Spontaneous pneumothorax is more common among smokers and persons with COPD.
E. Supplemental oxygen is sufficient therapy for the majority of patients with spontaneous pneumothorax.

______ 20. The respiratory alkalosis of hyperventilation syndrome often results in
A. cramping of the muscles of the hands and feet.
B. slowing of cardiac electrical conduction, causing bradycardia.
C. cramping of facial muscles causing characteristic grimace.
D. one of several cardiac dysrhythmias.
E. altered mental status, specifically, lethargy and depression.

©2008 Pearson Education, Inc.
Intermediate Emergency Care: 1985, 3rd ed.

Chapter 15

Gastrointestinal Emergencies

Review of Chapter Objectives

After reading this chapter, you should be able to do the following:

1. Describe the differences among:

a. Visceral pain **p. 550**
Visceral pain originates in the walls of hollow organs and is generally produced by inflammation, distension (stretching), or ischemia (inadequate blood flow). It is usually not well localized and appears as dull crampy pain.

b. Somatic pain
Somatic pain is generally sharp, well-localized pain.

c. Referred pain
Referred pain is pain originating from a region other than where it is felt.

2. Discuss the following sources of abdominal pain:

a. Appendicitis **pp. 550–551**
Appendicitis is an inflammation of the vermiform appendix. It generally presents with diffuse periumbilical pain that localizes to the right lower quadrant that may be sharp in nature.

b. Cholecystitis **p. 551**
Cholecystitis is the inflammation of the gallbladder. It produces upper right quadrant pain and may irritate the diaphragm, producing referred right shoulder pain. The pain may also be colicky and follow a meal high in fatty foods. Pale, cool, clammy skin and nausea and vomiting are common.

c. Pancreatitis **p. 551**
Pancreatitis is an inflammation of the pancreas due to alcoholism, or obstruction of the common bile and pancreatic ducts. Pancreatic enzymes become activated and begin to digest the pancreas. Pain varies depending on the amount of the pancreas involved and often localizes to the left upper quadrant though it may radiate to the back or epigastric regions.

d. Diverticulitis **pp. 551–552**
Diverticulitis is the result of inflamed large bowel outpouchings producing crampy left lower quadrant pain. That pain may become sharp and associated with anorexia, nausea, and vomiting.

e. Peptic ulcer disease **p. 552**
Ulcers are erosions of the stomach or small bowel due to stress, drug, bacterial infection, or the oversecretion of gastric acids. They produce burning or gnawing sensations located in the upper abdomen, often relieved by antacids or milk. Ulcers may produce GI hemorrhage.

f. Bowel obstruction **p. 552**
Bowel obstructions block the intestinal lumen and produce diffuse visceral pain with vomiting, sometimes containing bile or smelling like feces.

©2008 Pearson Education, Inc.

g. **Urinary tract infection** **p. 552**
Urinary tract infection affects the urethra and bladder producing painful urination and lower abdominal and referred flank pain. It is often accompanied by the sensation of a full bladder and urinary urgency and frequency.

h. **Kidney stones** **pp. 552–554**
The passage of a kidney stone is often accompanied by acute, severe, colicky flank pain that moves more anterior in the abdomen and groin as the stone passes. Nausea and vomiting are common.

i. **Pyelonephritis** **p. 554**
Pyelonephritis (or kidney infection) produces variable pain and symptoms but flank pain is most common and may be accompanied with malaise, nausea, vomiting, and difficult or painful urination.

j. **Pelvic inflammatory disease** **p. 554**
Pelvic inflammatory disease (PID) is an inflammation of the female reproductive organs most often caused by sexually transmitted disease. Signs include lower abdominal pain, pain with walking, or lower back pain. They may also experience vaginal discharge, nausea, vomiting, and fever.

k. **Abdominal aortic aneurysm** **pp. 554–555**
Abdominal aortic aneurysm (AAA) is a dilation of the aortic lumen due to a weakening of the vessel wall. It is accompanied by constant, severe abdominal pain that often radiates to the lower back, groin, or flank. If the defect ruptures, the pain becomes acute and severe. Most patients die with rupture before reaching the hospital.

l. **Dissecting aortic aneurysm** **p. 555**
Dissecting aortic aneurysm is a tear of the inner wall of the aorta that permits high pressure blood to separate the layers of the vessel. The developing hematoma disrupts the blood flow to arteries coming off the aorta. Pain is often described as tearing or ripping sensation that radiates into the chest.

m. **Ruptured ectopic pregnancy** **p. 555**
Ectopic pregnancy is fetal development outside the uterus (most commonly the fallopian tube). Rupture of the fallopian or other abdominal structure can lead to severe hemorrhage, shock, and death. The pain may be reported as sharp pain located in the lower abdomen that may radiate to the shoulder on the affected side. The patient may report a missed period or vaginal bleeding.

n. **Acute myocardial infarction** **p. 555**
See Chapter 13.

3. Discuss the following sources of gastrointestinal bleeding:

a. **Esophageal varices** **pp. 555–557**
Esophageal varices are enlarged veins in the esophagus and frequently result from kidney disease. Rupture can produce severe hemorrhage, shock, and death. Usually there is no pain though the patient may vomit bright red blood.

b. **Hemorrhoids, tumors, and polyps**
Hemorrhoids are engorged veins in the lower rectum, while tumors and polyps can occur anywhere in the GI tract. The passing of hard stool may abrade or rupture these structures, causing hemorrhage.

c. **Esophagitis/gastritis**
Esophagitis/gastritis is an inflammation of the esophagus or gastrointestinal tract that may produce some bleeding.

4. Describe the general assessment and management of the patient with gastrointestinal complaints. **pp. 550–560**

Begin your assessment of the patient with abdominal complaints with a scene size-up and initial assessment. Assure the scene is safe, then assure the ABCs. Conduct a thorough patient history (SAMPLE) followed by the OPQRST-ASPN history. Be sure to obtain a set of baseline vital signs noting that changes in vitals along with alterations in mental status may indicate early shock due to hemorrhage or other processes. A focused assessment of the abdomen should begin with the least invasive step, which is a visual inspection. This includes checking the patient appearance and

©2008 Pearson Education, Inc.
Intermediate Emergency Care: 1985, 3rd ed.

positioning as well as visually inspecting the abdomen for signs of distention or discoloration. Auscultation and percussion often do not provide useful information in the field. However, if you do auscultate, be sure to do so before palpating in order to avoid perturbation in abdominal sounds. Palpation with gentle pressure should start in the least affected quadrant and move toward the area of greatest pain. Remember to immediately stop palpation if you feel any pulsation. Further palpation may cause rupture of the affected blood vessel or organ.

General management of the patient with abdominal complaints would include maintaining the ABCs by providing high-flow, high-concentration oxygen, placing the patient in a position of comfort, giving psychological support, diligently managing airway to prevent aspiration since the patient may vomit, establishing IV access (with a large-bore IV), and providing fluid resuscitation with crystalloid as warranted if the patient appears hemodynamically unstable, and transporting to the most appropriate hospital. Monitor the patient to assure he/she remains hemodynamically stable and consult with medical direction as needed. Consider pain medication.

Case Study Review

Reread the case study in Chapter 15 and then read the following discussion. This case study demonstrates how EMT-Is react to a medical emergency involving severe pain of unknown origin. In addition to noting how the team reacts to the patient's presentation and assessment, note how clues to the nephrologic origin of his condition emerge from the assessment and history.

Rachel and Jack receive a call that is nonspecific but concerning: A man has fallen and cannot get up. Jack and Rachel have almost no information before arriving at the scene. They do not know the age of the patient, whether traumatic injury is involved, the nature of the underlying cause of the fall. In their first moments at the house they realize that they are dealing with a relatively young, apparently healthy man who is having an acute episode of severe pain and apparently is not able to move because of the pain.

Their initial actions center on historical questions about the pain and on an initial physical assessment. The patient tells them that the pain was of sudden onset and is very severe. His concerns about the possible cause of his problem give them an immediate clue: He tells them there is a family history of kidney stones, that his brother had one recently, and asks if he could be suffering from one. At the time this information is received, urine observed in the toilet, which may have blood in it (as it appears reddish yellow).

You aren't told whether there are any significant findings on physical exam, so the assumption is that the exam was largely benign. You do know that the patient's vital signs are consistent with pain and stress: a relatively high blood pressure (provided there is no history of chronic hypertension), tachycardia, and brisk respirations.

The team secures IV access and starts oxygen supplementation and transports to the emergency department. To help with the severe pain, Rachel gets permission to administer a total of 7 mg of morphine sulfate and the patient's pain decreases from 10 to 4 on a scale of 1 to 10.

At the Emergency Department, a diagnostic IVP shows complete ureteral obstruction due to an apparent radiopaque renal stone. Treatment centers on rest, gentle analgesia, and hydration to promote urine formation and flow. Finally, a visible stone is passed, David's pain subsides, and he can go home.

Content Self-Evaluation

Multiple Choice

______ 1. Pain generated from the walls of hollow organs and generally caused by inflammation, distension, or ischemia is called
A. referred.
B. visceral.
C. malaise.
D. somatic.
E. none of the above

©2008 Pearson Education, Inc.

______ 2. Well-defined sharp pain associated with specific dermatomes is called
A. referred.
B. visceral.
C. malaise.
D. somatic.
E. none of the above

______ 3. The irritation of outpouches of the large bowel is called
A. cholecystitis.
B. gastritis.
C. diverticulitis.
D. pyelonephritis.
E. none of the above

______ 4. Kidney infection, often associated with urinary infection, is called
A. cholecystitis.
B. gastritis.
C. diverticulitis.
D. pyelonephritis.
E. none of the above

______ 5. What percentage of patients with a rupturing AAA die before reaching the hospital?
A. 25%
B. 35%
C. 45%
D. 55%
E. 65%

______ 6. Which of the following signs and symptoms are consistent with an ectopic pregnancy?
A. hypotension
B. missed period
C. diffuse lower abdominal tenderness
D. shock
E. all of the above

______ 7. A common sign of lower gastrointestinal bleeding (LGIB) is the vomiting of either bright red or coffee-grounds-appearing blood.
A. True
B. False

______ 8. Under the investigation of the history of the present illness, a report of black tarry stool would likely be classified under which of the OPQRST-ASPN elements?
A. P
B. R
C. T
D. AS
E. PN

______ 9. Periumbilical ecchymosis is also called
A. Grey-Turner's sign.
B. Starling's sign.
C. CVA.
D. Cullen's sign.
E. none of the above

______ 10. Current research suggests that analgesics for abdominal pain will mask symptoms and should not be used.
A. True
B. False

©2008 Pearson Education, Inc.
Intermediate Emergency Care: 1985, 3rd ed.

Chapter 16

Toxicologic and Overdose Emergencies

Review of Chapter Objectives

After reading this chapter, you should be able to do the following:

1. Identify the need for appropriate personal protective equipment (standard precautions) and scene safety awareness concerns, and recognition of situations in which additional non-EMS resources need to be contacted in dealing with toxicologic and overdose emergencies. **p. 565**

Although specific protocols for managing toxicological emergencies may vary, certain basic principles apply to all situations. First and foremost, your safety and that of your crew is the primary concern. This means that the scene size-up begins right from time of dispatch, assuring law enforcement personnel are on the scene and the scene is safe to enter. Upon arrival assess the scene with a thorough evaluation, taking note of where you are and who is around you. Be alert for any potential danger to you, the rescuer. Remember, despite your natural urge to immediately assess and treat the patient, if you are incapacitated you will not be able to help anyone, and you will become a patient yourself. Be especially careful around patients who have abused drugs as they may be suicidal or have the potential for violence. They are often intoxicated, may act irrationally, and will not always be cooperative or happy to see you. Therefore look for signs of overdose such as empty pill bottles and used needles or other drug paraphernalia. Never put your hand blindly into a patient's pocket as it may contain used needles.

2. Describe the routes of entry of toxic substances into the body. **pp. 564–565**

There are four routes of entry into the body: ingestion, inhalation, surface absorption, and injection. Ingestion via the mouth is the most common route of entry for toxic exposure. Inhalation of a poison into the lungs results in rapid absorption from the alveolar air into the blood. Causative agents are in the form of gases, vapors, fumes, or aerosols. Surface absorption applies to cases in which entry is through the skin or mucous membranes. Injection applies when the toxic agent is injected under the skin, into muscle, or directly into the bloodstream.

3. Discuss the role of Poison Control Centers. **p. 564**

Poison Control Centers assist in the treatment of poison victims and provide information on new products and new treatment recommendations. They are usually based in major medical centers serving large populations, and many have computer systems that allow staff to rapidly and accurately access information. Centers are available to you 24 hours a day, 7 days a week: Take the time to memorize the telephone number of the center serving your area. Your center can help you determine the potential toxicity for your patient when you give them the following information: type of agent, amount and time of exposure, and physical condition of the patient. With this information, you may be able to start the current, definitive treatment in the field. The Poison Control Center can notify the receiving facility before you get the patient there.

©2008 Pearson Education, Inc.

4. Discuss the pathophysiology, assessment findings, need for rapid intervention and transport, and management of toxic emergencies. **pp. 568–575**

- **Pathophysiology:** With each route of entry, there is a general pattern of possible toxic effects depending on the type and amount of agent involved: Immediate effects involve the tissues exposed to the toxic agent during entry. Delayed, systemic effects are related to absorption into the bloodstream and circulation throughout the body. In ingestion, corrosive agents can cause immediate injury through burns of the lips, oral mucous membranes, tongue, throat, and esophagus. Delayed effects can arise from absorption via the small intestine into the blood with effects on distant organs and tissues. In inhalation, immediate injury can occur from irritation of the airways resulting in extensive edema and damaged tissue. Delayed, systemic effects occur when the agent travels through the bloodstream and interacts with distant organs and tissues. In surface absorption, immediate injury can occur in the involved skin or mucous membranes. Delayed effects again relate to absorption into the bloodstream. With injection, immediate injury is seen as irritation at the injection site, usually visible as red, irritated, edematous skin. Delayed, systemic effects are again due to distribution throughout the body via the bloodstream.
- **Assessment:** Certain basic principles of assessment apply to most toxicological emergencies. For instance, maintain a high index of suspicion that a poisoning or drug overdose may have occurred. During scene size-up, look for potential dangers to yourself and other rescuers, such as a threat of violence from suicidal patients and the threat of accidental injection from used needles that may be hidden on the patient's person or at the scene. In cases with chemicals and hazardous materials, it is crucial that you use the proper clothing and equipment. Be sure that such articles are distributed to team members who have been trained in their use.

  Assessment of the patient begins with a history if the patient appears to be able to give one. Critical questions include what kind of toxin the patient was exposed to and when exposure occurred (so you have clues for likelihood of immediate or delayed effects or both). Physical involves a rapid head-to-toe exam with full vital signs.
- **Time needs:** In accordance with your local protocols, relay information to Poison Control. Generally speaking, you never want to delay initiation of supportive or definitive care or transport because of delays in sending information to, or receiving information from, Poison Control. Time is of the essence, literally. Ongoing assessment is particularly important for this group of patients because they can deteriorate rapidly. Repeat initial assessment and vitals every 5 minutes for critical or unstable patients and every 15 minutes for stable patients. Specific assessment findings are given for each type of agent.
- **General management:** The preliminary steps of management include securing rescuer safety and removing the patient from any toxic environment. Support ABCs as you would with any other patient, keeping in mind that damage may have occurred to the mouth, pharynx, and/or airway in inhalation injury, and to the mouth and pharynx in ingestion incidents. The direct access to the cardiovascular system that occurs with injection cases may also complicate support of the ABCs.

  The first management step specific to toxicological emergencies is decontamination, that is, minimization of toxicity by reducing the amount of toxin absorbed into the body. Decontamination involves three steps: The first is reduction of intake of toxin (steps will be route-specific, such as removal from fume-filled atmosphere in inhalation, removal of clothes and cleansing of skin in surface absorption, removal of stinger in injection, etc.).

  The second step is reduction of absorption after toxin is in the body, and this usually applies to ingestion incidents. The most common method entails use of activated charcoal to bind molecules of the toxin to it and prevent absorption into the bloodstream. Gastric lavage (stomach pumping) is of limited use as a step to reduce absorption. Lavage must be done within about one hour of exposure to be effective, and its possible complications (aspiration and perforation) are significant. Lavage is uncommon except in specific circumstances, for example, when the toxin doesn't bind to activated charcoal or when the toxin has no antidote. The third step in decontamination is enhanced elimination of toxin from the body. Cathartics enhance gastric mobility and thus may shorten the time the toxin is in the GI tract. Know the limitations in use of cathartics in your area, especially among pediatric patients, in whom they can induce severe

©2008 Pearson Education, Inc.
Intermediate Emergency Care: 1985, 3rd ed.

electrolyte disturbances. Whole bowel irrigation with use of a gastric tube seems to be effective and carries few potential complications; however, its use is limited to only a few centers.

The third management step specific to toxicologic emergencies is use of an antidote, a substance that neutralizes the specific toxin and counteracts its effects in the body. There are not many antidotes, and few are 100% effective. Your best guide is to be thoroughly knowledgeable with your local protocols, the directions given by the Poison Control Center, and by counsel given by medical direction.

5. Differentiate among the most common poisonings, pathophysiology, assessment findings, and management of poisoning by ingestion, inhalation, absorption, injection, and overdose. **pp. 568–575**

Ingestion is the most common route of poisoning that you will see. Frequently ingested poisons include household products, petroleum-based agents such as gasoline and paint, cleaning agents such as alkalis and soaps, cosmetics, drugs (prescription, nonprescription, and illicit), plants, and foods. Some poisons can remain in the stomach for several hours, which may permit removal of the poison from the stomach and the body before systemic absorption can occur via passage through the small intestine. In at least one case, ingestion of aspirin, removal from the stomach is difficult because the ingested tablets bind together to form one large bolus. Useful questions for historical assessment include: (1) What did you ingest? (Obtain samples or containers whenever possible.) (2) When did you ingest the substance? (3) How much did you ingest? (4) Did you drink any alcohol? (5) Have you attempted to treat yourself (including induction of vomiting)? (6) Have you been under mental health care, and, if so, why? (Answer may indicate potential for suicide.) (7) What is your weight? Physical exam is especially important because history may be unavailable or unreliable. Your exam should provide physical evidence of intoxication and discover co-morbid conditions that may affect treatment or response. Pay particular attention to skin, eyes, mouth, chest, circulation status, and abdomen. Be aware that a patient may have ingested multiple substances. Management centers on prevention of aspiration, intubation where necessary (RSI may be required to avoid patient's clamping down on tube), use of high-flow oxygen, and IV access for volume replacement and possible IV drug administration. Remember that it is always important to have ongoing cardiac monitoring and reassessment of vital signs.

Toxic inhalations can be self-induced or due to accidental exposure. Commonly inhaled poisons include toxic gases, carbon monoxide, ammonia, chlorine, freon, toxic vapors, fumes, or aerosols (from products such as paint and other hydrocarbons, glue, etc.), carbon tetrachloride, methyl chloride, tear gas, mustard gas, amyl nitrite, butyl nitrite, and nitrous oxide. Inhaled toxins primarily cause direct injury in the respiratory system, and these problems may be most severe in patients who inhaled a chemical or propellant concentrated in either a paper or plastic bag.

Given the pathophysiology of inhaled toxins, you should look for signs/symptoms related to three major systems: the central nervous system (dizziness, headache, confusion, hallucinations, seizures, or coma), the respiratory system (tachypnea, cough, hoarseness, stridor, dyspnea, retractions, wheezing, chest pain or tightness, rales or rhonchi), and the heart (dysrhythmias). Management starts with protecting yourself from any toxins in the atmosphere and removal of the patient from the injurious environment. Follow these guidelines: Wear protective clothing, use appropriate respiratory protection, and remove the patient's contaminated clothing. Then you can perform the initial assessment, history, and physical examination focusing on the central nervous system, respiratory, and cardiac systems. Support ABCs as you would with any other patient, keeping in mind that damage may have occurred to the mouth, pharynx, and/or airway as a direct, immediate injury. Contact medical direction and your Poison Control Center according to your particular protocols.

For **surface absorption,** the most common contacts are with poisonous plants such as poison ivy, poison sumac, and poison oak. Many toxic chemicals can be absorbed through the skin. Organophosphates, which are used as pesticides, are easily absorbed through the skin and mucous membranes, as is cyanide. The signs and symptoms vary widely depending on the toxin involved. Whenever you suspect surface absorption, take the following general steps: (1) wear protective

©2008 Pearson Education, Inc.

clothing; (2) use appropriate respiratory protection; (3) remove the patient's contaminated clothing; (4) perform initial assessment, history, and physical exam; (5) initiate supportive measures; and (6) contact Poison Control Center and medical direction.

Females in the insect class *Hymenoptera*, honeybees, hornets, yellow jackets, wasps, and fire ants, are common causes of **injection injury.** In addition, spiders, ticks, snakes, and certain marine animals are known causes of toxic exposure by injection. In addition to intentional injections, most poisonings by injection involve bites and stings from insects and animals. Be alert for the possibility of allergic reactions or anaphylaxis. Over time, beware of delayed systemic reactions. General principles of field management include the following: (1) protection of all rescue personnel because the culprit organism may still be in the area; (2) removal of the patient from danger of repeated injection (particularly in the case of yellow jackets, wasps, or hornets); (3) whenever possible and safe, obtain the injury-causing organism and bring it to the emergency department; (4) perform initial assessment and rapid physical exam; (5) prevent or delay further absorption of the poison; (6) initiate supportive measures as needed; (7) watch for anaphylaxis; (8) transport as rapidly as possible; and (9) contact Poison Control Center and medical direction per protocols.

6. Define substance abuse and drug overdose and differentiate among the most common drugs of abuse, including alcohol, and their assessment and management. pp. 571–575

Substance or **drug abuse** is use of a pharmacological product for purposes other than medically defined reasons. **Drug overdose** is the over-administration of a drug such that it causes unfocused effects.

The most commonly abused drugs include: (1) alcohol in its fermented and distilled forms; (2) barbiturates such as phenobarbital and thiopental; (3) cocaine (both crack and rock forms); (4) narcotics/opiates such as heroin, codeine, meperidine, morphine, hydromorphone, pentazocine, methadone, Darvon, and Darvocet; (5) marijuana and hashish (also called grass or weed on the street); (6) amphetamines such as Benzedrine, Dexedrine, and Ritalin (called speed on the street); (7) hallucinogens including LSD, STP, mescaline, psilocybin, and PCP (also called angel dust); (8) sedatives from different chemical families such as Seconal, Valium, Librium, Xanax, Halcion, Restoril, Dalmane, and phenobarbital; and (9) the benzodiazepines, Valium, Librium, Xanax, Halcion, Restoril, Dalmane, Centrax, Ativan, and Serax.

In addition to the specific drugs discussed below, it is notable that many groups of drugs produce definable toxic syndromes. Knowledge of these syndromes is useful because it helps you cluster information for compounds that produce similar clinical pictures. (1) Anticholinergic toxidrome is caused by belladonna alkaloids, atropine, scopolamine, synthetic anticholinergics, and incidental anticholinergics such as antihistamines, tricyclic antidepressants, and phenothiazines. Signs and symptoms include dry skin/mucous membranes, blurred near vision, fixed dilated pupils, tachycardia, hyperthermia and flushing, lethargy, and CNS signs, respiratory failure, and cardiovascular collapse. Management is as described for the tricyclics below. (2) Narcotic toxidrome is due to illicit drugs such as heroin and opium, prescription narcotics such as meperidine and methadone, and combination medications including narcotic agents such as hydromorphone, diphenoxylate (Lomotil), and oxycodone. Assessment findings include CNS depression, pinpoint pupils, slowed respirations, hypotension, positive response to naloxone. Note that pupils may be dilated and excitement may predominate the clinical picture. Management is described below. (3) The sympathomimetic toxidrome is caused by aminophylline, amphetamines, caffeine, cocaine, ephedrine, dopamine, methylphenidate (Ritalin), and phencyclidine. Features include CNS excitation, hypertension, seizures, and tachycardia (hypotension with caffeine). Management is discussed below.

a. Cocaine

Cocaine has sympathomimetic effects, and assessment findings include CNS excitation, dilated pupils, hyperactivity, hypertension, seizures, tachycardia, and hypotension if taken with caffeine. Benzodiazepines may be required for seizures or diazepam 5–10 mg can be given as a seizure precaution; beta blockers are contraindicated because their unopposed alpha receptor stimulation can cause cardiac ischemia, increased hypertension, and hyperthermia. General measures include ABCs, respiratory support and oxygenation, ECG monitoring, IV access, and treatment of any life-threatening dysrhythmia.

©2008 Pearson Education, Inc.
Intermediate Emergency Care: 1985, 3rd ed.

b. **Marijuana and cannabis compounds**
Marijuana and related compounds can be smoked (inhaled) or taken orally, and pertinent signs and symptoms include euphoria, dry mouth, dilated pupils, and altered sensation. Management centers on ABCs, reassurance and speaking in a quiet voice, and ECG monitoring if indicated.

c. **Amphetamines and amphetamine-like drugs**
Amphetamines are CNS stimulants that can be taken orally or injected. Assessment findings include exhilaration, hyperactivity, dilated pupils, hypertension, psychosis, tremors, and seizures. Management centers on ABCs, oxygenation and ECG monitoring, IV access, treatment of any life-threatening dysrhythmia, and diazepam 5–10 mg as a seizure precaution. Diazepam and haloperidol in combination may be useful in controlling hyperactivity.

d. **Barbiturates**
The barbiturates, which are CNS depressants, can be taken orally or injected. Signs and symptoms include lethargy, emotional lability, incoordination, slurred speech, nystagmus, coma, hypotension, and respiratory depression. Management focuses on ABCs and respiratory support with oxygenation, IV access, ECG monitoring, and contact with Poison Control. Alkalinization of urine and diuresis may improve elimination of barbiturates from the body.

e. **Sedative-hypnotics**
Sedative-hypnotics are generally taken orally, and they are also CNS depressants. Assessment findings include altered mental status, hypotension, slurred speech, respiratory depression, shock, bradycardia, and seizures. Management centers on ABCs with respiratory support and oxygenation, IV access, ECG monitoring, and possible use of naloxone dependent on agent taken and advice of medical direction.

f. **Narcotics/opiates**
The narcotics can be taken orally or by injection. Pertinent assessment findings include CNS depression, constricted pupils, respiratory depression, hypotension, bradycardia, pulmonary edema, and coma. General management centers on ABCs with respiratory support and oxygenation, IV access, and ECG monitoring. You may use the antidote naloxone, which can be titrated to relieve symptoms of toxicity without provoking withdrawal symptoms in addicts. General instructions involve use of 1–2 mg naloxone IV or endotracheally per medical direction until respiration improves. Larger doses (2–5 mg) may be required in the management of Darvon overdose and alcoholic coma.

g. **Drugs abused for sexual purposes/sexual gratification**
This group includes a number of miscellaneous agents that are used to stimulate and enhance sexual experience but do not have medically approved indications for such use. MDMA, popularly known as Ecstasy, is an example. Ecstasy is a modified form of methamphetamine and has similar, although milder, effects. Look for its use on college campuses and in nightclub settings. Initial signs and symptoms of use include anxiety, tachycardia, nausea, and hypertension, followed by relaxation, euphoria, and feelings of enhanced emotional insight. Studies indicate prolonged use may cause brain damage. Cases that can lead to death have the following assessment findings: confusion, agitation, tremor, high temperature, and diarrhea. No specific treatment exists, so supportive measures should be taken. Flunitrazepam, or Rohypnol, is illegal in the U.S. but has been used as a "date rape drug" when slipped into a woman's drink. The drug is a strong benzodiazepine that causes sedation and amnesia. When this drug is suspected, treat as for other benzodiazepines but remember to look for consequences of sexual assault and be sure to treat them as well.

7. Given several scenarios of poisoning or overdose, provide the appropriate assessment, treatment, and transport. pp. 564–565

Remember that the basic assessment of a patient with a toxicologic emergency includes careful scene size-up, protection of rescue personnel, and rapid response to any needs to support the ABCs. Treatment may include the use of antidotes, where available. Rapid transport is standard. Detailed specifics for many drugs and toxic substances are given in other objectives for this chapter.

©2008 Pearson Education, Inc.

Case Study Review

Reread the case study in Chapter 16 and then read the following discussion. This case study demonstrates how a drug overdose that presents with a relatively normal patient can proceed to a serious emergency and death. Here it is most appropriate to move quickly to gather as much information as you can and move to what care you can offer as quickly as possible.

Christa and Jack use information from a previous call to prepare themselves for what they might find on this call. The history of overdose, the prescription of valium, and the report of an overdose all suggest this could be a serious emergency. Jack is right when he states, "Well, you can put those new Intermediate skills to work!"

Police on the scene suggest the scene is secure and the threat of violence is now remote. A quick history identifies a clear picture of the nature and degree of overdose (often not the case). Christa treats the patient for both the overdose and the emotional affect that brought it on. She does her best to calm, comfort, and reassure the patient. She confirms the amount of medication taken and begins her assessment. Jack completes the vital signs and the team now has the information needed for contact with both the Poison Control Center and medical direction. The information from Poison Control is valuable in determining the patient's priority for care and transport and helps the team begin to plan their care. Medical direction gives permission for activated charcoal to help absorb and deactivate the medication. In the past we would have given ipecac to force vomiting but research has determined that this endangers the airway and does not remove significant amounts of the toxin. Jack and Christa will monitor and protect the airway as they prepare and then transport the patient.

Content Self-Evaluation

Multiple Choice

_____ 1. The most common route of entry for toxic substances is
- A. inhalation.
- B. ingestion.
- C. surface absorption.
- D. injection.
- E. adsorption.

_____ 2. The three principles of decontamination are
- A. removal of patient from toxic environment, reduction in intake of toxin, and increase in elimination of toxin from body.
- B. removal of patient from toxic environment, removal of patient's clothing and washing of patient's body, and increase in elimination of toxin from body.
- C. removal of patient from toxic environment, reduction in intake of toxin, and use of antidote, if one exists.
- D. removal of patient's clothing and washing of body, reduction in intake of toxin, and reduction in absorption of toxin already in body.
- E. reduction in intake of toxin into the body, reduction of absorption of toxin already in the body, and increase in elimination of toxin from the body.

_____ 3. All of the following statements are correct when treating ingestion emergencies EXCEPT:
- A. Maintaining the ABCs is the top priority along with monitoring of all vitals.
- B. Prevention of aspiration is a major objective, and intubation may be necessary.
- C. An IV at keep-vein-open rate is recommended for all potentially dangerous ingestion incidents.
- D. Induce vomiting unless it is against local protocol or you are told not to do so by Poison Control.
- E. Follow general treatment guidelines with decontamination procedures.

©2008 Pearson Education, Inc.
Intermediate Emergency Care: 1985, 3rd ed.

_____ 4. The most effective prehospital means of reducing absorption of toxins in the body is
A. gastric lavage (stomach pumping).
B. activated charcoal.
C. syrup of ipecac.
D. whole bowel irrigation.
E. chelating agents.

_____ 5. Which of the following is not a question commonly asked of a poisoning patient during the focused history?
A. How much of the agent(s) did you ingest?
B. How long ago did you ingest the agent(s)?
C. Were any people with you when you ingested the agent(s)?
D. Did you drink any alcohol?
E. Have you attempted to treat yourself in any way?

_____ 6. The physical exam is crucial in toxicological emergencies, and it has two purposes: (1) documenting physical evidence of intoxication and (2) detecting any underlying illness or condition that might affect either patient's symptoms or outcome of exposure.
A. True
B. False

_____ 7. All of the following are respiratory signs or symptoms of a toxic inhalation exposure EXCEPT
A. huffing.
B. chest tightness.
C. cough.
D. tachypnea.
E. dizziness.

_____ 8. In common toxic drug ingestions, the use of benzodiazepines is frequently recommended to calm a patient who has taken
A. alcohol, narcotics, and barbiturates.
B. alcohol, hallucinogens, and barbiturates.
C. cocaine, amphetamines, and hallucinogens.
D. cocaine, alcohol, and amphetamines.
E. cocaine, amphetamines, and barbiturates.

_____ 9. The first priorities, in proper order, with surface-absorption exposures are to remove the patient from the toxic environment, perform the initial assessment, and then ensure your safety.
A. True
B. False

_____ 10. Flumazenil is an antidote for which of the following ingested substances?
A. arsenic
B. benzodiazepines
C. cyanide
D. ethylene glycol
E. methyl alcohol

Special Project

Analyzing an Emergency Scene

Use your experience and what you have learned in this chapter to answer the questions about the following scenario.

You are called to the apartment of an elderly gentleman after his son phoned 911 to report that when he telephoned his father for a nightly check, his father had slurred speech and sounded confused. The son told dispatch that his father had felt "under the weather" with a cold recently but had otherwise been in his usual, somewhat fragile, state of health. No specifics were given.

©2008 Pearson Education, Inc.

You find the patient alone in his apartment. He is an unkempt, confused gentleman who repeatedly introduces himself and asks your names. He looks moderately uncomfortable, has nasal congestion and a mild cough, and says he has been "a bit ill" for several days. He states that he took a long nap, and then got up and took his pills. He says he doesn't need any help, he just needs to sit a bit to clear his head. When asked what pills he took, and how long ago, he says he "thinks" he just took the bedtime pills, but he may also have taken the afternoon ones because he might have slept through the normal time to take them. He doesn't know where the pharmacy bottles are because his visiting nurse makes up his pill case once a week. You note on the nightstand next to the bed a pill case, one of those that has the days of the week and several times per day marked on it with a compartment for each dosing time. You observe that several compartments for each day have tablets or capsules, often multiple.

1. What kind of toxicological emergency might this situation represent, and would you suspect accidental or intentional circumstances?

As you start your physical assessment, the patient says, "Oh, my, I'm dizzy," and sits awkwardly on the floor. His pulse is difficult to determine, but it is weak, slow, and possibly irregular.

2. What are your initial interventions?
3. What priorities do you give to calling the Poison Control Center, medical direction, and initiating transport?
4. What, if anything, do you take with you from the apartment?

©2008 Pearson Education, Inc.
Intermediate Emergency Care: 1985, 3rd ed.

Chapter

17 Allergic Reactions and Anaphylaxis

Review of Chapter Objectives

After reading this chapter, you should be able to do the following:

1. Discuss the pathophysiology of allergy and anaphylaxis. **pp. 578–581**

The signs and symptoms associated with allergy and anaphylaxis are due to the physiologic changes triggered by the chemical mediators of the immune response that are released from the basophils and mast cells. Histamine is the primary mediator of all allergic reactions. It is a potent substance that causes bronchoconstriction, vasodilation and increased vascular permeability, and increased intestinal motility. Other chemical substances are also released that have effects similar to or synergistic with histamine, such as SRS-A (slow-reacting substance of anaphylaxis), which results in an asthmalike attack or asphyxia.

2. Describe the common routes of substance entry into the body. **p. 580**

Allergens can enter the body through various routes including oral ingestion, inhalation, topically, and through injection or envenomation. The vast majority of anaphylactic reactions result from injection or envenomation.

3. Define the immune system, allergic reaction, anaphylaxis, antigen, and antibody. **pp. 578–579**

The immune system is an intrinsic body system that identifies and removes substances from the body that are recognized as foreign. An **allergic reaction** is an exaggerated immune response to a foreign protein or other substance, while **anaphylaxis** is an unusual or exaggerated allergic reaction to a foreign protein or other substance.

An **antigen** is any substance that is capable, under appropriate conditions, of inducing a specific immune response. An **antibody** is a member of a unique class of chemicals that are manufactured by specialized cells of the immune system. The antibody is the principle agent of a chemical attack on an invading substance. Following exposure to an antigen, antibodies are released from cells of the immune system. The antibodies attach themselves to the invading substance so it can be removed from the body by other cells of the immune system.

4. List common antigens most frequently associated with allergies and anaphylaxis. **p. 580**

Any substance that is capable, under appropriate conditions, of inducing a specific immune response is known as an antigen. Most antigens are proteins. The following agents are among those that commonly trigger anaphylaxis: antibiotics, foods, or insect stings. Refer to Table 17-1 on text page 579 for a more complete list.

5. Describe the physical manifestations of anaphylaxis. **p. 581**

The signs and symptoms of anaphylaxis begin within 30 to 60 seconds following exposure for the vast majority of patients. The more rapid the onset, the more severe the patient presentation.

©2008 Pearson Education, Inc.

Respiratory manifestations of anaphylaxis include laryngeal edema and bronchoconstriction. Cardiovascular symptoms include tachycardia plus massive vasodilation resulting in profound hypotension. The combination of respiratory and cardiovascular signs will lead to a rapid deterioration of the patient's mental status. Generalized flushing and urticaria (hives) are common, as is angioedema about the head, face, and neck. Nausea, vomiting, and diarrhea may accompany hypermotility of the gastrointestinal tract.

6. Identify and differentiate between the signs and symptoms of allergic reaction and anaphylaxis. p. 583

Allergic reactions can range from a mild skin rash to a severe life-threatening multisystem response. Allergic reaction, also known as hypersensitivity, takes two forms, delayed or immediate. Delayed hypersensitivity is the result of cellular immunity and does not involve antibodies. It may occur hours to days after exposure and is very common. Delayed hypersensitivity usually presents as a skin rash and is often due to exposure to certain drugs and chemicals, for instance, poison ivy. Other signs and symptoms may include mild bronchoconstriction, mild intestinal cramps, or diarrhea, while the patient's mental status and vital signs will remain normal.

Immediate hypersensitivity is antibody-mediated immunity and often has a genetic link. The range of clinical presentation is widely variable. Examples of these reactions include hay fever, drug and food allergies, eczema, and asthma. Allergens can enter the body by various routes, but as a rule, those that enter by injection tend to have more rapid and more severe effects. Immediate hypersensitivities may be merely annoying, like the itching eyes and runny nose of hay fever, or may pose a real and immediate life threat, as seen in the anaphylactic reaction described in the case study at the beginning of this chapter.

The signs and symptoms of anaphylaxis begin within seconds following exposure. The more rapid the onset of symptoms, the more severe the patient presentation. Respiratory manifestations of anaphylaxis include laryngeal edema and bronchoconstriction. Cardiovascular symptoms include tachycardia plus massive vasodilation resulting in profound hypotension. A rapid deterioration of the patient's mental status accompanies the cardiovascular collapse. Generalized flushing and urticaria are common, as is angioedema about the head, face, and neck. Nausea, vomiting, and diarrhea may accompany hypermotility of the gastrointestinal tract. Refer to Table 17-2 on text page 583 for a comparison of signs and symptoms of mild allergic reactions and severe allergic reactions or anaphylaxis.

7. Explain the various treatments and pharmacological interventions used in the management of allergic reactions and anaphylaxis. pp. 582–584

The first priority in the management of allergic reactions and anaphylaxis is to establish and maintain the patient's airway. Administer oxygen immediately along with ventilatory support as needed. You should be prepared to intubate, recognizing that laryngeal edema may change the size and appearance of the airway.

Establish vascular access as soon as possible and be prepared to run crystalloid solutions wide open if the patient is hypotensive.

Epinephrine is the drug of choice for severe allergic reaction and anaphylaxis. In mild to moderate cases, administer 0.3–0.5 mg of 1:1,000 epinephrine subcutaneously. Remember that the effects of epinephrine wear off quickly, so be prepared to repeat boluses in 3 to 5 minutes. As is always the case, your management approach should always be dictated by local protocols.

8. Correlate abnormal findings in assessment with the clinical significance in the patient with an allergic reaction or anaphylaxis. pp. 581, 583

The central physiological action in severe allergic reaction and anaphylaxis is the massive release of histamine and other chemical mediators of the immune system. The resultant bronchospasm, airway edema, peripheral vasodilation, and increased capillary permeability can take a patient from his or her usual state of health to the brink of death in mere seconds. This chemically caused transformation is readily evident in the patient's clinical presentation: air hunger, dyspnea, angioedema, tachycardia, and hypotension. Your timely intervention is imperative to your patient's survival.

©2008 Pearson Education, Inc.
Intermediate Emergency Care: 1985, 3rd ed.

9. Given several preprogrammed and moulaged patients, provide the appropriate assessment, care, and transport for the allergic reaction and anaphylaxis patient. **pp. 579–584**

Throughout your classroom, clinical, and field training, you will encounter a variety of real and simulated patients with allergic reactions or anaphylaxis emergencies. Use the information provided in this chapter of your text, as well as the application of this information as demonstrated by your instructors, preceptors, and mentors to enhance your ability to assess, manage, and transport these patients.

Case Study Review

Reread the case study in Chapter 17 and then read the following discussion. This case study draws attention to the typical presentation and management for a patient experiencing severe anaphylaxis.

In this case study, an injection of a radiocontrast dye was administered just 15 minutes earlier. The patient's immediate response was a red rash and generalized itching that quickly progressed to marked respiratory compromise and cardiovascular collapse. The clinic staff had administered oxygen via a nasal cannula and was setting up an IV.

With the arrival of Steve and Beth on-scene, appropriate emergency care was quickly initiated; the nasal cannula was replaced with high-flow oxygen via nonrebreather mask, keeping an ET kit readily accessible. Beth established vascular access and initiated fluid resuscitation (of 500 mL) to compensate for massive vasodilation, while Steve administered epinephrine subcutaneously to counteract the immune system response. Although the patient showed improvement within 2 minutes of the epinephrine administration, Steve knew that the medication wears off quickly and watched the patient carefully. Diphenhydramine was also administered to block the histamine receptors. All of these efforts were effective in reversing the anaphylaxis, however the persistent hypotension and tachycardia suggest the need for some additional fluid (250 mL bolus).

Content Self-Evaluation

Multiple Choice

______ 1. The unique class of chemicals that are manufactured by specialized cells of the immune system to attack invading foreign proteins is
- A. allergens.
- B. antigens.
- C. toxins.
- D. antibodies.
- E. pathogens.

______ 2. Any substance that is capable, under appropriate conditions, of inducing a specific immune response is a(n)
- A. immunoglobulin.
- B. antigen.
- C. toxin.
- D. antibody.
- E. pathogen.

______ 3. Anaphylaxis is best defined as an exaggerated, sometimes potentially life-threatening response by the immune system to a foreign substance.
- A. True
- B. False

______ 4. All of the following are common allergens EXCEPT
- A. insect stings.
- B. drugs.
- C. antibodies.
- D. seafood.
- E. radiology contrast materials.

©2008 Pearson Education, Inc.

_____ 5. The vast majority of anaphylactic reactions occur as a result of
A. inhalation.
B. ingestion.
C. injection.
D. topical exposure.
E. genetics.

_____ 6. The primary chemical mediator of an allergic reaction is
A. heparin.
B. histamine.
C. SRS-A.
D. basophil.
E. the mast cell.

_____ 7. The principle body systems affected by anaphylaxis include all of the following EXCEPT
A. respiratory.
B. vascular.
C. gastrointestinal.
D. renal.
E. skin.

_____ 8. Urticaria, a wheal and flare reaction characterized by red raised bumps that appear on the skin, is due to
A. bronchodilation.
B. vasodilation.
C. increased intestinal motility.
D. increased vascular permeability.
E. secretion of gastric acids.

_____ 9. The primary drug for the management of anaphylaxis is
A. ipecac.
B. diphenhydramine.
C. epinephrine.
D. methylprednisolone.
E. albuterol.

_____ 10. The first priority when responding to a patient with an anaphylactic reaction is to
A. protect the airway.
B. administer diphenhydramine.
C. stabilize the cervical spine.
D. ensure scene safety.
E. establish vascular access.

©2008 Pearson Education, Inc.
Intermediate Emergency Care: 1985, 3rd ed.

Chapter 18

Neurologic Emergencies

Review of Chapter Objectives

After reading this chapter, you should be able to do the following:

1. **Define and discuss the epidemiology (including the morbidity/mortality and preventative strategies), pathophysiology, assessment findings, and management for the following neurologic problems.**

a. Stroke **pp. 589–597**

Stroke is a general term for injury or death of brain tissue, usually due to interruption of blood flow to that region of the cerebrum. The term "brain attack" is being used more frequently because of some similarities between stroke and heart attack, the latter also being due to oxygen deprivation. You should also realize that there are more treatment similarities to heart attacks. Strokes due to thromboembolic causes may be aborted or minimized with use of thrombolytic agents now used with heart attack (such as tissue plasminogen activator, tPA). The importance to you is that prompt recognition and transport of stroke patients is greater than ever. Stroke patients who may be candidates for thrombolytic therapy must receive definitive treatment within 3 hours of onset.

Strokes are the third most common cause of death and a frequent cause of considerable disability among middle-aged and elderly persons. Major risk factors include atherosclerosis, heart disease, hypertension, diabetes, abnormal blood lipid levels, use of oral contraceptives, and sickle cell disease. Strokes can be caused either by occlusion of an artery or by hemorrhage. Both interrupt blood flow to distal tissues. An occlusive stroke is any caused by blockage of the artery, resulting in ischemia to brain tissue that may progress to infarction if oxygen deprivation continues long enough. Infarcted brain tissue swells, further damaging nearby tissue that might have only a marginal blood supply itself. If swelling is sufficiently severe, herniation (protrusion of tissue through the foramen magnum, the opening at the base of the skull through which the spinal cord emerges from the cranium) can occur. Occlusive strokes are either thrombotic or embolic in origin.

Thrombotic strokes are due to a thrombus, or blood clot, that forms in and then obstructs a cerebral artery. Thrombosis is often related to atherosclerotic change in the artery. Unsurprisingly, the signs and symptoms of a thrombotic stroke are often gradual in onset. The stroke often occurs at night and is characterized by the patient waking with altered mental status and/or loss of speech, sensation, or motor function. An embolic stroke is caused by a solid, liquid, or gaseous mass that is carried to the site of obstruction from a remote site. The most common brain emboli are blood clots that often arise from diseased blood vessels in the neck (namely, the carotid artery) or from abnormal cardiac contraction. Atrial fibrillation often results in atrial dilation, a precursor to clot formation. Other types of emobli include air, tumor tissue, and fat. Typically, embolic strokes present with sudden onset of severe headaches. Hemorrhagic strokes are due to bleeding within brain tissue, and they can be categorized as intracerebral or subarachnoid (see Figure 18-2, text page 591) discussed in detail below under intracranial hemorrhage.

©2008 Pearson Education, Inc.

Prompt and proper assessment of a stroke in progress is very important. Signs and symptoms will depend on the type of stroke and the area of the brain affected by it. Onset of symptoms may be acute, and the patient may be unconscious. You may observe stertorous breathing due to paralysis of part of the soft palate. Respiratory expirations may be puffs of air out of the cheeks and mouth. The patient's pupils may be unequal. If so, the larger pupil will be on the side of the hemorrhage. Paralysis, when present, usually involves one side of the face, one arm, or one leg. Speech disturbances may be noted, and the patient's skin may be cool and clammy.

Common signs and symptoms of stroke include the following.

one-sided facial drooping
headache
confusion and agitation
dysphasia (difficulty in speech)
aphasia (inability to speak)
dysarthria (impairment of tongue and muscles making speech difficult)
vision problems such as blindness in one eye or double vision
hemiparesis (one-sided weakness)
hemiplegia (one-sided paralysis)
paresthesias
inability to recognize by touch
gait disturbances or uncoordinated motor movements
dizziness
incontinence
coma

Management of stroke emphasizes early recognition, supportive measures, prompt, rapid transport, and notification of the emergency department (see algorithm in Figure 18-8, text page 596). Remember that aggressive airway management is vital in these patients. Other field measures include the following: (1) assurance of scene safety, including body substance isolation, (2) airway management including suction as needed, (3) ventilation assistance as needed: If the patient is apneic or breathing is inadequate, provide positive-pressure ventilation at 20/minute. Hyperventilation eliminates excessive CO_2 levels. Avoid over-hyperventilation because excessively low CO_2 levels can cause profound cerebral vasoconstriction. If breathing is adequate, give oxygen via nonrebreather mask at 15 L/minute, (4) complete a detailed patient history, (5) keep patient supine or in recovery position. If the patient has congestive heart failure, place patient in semi-upright position as needed. If patient has altered mental status and you suspect potential for airway compromise, keep him or her in left lateral recumbent, or recovery position, (6) determine blood glucose level; if hypoglycemia is present, consider 50% dextrose by IV push, (7) start an IV of normal saline or lactated Ringer's at a keep-vein-open rate or place a saline or heparin lock (avoiding dextrose solutions, which may increase intracranial pressure due to osmotic effect), (8) monitor cardiac rhythm, (9) protect paralyzed extremities, (10) reassure patient and explain all procedures as patient may be able to understand even if he or she cannot respond, and (11) transport without excessive movement or noise.

b. Intracranial hemorrhage **p. 591**

Hemorrhagic strokes are due to blood within brain tissue, and they can be categorized as intracerebral or subarachnoid. These intracranial hemorrhages often occur with sudden onset of a severe headache. Most intracranial hemorrhages occur in a hypertensive patient when a small vessel deep within brain tissue ruptures. Subarachnoid hemorrhages most commonly result from either congenital blood vessel anomalies or from head trauma. Congenital anomalies include aneurysms and arteriovenous malformations. Aneurysms tend to be on the brain's surface and may either hemorrhage into brain tissue or into the subarachnoid space. Hemorrhage within brain tissue may tear and separate normal brain tissue. Release of blood into the ventricles containing CSF may paralyze vital centers. If blood impairs drainage of CSF, the resultant increase in intracranial pressure may cause herniation of brain tissue.

c. Transient ischemic attack **pp. 594–595**

A transient ischemic attack (TIA) is a temporary manifestation of the signs and/or symptoms of stroke that is due to temporary interference with blood supply to the affected part of the

©2008 Pearson Education, Inc.
Intermediate Emergency Care: 1985, 3rd ed.

brain. These symptoms may persist for a few minutes or for hours, but they almost always resolve within 24 hours. After the attack (because it reflects ischemia, not infarction), there is no evidence of brain or neurological damage. The most common cause is carotid artery disease (provoking an embolic event). Other causes can be small emboli of different origin, decreased cardiac output, hypotension, overmedication with antihypertensive medications, or cerebrovascular spasm. Part of the importance of recognizing TIAs is that they may be the precursor to a stroke. One third of TIA patients suffer a stroke soon afterward. A TIA is typically sudden in onset, with specific signs and symptoms depending on the part of the brain involved.

In the prehospital setting, it is virtually impossible to distinguish a TIA from a stroke. While taking the history, try to get the following information: previous neurological symptoms, if any; initial symptoms and their progression; changes in mental status; precipitating factors, if any; dizziness; palpitations; history of hypertension, cardiac disease, sickle cell disease, or previous TIA or stroke. Because TIAs and strokes are generally indistinguishable in the field, the management is the same. (See Stroke, above.)

d. Seizures **pp. 597–601**

A seizure is a temporary alteration in behavior due to a massive discharge of one or more groups of neurons in the brain. Seizures can be induced in anyone under certain stressful conditions such as hypoxia or rapidly decreasing blood glucose. Febrile seizures often occur in young children with a sudden increase in body temperature. Structural diseases of the brain such as tumors, head trauma, toxic eclampsia, and vascular disorders can also cause a seizure. Recurrent seizures without such a known cause are termed epilepsy. Epilepsy affects about 2.5 million persons, who may present with a neurological emergency or have another condition complicated by their seizure disorder. Most cases of epilepsy are idiopathic, that is, without known cause, whereas others arise secondary to damage from strokes, head trauma, tumor, surgery, or radiation, etc.

Assessment begins with history according to the patient or bystanders, as well as physical impression. Remember that many people think the only kind of seizure is a "grand mal," so a bystander who does not know the patient may suggest he is on drugs, or that he fainted, or give other information that is misleading. In addition, other medical conditions can present similarly to a seizure: Examples are migraine headaches, cardiac dysrhythmias, hypoglycemia, or orthostatic hypotension. Hyperventilation, as well as a number of CNS conditions, can cause stiffness in the extremities. Decerebrate movements can be caused by increased intracranial pressure. Thus, there is often more potential harm than good in administering an anticonvulsant.

The patient history should include an attempt to ascertain the following information: (1) history of seizures, and, if so, particulars of type, nature, and frequency, (2) recent history of head trauma, (3) possibility of alcohol or other drug use, (4) recent history of fever, headache, or stiff neck, (5) history of diabetes, heart disease, or stroke, and (6) current medications. During physical exam, look for evidence of head injury or injury to the tongue and for evidence of alcohol or drug abuse. Be sure to document any dysrhythmias.

Active management may not be needed for many types of seizures, including short generalized tonic-clonic seizures that have ended before you arrive. Management for most generalized seizures in process is supportive: Manage the airway, make sure the patient does not injure him- or herself, and monitor for possible hyper- or hypothermia, depending on environmental conditions. General procedures include the following: (1) assurance of scene safety, (2) maintenance of airway (DO NOT force objects between the patient's teeth or push objects into the mouth that may initiate vomiting), (3) administration of high-flow oxygen, (4) establishment of IV access, running normal saline or lactated Ringer's solution at keep-vein-open rate, (5) determination of blood glucose level, with 50% glucose given in hypoglycemia, (6) physical protection of patient from surroundings, (7) maintenance of temperature, (8) postictal positioning on left side with suction if required, (9) monitoring of cardiac rhythm, (10) consideration of an anticonvulsant if seizure is prolonged (greater than 5 minutes), (11) transport the patient in supine or lateral recumbent position in quiet, reassuring atmosphere.

Status epilepticus, two or more generalized seizures without intervening return of consciousness, can be a life-threatening emergency. The most common cause in adults with epilepsy is failure to comply with medication regimen. Status is a major emergency because it involves a prolonged period of apnea with the possibility of CNS hypoxia. The most valuable intervention is to protect the airway and to deliver 100% oxygen, preferably by BVM device.

©2008 Pearson Education, Inc.

After airway and breathing have been addressed, start an IV with normal saline at keep-vein-open rate, monitor cardiac rhythm, give 25 g 50% dextrose IV push if hypoglycemia is present, give 5–10 mg diazepam IV push for an adult, and continue to monitor airway. Note that some patients will require large doses of diazepam, and this may cause respiratory depression. Depression, if significant, can be reversed with flumazenil, although this may also result in the return of seizures.

e. Syncope **pp. 601–602**

Syncope, or fainting, is characterized by a sudden, temporary loss of consciousness caused by insufficient blood flow to the brain, with recovery almost immediate upon supine positioning. Syncope is very common, accounting for roughly 3% of all emergency department visits. It can occur at any age. Symptoms may include prior feelings of dizziness or lightheadedness or there may be no warning at all. By definition, if return of consciousness does not occur within a few moments, the event is NOT syncope, it is something more serious. (Review Table 18-1, text page 599, for help in distinguishing between syncope and seizure.)

There are three pathophysiologic mechanisms for syncope: cardiovascular, noncardiovascular, and idiopathic. Cardiovascular causes include dysrhythmias or mechanical problems such as an abnormally functioning heart valve. Noncardiovascular causes include metabolic, neurological, or psychiatric conditions. For instance, hypoglycemia, a transient ischemic attack (TIA), or an anxiety attack may all precipitate syncope. Idiopathic, as always, means there is no known cause even after careful evaluation. Management begins with an attempt to find and treat the underlying cause. If no cause is established, the patient should be transported to an appropriate emergency department for evaluation. Field management is somewhat similar to that for seizure: assure scene safety, maintain open airway, administer high-flow oxygen and assist ventilations as needed, check circulatory status (heart rate and rhythm, blood pressure), check and continue monitoring mental status, start IV with normal saline or lactated Ringer's at keep-vein-open rate, determine blood glucose level, monitor cardiac rhythm, and transport in reassuring environment.

f. Headache **p. 602**

Headaches, either acute or chronic, are a tremendously common complaint: You've probably had problems with a headache at least once. Nearly 45 million Americans suffer from chronic headaches. There are three general categories of headache: vascular, tension, and organic. Headaches of vascular origin include migraines and cluster headaches. Migraines occur more commonly in women, whereas cluster headaches occur more commonly in men. Migraines are typically characterized by intense, throbbing pain, sensitivity to light or sound, nausea, vomiting, and sweating. Migraines may last from several minutes to several days. They typically present as one-sided headaches and they may be preceded by an aura. Cluster headaches usually occur as a series of one-sided headaches that are sudden in onset, intense, and continue for roughly 15 minutes to 4 hours. Symptoms may include nasal congestion, drooping eyelid, and an irritated eye. Tension headaches account for a significant percentage of headaches. Most personnel in emergency medicine, have, or will, have a tension headache. Some people experience them on a daily basis. These persons may wake with a headache that worsens over the course of the day. The typical tension headache has a dull, achy pain that feels as if forceful pressure is being applied to the neck or head. The last class of headache, organic headaches, is less common. They occur in association with tumor, infection, or other diseases of the brain, eye, or other body system.

Because headaches can herald serious illness or precede a catastrophic event such as a ruptured aneurysm, it is always important to keep these possible underlying causes in mind when you speak with a patient complaining of headache. A continuous throbbing headache, particularly if over the occiput, accompanied by fever, confusion, and stiffness of the neck is classic for meningitis. Sudden onset pain, often described as "the worst pain of my life," or changes in pain pattern should all be considered possible signs of conditions as grave as intracranial hemorrhage. In general, any headache of acute onset or of changing pattern demands immediate attention on your part.

A complete and thorough history is important in evaluating the patient with headache. Questions that may evoke valuable information include the following: What were you doing when the pain started? Does anything make the pain worse (such as light, sound, or movement)? What is the quality of the pain, throbbing, crushing, tension? Does pain radiate to the neck, arm, back, or jaw? What is the severity of the pain on a scale of 1–10 and has severity changed? How long has

©2008 Pearson Education, Inc.
Intermediate Emergency Care: 1985, 3rd ed.

the headache been present (is it acute or chronic)? You will see that the same line of questioning about pain is used in other settings, too, as with patients who complain of abdominal pain.

Management is supportive and generally includes the following: (1) assurance of scene safety, (2) protection of airway, (3) placement of patient in position of comfort (often accomplished by patients themselves), (4) high-flow oxygen with ventilation assistance as needed, (5) IV with normal saline or lactated Ringer's at keep-vein-open rate, determination of blood glucose, monitoring of cardiac rhythm, (6) transport with reassurance in an environment that is calm and quiet, (7) consideration of use of antiemetics or analgesics. Antiemetics that might be helpful for migraine include prochlorperazine (Compazine) and abortive agents such as sumatriptan (Imitrix).

2. Describe and differentiate the major types of seizures. **pp. 597–598**

Seizures can be clinically grouped as generalized or partial on a pathophysiologic basis. Generalized seizures begin with an electrical discharge in a small part of the brain but the abnormal activity spreads to involve the entire cerebral cortex. In contrast, partial seizures may remain confined to a small area, causing localized malfunction, or they may spread and become secondarily generalized seizures.

Generalized seizures include tonic-clonic (also commonly called grand mal) and absence seizures. A tonic-clonic seizure is a generalized motor seizure that produces a temporary loss of consciousness. Usually, it includes a tonic phase (in which muscle tone is increased) and a clonic phase (in which muscles in the extremities jerk rhythmically). In some cases, temporary paralysis of the intercostal muscles causes an interruption in breathing and cyanosis may become evident. When respirations resume, you may see copious amounts of frothy oral secretions. Incontinence is also common during a seizure, and you may note agitation or confusion, drowsiness, or even coma following a seizure, depending on the norm for that patient. Absence seizures present very differently. They are characterized by a sudden onset of a brief (typically 10- to 30-second) loss of consciousness or awareness. Loss of consciousness may be so brief that the casual observer misses it altogether. These idiopathic seizures of childhood rarely occur after age 20. Note that absence seizures may not respond to your normal treatment modalities.

Pseudoseizures, also called hysterical seizures, are not true electrical seizures. Rather, they represent psychiatric phenomena. The patient typically presents with sharp, bizarre movements that may be interrupted with a terse command such as "Stop it!"

Partial seizures may be either simple or complex. Simple seizures involve local motor, sensory, or autonomic dysfunction in one area of the body; there is no loss of consciousness. You should remember, however, that they may spread in area of involvement and progress to a generalized, tonic-clonic seizure. Complex seizures, which usually originate in the temporal lobe, are often characterized by an aura and focal findings such as alterations in mental status or mood. Patients in the midst of such a seizure may appear intoxicated or mentally unstable: They may be confused, stagger, have purposeless movements, or show sudden personality changes. These seizures typically last 1–2 minutes, and the patient will slowly come back to baseline after that period.

3. Describe the phases of a generalized seizure. **pp. 597–598**

Although patients are individuals with their own seizure patterns, many tonic-clonic seizures progress through seven phases: (1) aura, a subjective sensation that serves as a warning to those patients who experience it, (2) loss of consciousness, during the aura sensation, if there is one, (3) tonic phase, (4) hypertonic phase, during which you will see extreme muscular rigidity, including hyperextension of the back, (5) clonic phase of muscle spasms (often including the jaws) marked by rhythmic movements, (6) post-seizure, during which the patient is in a coma, and (7) postictal, during which the patient awakens.

4. Given several preprogrammed nontraumatic neurological emergency patients, provide the appropriate assessment, management, and transport. **pp. 589–603**

As a prehospital care provider you will frequently see patients who have the neurologic problems or conditions discussed in this chapter. Review the objectives above to familiarize yourself with assessment and care in the setting of common neurologic emergencies.

©2008 Pearson Education, Inc.

Case Study Review

Reread the case study in Chapter 18 and then read the following discussion. This case study demonstrates how EMT-Is react to a relatively common neurological emergency, a stroke. While the dispatch information does not identify such, the presentation quickly identifies the nature of the illness and they begin their care. The case study demonstrates that important quick recognition and rapid transport can influence the outcome of this type of call.

Jason and Scott are dispatched to an "unknown medical." This gives them little information to think about as the cause of the emergency so they must take a rather generic approach. They will be guided by the patient history and the investigation of the chief complaint. Here, the patient's wife describes the gradual onset of her husband's problem that is right-sided, with the exception of his left eye. This is very suggestive of a stroke. Their physical exam confirms this, including his right-sided reduced strength, inability to speak (yet he does answer questions with nods). The Intermediates employ the Cincinnati Stroke Scale and evaluate facial droop and abnormal speech. They also ask Mr. Willis to hold both arms out in front, palms up for 10 seconds with his eyes closed. They note that the right arm drifts downward and the palm rotates downward as well. All these signs are strongly suggestive of stroke.

Once Jason and Scott recognize the stroke they decide to both move quickly and to identify as much information to determine the nature of the stroke and other medical history elements that indicate or contraindicate fibrolytic therapy. Time is of the essence as there is a 3-hour window in which the fibrolytic agents are most effective. And some of that time has been already consumed during which Mrs. Willis recognized the problem, the EMT-Intermediate team responded, and the team has now assessed the patient. Mr. Willis will be transported to a facility with the equipment and trained personnel to rapidly provide his care.

Jason and Scott will ask questions to help identify any contraindications to the fibrolytic therapy. They will investigate any recent surgeries, bleeding disorders, medications like aspirin, all of which suggest a higher complication rate with the stroke therapy. They will also document their assessment findings to help the receiving hospital personnel better and more quickly identify the nature and extent of the stroke. They do their job well; Mr. Willis quickly receives his therapy and much of the stroke signs and symptoms resolve.

Content Self-Evaluation

Multiple Choice

______ 1. The two mechanisms that generally cause altered mental status are
A. occlusive and hemorrhagic strokes.
B. systemic diseases and drugs or toxic agents.
C. structural lesions and toxic-metabolic states.
D. head trauma and CNS disease.
E. toxic-metabolic states and brain tumors.

______ 2. The type of stroke caused by a rupturing cerebral artery is a(n) ______ stroke.
A. occlusive
B. embolic
C. thrombotic
D. hemorrhagic
E. aneural

______ 3. Which type of stroke is caused by an obstruction that travels to the brain?
A. embolic
B. hemorrhagic
C. transient
D. fibrinolytic
E. none of the above

©2008 Pearson Education, Inc.
Intermediate Emergency Care: 1985, 3rd ed.

_____ 4. Which of the following is not one of the critical criteria in the treatment of stroke with fibrinolytic agents?
A. Early identification of the stroke
B. Early notification of the EMS system
C. Identification of the patient as a fibrinolytic therapy candidate
D. Rapid transport to the proper facility
E. Therapy must be offered within 45 minutes of onset.

_____ 5. Which is not an element of the Los Angeles Prehospital Stroke Screen?
A. facial droop
B. eye opening
C. arm drift
D. abnormal speech
E. all of the above

_____ 6. Twenty-four hours after a transient ischemic attack (TIA) the patient will usually display no neurologic signs.
A. True
B. False

_____ 7. If a stroke patient is apneic or breathing inadequately, hyperventilation should be avoided because it
A. causes profound cerebral vasoconstriction.
B. causes a reflex increase in respiration rate.
C. eliminates excess CO_2 levels.
D. increases CO_2 levels toward normal range.
E. increases the ability of brain cells to take up any available oxygen.

_____ 8. Among the many types of epileptic seizures, the most likely to require intervention on your part are
A. absence seizures.
B. status epilepticus
C. petit mal seizures.
D. simple partial seizures.
E. complex partial seizures.

_____ 9. The phase of a seizure in which a patient experiences alternating contraction and relaxation of the muscles is the _____ phase.
A. tonic
B. clonic
C. aural
D. hypertonic
E. postictal

_____ 10. All of the following are characteristics of a complex partial seizure EXCEPT
A. distinctive auras.
B. loss of contact with surroundings.
C. confusion.
D. clonic movements.
E. making unintelligible sounds.

©2008 Pearson Education, Inc.

Chapter

19 Diabetic Emergencies

Review of Chapter Objectives

After reading this chapter, you should be able to do the following:

1. Describe the pathophysiology of diabetes mellitus. **pp. 607–608**

Juvenile onset or Type I diabetes mellitus is a serious disease characterized by very low production of insulin by the beta cells of the pancreas. In many cases, there is no insulin being produced. It is called juvenile onset diabetes because of the average age of the patient at the time of diagnosis. Type I diabetes is also known as insulin-dependent diabetes mellitus (IDDM) because patients require regular injections of insulin to control their disease. Heredity appears to be an important factor in determining which people will develop Type I diabetes. The cause of Type I diabetes is not clear. Other factors attributed to triggering juvenile onset diabetes are viral infection, an autoimmune response, or genetically determined premature deterioration of beta cells. The immediate cause of Type I diabetes is the destruction of pancreatic beta cells.

Type II diabetes mellitus, also known as non-insulin-dependent diabetes (NIDDM), is responsible for almost 90 percent of all cases of diabetes. Type II diabetes usually begins in later life and is often associated with obesity, so it is known as adult onset diabetes. Type II diabetes is associated with a moderate decline in insulin production accompanied by a marked decrease in the utilization of the insulin within the body. The cause is not clearly understood, although obesity is believed to play a role in its development. Increased weight, along with the increased size of fat cells, causes a relative deficiency in the number of insulin receptors, thus making the fat cells less responsive to insulin. Type II diabetes is usually managed through a combination of diet, exercise, and the administration of medications to reduce either blood glucose or enhance the efficiency of insulin. Occasionally insulin administration is required.

2. Differentiate between normal glucose metabolism and diabetic glucose metabolism. **pp. 608–610**

Metabolism, which means "to change," is a term used to refer to all of the chemical and energy transformations within the body. Two kinds of change take place in the cell. One kind builds complex molecules from simple ones (anabolism), such as the synthesis of glycogen from glucose. The other kind breaks down complex molecules into simpler ones (catabolism), such as occurs with the breakdown of glucose into carbon dioxide, water, and energy (in the form of ATP). When materials are abundant after meals and the glucose is high, insulin enables cells to use glucose directly and to store energy as glycogen, protein, and fat. Insulin stimulates glucose pathways. In contrast, glucagon, the dominant hormone during periods of low blood glucose, stimulates catabolic pathways to produce usable energy from the body's stores.

The rate at which glucose can enter the cell is dependent upon insulin levels. Insulin combines with insulin receptors on the surface of the cell membrane, allowing glucose to enter the cell by increasing the permeability of the cell membrane. The rate at which glucose can be transported into the cells can be accelerated tenfold by insulin.

©2008 Pearson Education, Inc.

Sometimes the body cannot use glucose as its primary energy source, as is the case in patients with diabetes mellitus. Without insulin, the amount of glucose that can be transported into the cells is far too small to meet the body's energy demands. Without insulin, the glucose remains in the bloodstream, resulting in hyperglycemia. Carbohydrate depletion is also seen in other conditions, such as a high-fat, low-carbohydrate diet or starvation (which can be associated with some eating disorders). Under these conditions, the body slowly switches from glucose to fat as the primary energy source. Adipose cells break down fats into their component free fatty acids, and the blood concentration of these acids rises considerably.

Most of the fatty acids are used directly by the body's cells as an energy source. The liver takes in some, where the catabolism of fatty acids produces acetoacetic acid. When more acetoacetic acid is released by the liver than can be effectively utilized by body cells, it accumulates in the bloodstream along with two other closely related substances, acetone and β-hydroxybutyric acid. The three substances are collectively called ketone bodies. Their presence in excessive quantities is called ketosis.

3. Describe the mechanism of ketone body formation and its relationship to ketoacidosis. pp. 609–610

When the body's carbohydrate stores begin to become depleted, small amounts of glucose can be formed by the breakdown of protein and fat through the process of gluconeogenesis. The byproducts of amino acid breakdown include carbon dioxide and water and the formation of urea. The breakdown of fat results in the formation of carbon dioxide, water, and ketone bodies.

The normal blood ketone level in humans is low because ketones are usually metabolized as rapidly as they are formed. If there are low levels of glucose stored in the cells, the ability of the body to oxidize the ketones is soon exceeded and ketones begin to build up in the bloodstream, resulting in a condition known as ketosis. This results in an increased amount of acid in the body fluids. The resulting metabolic acidosis is often severe and can be fatal.

4. Discuss the physiology of the excretion of potassium and ketone bodies by the kidneys. pp. 609–610, 616–618

Whenever the flow rate of fluid inside the tubules of the kidney rises, as in osmotic diuresis, an increase in excretion of potassium occurs. This leads to the potential for significant hypokalemia and its effects, such as potentially life-threatening cardiac dysrhythmias. In ketotic states, ketone bodies are excreted through respiration and will also spill into the urine.

5. Describe the relationship of insulin to serum glucose levels. pp. 608–610, 613–618

Insulin is a glucagon antagonist and lowers the blood glucose level by promoting energy storage. Insulin increases the rate at which various body cells take up glucose by changing the permeability of the cell membranes. These changes also make the cell more permeable to potassium, magnesium, and phosphate ions, as well as many amino acids. Because the liver rapidly breaks down insulin, the hormone must be secreted constantly.

Homeostasis of blood glucose is remarkably effective. In non-diabetics, when blood glucose is high, as after a meal, the beta cells of the pancreas release insulin. Insulin enables cells to use glucose directly as well as to store energy as glycogen, protein, and fat. If you were to draw a venous blood sample to measure fasting blood glucose levels, you'd find the level in healthy individuals is usually between 80–90 mg glucose/dL blood. In the first 60–90 minutes after a meal the level will increase to approximately 120–140 mg/dL before dropping off to near-fasting levels as insulin is released to move the glucose from the bloodstream into the cells. Conversely, when blood glucose levels are low, the alpha cells of the pancreas release glucagon to raise the blood glucose level.

6. Describe the effects of decreased levels of insulin on the body. pp. 613–614

Insulin deficiency contributes to the development of hyperglycemia. Without insulin to facilitate the movement of large glucose molecules across cell membranes, the blood glucose level rises even as the intracellular level of glucose plummets. At the same time, the alpha cells of the pancreas release glucagon to increase blood glucose by stimulating the breakdown of glycogen, as well as

©2008 Pearson Education, Inc.
Intermediate Emergency Care: 1985, 3rd ed.

stimulating the breakdown of body proteins and fats with subsequent chemical conversion to glucose (gluconeogenesis).

7. Describe the effects of increased serum glucose levels on the body. **pp. 616–618**

With a rise in blood glucose levels, as is the case in Type I diabetes, the body's cells cannot take up circulating glucose. Glucose then spills into urine, leading to a large water loss, via osmotic diuresis, and significant dehydration. This can lead to significant loss of potassium and hypokalemia.

8. Discuss the pathophysiology, assessment findings, and management of the following endocrine emergencies:

a. Hypoglycemia **pp. 614–616**

Hypoglycemia, or low blood glucose, is a potentially life-threatening medical emergency. Sometimes called insulin shock, it can occur if a patient accidentally or intentionally injects too much insulin, eats an inadequate amount of food after taking insulin, or has overexercised and burned up all available glucose. Untreated, the insulin will cause the blood glucose to drop to a very low level. The longer the period of hypoglycemia persists, the greater the risk that the brain cells will be permanently damaged or even killed.

The signs and symptoms of hypoglycemia are many and varied. An abnormal mental status is the most important and often the earliest sign. In the earliest stages of hypoglycemia, the patient may appear restless or impatient or complain of hunger. As the blood sugar falls lower, he or she may display inappropriate anger or display a variety of bizarre behaviors. Physical signs may include diaphoresis and tachycardia. If the blood sugar falls to a critically low level, the patient may sustain a hypoglycemic seizure or become comatose. In contrast to diabetic ketoacidosis, hypoglycemia can develop quickly. When encountering a patient behaving bizarrely, you should always consider hypoglycemia.

In suspected cases of hypoglycemia, perform the initial assessment quickly. Inspect the patient for a Medic-Alert bracelet. If possible, determine the blood glucose level. If the blood glucose level is noted to be less than 60 mg/dL, draw a red-top tube of blood and start an IV of normal saline. Next, administer 50–100 milliliters (25–50 grams) of 50 percent dextrose intravenously. If the patient is conscious and able to swallow, complete glucose administration with orange juice, sodas, or commercially available glucose pastes.

If the blood glucose cannot be obtained and if the patient is unconscious, you should start an IV of normal saline and administer 50–100 milliliters (25–50 grams) of 50 percent dextrose. Expedite transport to the nearest medical facility. If you suspect alcoholism, administer 100 mg of thiamine prior to the administration of dextrose.

b. Diabetic ketoacidosis **pp. 616–618**

Diabetic ketoacidosis is a serious, potentially life-threatening complication of diabetes mellitus. It occurs when profound insulin deficiency is coupled with increased glucagon activity.

The onset is slow, lasting from 12 to 24 hours. In its early stages, the signs and symptoms include intensified thirst, excessive hunger, increased urination, and malaise. Increased urination results from the osmotic diuresis accompanying glucose spillage into the urine. Intensified thirst is caused by the body's attempt to replace the fluids lost by increased urination. Nausea, vomiting, marked dehydration, tachycardia, and weakness characterize diabetic ketoacidosis. The skin is usually warm and dry. Coma is not uncommon. The breath may have a sweet or acetone-like character due to the increased ketones in the blood. Very deep, rapid respirations, called Kussmaul's respirations, also occur. Kussmaul's respirations represent the body's attempt to compensate for the metabolic acidosis produced by the ketones and organic acids present in the blood. It may be complicated by several electrolyte imbalances. The most significant is decreased potassium. Decreased potassium (hypokalemia) can lead to serious dysrhythmias or even death.

The approach used with the patient suffering from diabetic ketoacidosis is essentially the same as with any unconscious patient. You should first complete your initial assessment of airway, breathing, and circulation. You will then complete your focused history and physical exam. Pay particular attention to the presence of a Medic-Alert bracelet and/or insulin in the refrigerator. Also, obtain a history from bystanders. The fruity odor of ketones occasionally can be detected on the breath. If possible, complete the rapid test for blood glucose.

©2008 Pearson Education, Inc.

It is not uncommon for patients in ketoacidosis to have blood glucose levels well in excess of 300 mg/dL. The field management of such cases is focused on maintenance of ABCs and fluid resuscitation to counteract the patient's dehydration. Treatment should include drawing a red-top tube (or the tube specified by local protocols) of blood. Following this, you should administer one to two liters of normal saline per protocol. If transport time is lengthy, the medical direction physician may request intravenous or subcutaneous administration of regular insulin.

If the blood glucose level cannot be quickly determined, draw a red-top tube of blood for analysis and start an IV of normal saline. Following this, administer 50 mL (25 grams) of 50 percent dextrose solution. This additional glucose load will not adversely affect the ketoacidotic patient because it is negligible compared to the total quantity present in the body. If the patient is alcoholic, consider administering 100 mg of thiamine. Transportation to an appropriate facility should be expedited.

c. Hyperglycemia **pp. 616–618**

Diabetes mellitus results from either inadequate amounts of circulating insulin or inadequate utilization of insulin. This means that there is an excess of blood glucose while there is an intracellular deficit. In diabetes, glucose builds up in the bloodstream, especially after meals. The blood glucose level rises higher and returns to normal more slowly in the diabetic than in the nondiabetic. An oral glucose tolerance test uses this phenomenon in the diagnosis of diabetes. The diabetic's inadequate insulin level and impaired glucose tolerance are partly due to the decreased entry of glucose into the cells, thus leaving more glucose in the bloodstream.

The second cause of hyperglycemia in the diabetic results from difficulties with the function of the liver. When blood glucose levels are high, insulin secretion is normally increased and the breakdown of glycogen is decreased. In the diabetic, however, insulin secretion is decreased, and the alpha cells secrete glucagon to stimulate glycogenolysis by the liver, thus raising the blood glucose level.

In Type I diabetes the decreased insulin secretion is accompanied by a steady accumulation of glucose in the blood. Hyperglycemia acts like an osmotic diuretic and glucose "spills over" into the urine (glycosuria) pulling large amounts of water with it (polyuria). The body's attempt to dilute the concentration of glucose in the bloodstream results in intracellular dehydration and stimulates thirst (polydipsia). As the cells become glucose-depleted, they begin to use proteins and fats as an energy source resulting in weight loss and the formation of harmful byproducts, such as ketones and organic free fatty acids. The body's response to this state of cellular starvation is to trigger hunger in the patient (polyphagia). If the acids and ketones continue to collect in the blood, severe metabolic acidosis occurs and coma ensues, resulting in serious brain damage or death.

Type II diabetes does not usually result in diabetic ketoacidosis. It can, however, develop into a life-threatening emergency termed hyperglycemic hyperosmolar nonketotic (HHNK) coma. In Type II diabetes, when blood glucose levels exceed 600 mg/dL, the high osmolality of the blood causes an osmotic diuresis and marked dehydration of body cells. However, sufficient insulin is produced to prevent the manufacture of ketones and the complications of metabolic acidosis. In this respect, the condition differs from diabetic ketoacidosis.

Case Study Review

Reread the case study in Chapter 19 and then read the following discussion. This case study draws attention to the assessment and management of a commonly encountered patient presentation, altered mental status, which is subsequently determined to be due to the potentially life-threatening endocrine emergency, hyperglycemia, and diabetic ketoacidosis.

Rick and Pam respond to a typical medical emergency with only limited and general information about the call. They will count on the investigation of the chief complaint and patient history to guide them to the medical problem and, eventually, the field diagnosis. The history of a general illness developing over two weeks and the physical findings of cool and dry skin rules out fever and dry lips and mucous

©2008 Pearson Education, Inc.
Intermediate Emergency Care: 1985, 3rd ed.

membranes only suggest dehydration. The vital signs also do not help with a diagnosis. Only after the patient's daughter reveals the history of diabetes is the cause of the problem suggested. The history of frequent urination and thirst (polyuria and polydipsia) further supports the diagnosis. It is quickly confirmed when the glucometer reads 682. Had this history not been given or available, Rick and Pam would probably have tried the glucose test just to rule out a diabetic cause to the problem and assure the glucose level was within normal limits. The fluid infusion will help rehydrate the patient and her electrolytes will be stabilized in the emergency department.

Content Self-Evaluation

MULTIPLE CHOICE

_____ 1. Which of the following is an exocrine gland?
- A. pituitary
- B. thymus
- C. pancreas
- D. parathyroid
- E. adrenal

_____ 2. The term describing the sum of cellular processes that produce energy and molecules needed for growth and repair is
- A. anabolism.
- B. catabolism.
- C. metabolism.
- D. homeostasis.
- E. physiology.

_____ 3. Diabetes mellitus is caused by the inadequate production or activity of
- A. polypeptide.
- B. glucagon.
- C. somatostatin.
- D. cortisol.
- E. insulin.

_____ 4. Insulin's primary function is to
- A. metabolize glucose at the cellular level.
- B. free glucose from muscle storage sites.
- C. transport glucose across the cell membrane.
- D. store glucose at the cellular level.
- E. enhance the function of glucagon.

_____ 5. Osmotic diuresis, a characteristic of untreated diabetes, is the basis of
- A. polydipsia and polyphagia.
- B. weight loss.
- C. weakness.
- D. polyuria.
- E. polyphagia.

_____ 6. The most important sign or symptom associated with hypoglycemia is
- A. tachycardia.
- B. cool, clammy skin.
- C. altered mental status.
- D. polydipsia.
- E. polyphagia.

_____ 7. You should always consider administering 50 percent dextrose with an altered mental status in a known diabetic, even in the absence of a blood glucose level.
- A. True
- B. False

_____ 8. You should administer 50% dextrose if the blood glucose level falls below
- A. 200 mg/dh.
- B. 150 mg/dh.
- C. 60 mg/dh.
- D. 30 mg/dh.
- E. 10 mg/dh.

©2008 Pearson Education, Inc.

______ 9. All of the following are signs and symptoms of diabetic ketoacidosis EXCEPT
A. abdominal pain.
B. deep rapid respirations.
C. decreased mental function.
D. cold, clammy skin.
E. tachycardia.

______ 10. Diabetic ketoacidosis, characterized by high blood glucose and metabolic acidosis, occurs as a result of all of the following EXCEPT
A. profound insulin deficiency.
B. increased glucagon activity.
C. cessation of insulin injections.
D. physiologic stress.
E. overexertion.

______ 11. Kussmaul's respirations are a primary compensatory mechanism for reducing acidosis in the patient with diabetic ketoacidosis.
A. True
B. False

______ 12. Which of the following signs or symptoms is likely to be present in the patient experiencing diabetic ketoacidosis?
A. acetone breath odor
B. apathy
C. diplopia
D. drooling
E. diaphoresis

______ 13. Kussmaul's respirations are seen in which of the following conditions?
A. diabetic ketoacidosis
B. hyperglycemic hyperosmolar nonketotic coma
C. hypoglycemia
D. insulin shock
E. thyrotoxicosis

______ 14. In contrast to hypoglycemia, diabetic ketoacidosis develops quickly and may cause a rapidly developing bizarre behavior.
A. True
B. False

______ 15. Hyperglycemic hyperosmolar nonketotic acidosis differs from diabetic ketoacidosis because significant production of ketone bodies is prevented by the action of
A. polypeptide.
B. glucagon.
C. somatostatin.
D. cortisol.
E. insulin.

©2008 Pearson Education, Inc.
Intermediate Emergency Care: 1985, 3rd ed.

Chapter 20

Environmental Emergencies

Review of Chapter Objectives

After reading this chapter, you should be able to do the following:

1. **Define environmental emergency.** **p. 623**

   An environmental emergency is a medical condition caused by or exacerbated by environmental factors such as weather, terrain, or other local factors.

2. **Identify risk factors most predisposing to environmental emergencies.** **pp. 628–629, 632**

   General risk factors that place an individual at greater risk for an environmental emergency include age (very young and very old), poor general health, fatigue, predisposing medical conditions, and certain prescription or over-the-counter medications. Among drowning and near-drowning cases, alcohol use by an adult victim or the supervising adult is common.

3. **Identify environmental factors that may cause illness or exacerbate a preexisting illness or complicate treatment or transport decisions.** **pp. 623–628**

   Environments with certain characteristics are more likely to have emergencies: For instance, deserts may have tremendous variation in temperature between the hottest part of the day and overnight. Other such factors include current season, local weather patterns, atmospheric (high altitude) or hydrostatic (underwater) pressure, and the type of terrain. Rough or isolated terrain may significantly increase time for EMS response and for transport to the appropriate treating facility.

4. **Identify normal, critically high, and critically low body temperatures.** **pp. 626–627, 628**

   In the core of the body, temperature usually varies within 1° of 98.6°F (37°C). Heat exhaustion occurs at core temperatures above 100°F (37.8°C), and heatstroke can occur at 105°F (40.6°C) and higher. In contrast, mild hypothermia is associated with core temperatures of roughly 90–95°F (32–35°C). Severe hypothermia develops when core temperature drops below 90°F (32°C). The upper and lower core-body temperatures compatible with survival are roughly 114°F and 86°F, respectively.

5. **Describe several methods of temperature monitoring.** **pp. 626, 629, 630, 631, 632, 633**

   Core body temperature can be monitored with a tympanic or rectal thermometer. Peripheral body temperature, which is usually a little bit lower, can be measured with use of an oral thermometer or a thermometer placed under the armpit (an axillary temperature). Approximate peripheral temperature or change in peripheral temperature can often be discerned by touch.

©2008 Pearson Education, Inc.

6. Describe the body's compensatory processes for overheating and for excess heat loss. **pp. 626–628**

The human body does not generate "cold," it generates heat, and this process is called thermogenesis. There are three types of thermogenesis: The most basic and vital type is thermoregulatory thermogenesis, in which the nervous system and endocrine system work together to control the rate of cellular metabolism, which directly changes the rate of internal heat production. In work-induced thermogenesis, heat is produced through the work of skeletal muscles during exercise. In a cool or cold environment, muscles will produce some additional heat through shivering. The last type of heat generation is diet-induced thermogenesis, and it reflects the heat generated by cells as they process food and nutrients and eventually metabolize the breakdown products.

The body's thermal regulation is achieved through coordination of the nervous and endocrine systems. This is intuitively logical because these two systems are the control systems for all major body functions. Cells in the hypothalamus, a structure at the base of the brain, have the ability to act as a thermostat. As nerve cells, they sense the temperature of the core blood passing by them and they can receive messages from temperature sensors located in other parts of the body. Additional sensor cells for core temperature are located in the spinal cord, abdomen, and around the great veins in the chest. Peripheral sensors are in the skin and subcutaneous tissue.

On a cool day, peripheral temperature may drop. When the hypothalamic cells get the message, the cells act as endocrine cells, producing and secreting a hormone into the blood that acts to increase work-induced thermogenesis. Heat is produced through shivering. Also piloerection, or "goose bumps," the standing of small hairs, results in decreased air flow over the skin surface. If the environment is so cold that both peripheral and core temperature drop, the hypothalamic cells secrete hormones that increase heat production through all three means: thermoregulatory, work-induced, and diet-induced thermogenesis. (In the last, body cells burn fats and thus produce more heat.) In addition, core temperature, which is critical for survival, is maintained in part by reducing blood flow (and thus, heat) to the most peripheral tissues, the skin and subcutaneous tissues. In contrast, when the thermostat cells sense peripheral temperature is too high (as when you exercise vigorously), they stop releasing the hormone that stimulates thermogenesis. Not only is heat production slowed, but mechanisms to dissipate heat into the external environment are also activated. These include dilation of blood vessels in the skin and subcutaneous tissue (why people flush in the heat) and sweating.

This method of control, in which the production of a substance (in this case, heat) is turned off by the presence of that substance, is called negative feedback. Heat feeds back on the thermostat cells to turn off production of more heat. Think about the thermostat and furnace in a house. They work in a very similar fashion.

Thermogenesis consumes nutrient fuel for cells—fats, proteins, and carbohydrates—and it results in waste products such as carbon dioxide and water (from cellular respiration and fat breakdown) and urea (from protein breakdown). Extensive skeletal muscle use may also result in lactic acid accumulation. Heat dissipation through sweating consumes water, urea, and salts that are lost onto the skin surface.

7. List the common forms of heat and cold disorders. **pp. 628–638**

The common heat disorders are variants of hyperthermia, elevated core body temperature: In terms of increasing severity, these conditions are heat (muscle) cramps, heat exhaustion, and heatstroke. Cold disorders are frostbite, trench foot, and hypothermia.

8. Define heat illness and hyperthermia and list the common predisposing factors and preventive measures. **pp. 628–629, 632**

Heat illness is increased core body temperature (CBT) due to inadequate thermolysis (heat dissipation). Hyperthermia is a state of unusually high core body temperature.

Important predisposing factors for hyperthermia include age, general health, and medications. Both the very young and the very old have less responsive heat regulating systems and can tolerate less variation in their core body temperature. Persons who have diabetes with autonomic neuropathy are at higher risk for hyperthermia because damage to the autonomic nervous system may interfere with proper messaging to the CNS about temperature and may interfere with the

©2008 Pearson Education, Inc.
Intermediate Emergency Care: 1985, 3rd ed.

heat-dissipating processes of vasodilation and sweating. Several groups of medications can affect body temperature. Diuretics predispose to dehydration, which impairs ability to sweat. Beta blockers interfere with vasodilation, impair ability to increase heart rate in response to volume loss, and may interfere with temperature messages to the CNS. Psychotropics and antihistamines interfere with thermoregulation within the CNS. Additional factors include acclimatization to local conditions, length and intensity of heat exposure, and environmental factors such as humidity and wind. Preventive measures for heat disorders include three major elements. First, maintenance of adequate fluid intake is vital, and remember that thirst alone is an inadequate indicator for dehydration. Second, you should allow yourself time for acclimatization to the hot environment, which results in more perspiration with lower salt concentration, thus conserving body-fluid volume. Last, it is important to limit exposure to hot environments.

9. Identify the signs, symptoms, and treatment for heat cramps, heat exhaustion, and heatstroke. pp. 629–631

Heat cramps are caused by overexertion and dehydration in a hot environment. They occur when the temperature- and exercise-induced sweating (which consumes water and electrolytes including sodium) depletes the body of so much water and electrolytes that the actively exercising skeletal muscle fibers cramp. Signs and symptoms include cramping in fingers, arms, legs, or abdominal muscles. Patients are generally mentally alert with a feeling of weakness, but they may be dizzy or faint. Vital signs are stable, although temperature may be normal or slightly elevated. Skin is likely to be moist and warm. Note that heat cramps may be painful but they are NOT considered to be an actual heat illness. The general predisposing factors and preventive measures for all heat-related disorders are discussed with objective 8. Treatment for heat cramps is usually easily accomplished. First, remove the patient from the hot environment to a cooler one such as a shady area or an air-conditioned ambulance. For severe cramps, you can administer an oral saline solution (approximately 4 tsp salt/gallon water) or a sports electrolyte drink. Do NOT use salt tablets, which are not absorbed readily and can irritate the stomach causing ulceration or hypernatremia. If the patient cannot take liquids readily, an IV of normal saline may be needed. Palliative care may include muscle massage or moist towels over patient's head and the cramping muscles.

Heat exhaustion, which is considered a mild heat illness, is an acute reaction to heat exposure, and it is the most common heat-related illness seen by EMS providers. The loss of water and electrolytes (notably sodium) from working in a hot environment, combined with general vasodilation as a heat-dissipating mechanism, leads to a decreased circulating blood volume, venous pooling, and reduced cardiac output. The presenting symptoms are due to dehydration and sodium loss secondary to sweating. Because the symptoms are not unique to heat exhaustion, diagnosis requires presentation in the appropriate environmental setting. Remember that untreated heat exhaustion can progress to heatstroke. The signs and symptoms of heat exhaustion include increased body temperature (over 100°F, 37.8°C), cool clammy skin with heavy perspiration, rapid, shallow breathing, and a weak pulse. Signs of active thermolysis may include diarrhea and muscle cramps. The patient will feel weak and, in some cases, may lose consciousness. There also may be CNS symptoms such as headache, anxiety, paresthesia, and impaired judgment or even psychosis. The general predisposing factors and preventive measures for all heat-related disorders are discussed with objective 8. Treatment includes removal of the patient from the hot environment and placement in a supine position. For severe cramps, you can administer an oral saline solution (approximately 4 tsp salt/gallon water) or a sports electrolyte drink. Do NOT use salt tablets, as discussed above. If the patient cannot take liquids readily, an IV of normal saline may be needed. Remove some clothing and fan the patient to increase heat dissipation. Be careful not to cool the patient to the point of chilling him or her. Stop fanning if shivering develops, and consider covering the patient lightly. If shock is suspected, treat accordingly. If symptoms do not resolve, consider the possibility of increased core body temperature and evolution of heatstroke.

Heatstroke is a true environmental emergency, one in which the body's hypothalamic temperature regulation is lost and there is uncompensated hyperthermia resulting in cell death and damage to the brain, liver, and kidneys. Generally, heatstroke is characterized by body temperature above 105°F (40.6°C), CNS disturbances, and (usually) cessation of perspiration.

©2008 Pearson Education, Inc.

It is thought that sweating stops either because of destruction of sweat glands or because of sensory overload resulting in their temporary dysfunction. Patients may present with signs and symptoms including cessation of sweating, hot skin that is either moist or dry (depending on whether sweat has dried), very high core temperatures, deep respirations that become shallow and rapid respirations that may later slow, a rapid, full pulse that may slow later, hypotension with low or absent diastolic reading, confusion or disorientation or unconsciousness, and possible seizures. Field management centers on immediate cooling of the patient's body and replacement of fluids. First, remove the patient from the environment; if this is not done, other measures will be only minimally useful. Initiate rapid active body cooling to a target temperature of 102°F (39°C). This can be accomplished en route to the hospital. Remove the patient's clothing and cover with sheets soaked in tepid water. If necessary, either fanning or misting may be used. Be sure you avoid overcooling because this can trigger reflex hypothermia. Tepid water avoids the risk of producing reflex peripheral vasoconstriction and shivering that can be produced by exposure to cold water. In addition, use high-flow oxygen and assist respirations if they are shallow. Use pulse oximetry if available. Administer fluid therapy orally (if possible) or IV. In many cases, orally will suffice. Remember in this setting that electrolyte replacement is not nearly as necessary as water/volume replacement. If IVs are needed, start one or two and make the initial infusion with the line(s) wide open. Be sure to monitor the ECG because dysrhythmias can develop at any time. Avoid vasopressors and anticholinergic drugs because they may inhibit sweating and can contribute to development of a hyperthermic state in high-humidity, high-temperature environments. Lastly, monitor body temperature for trends toward target temperature or for other shift. If you work in a hot climate, try to make sure your thermometers measure above 106°F and below 95°F.

10. Discuss the role of dehydration and the role of fluid therapy in heat disorders. pp. 629–631

Dehydration often accompanies heat disorders because it inhibits vasodilation and heat dissipation (thermolysis). Dehydration leads to orthostatic hypotension and the following symptoms: nausea, vomiting, abdominal distress, vision disturbances, decreased urine output, poor skin turgor, and signs of hypovolemic shock. These may present along with the signs and symptoms of heatstroke. When assessment suggests dehydration, rehydration is critical. IV fluids may be needed, especially when the patient has altered mental status or is nauseated. An adult with moderate to severe dehydration may require 2–3 liters of IV fluids or more.

Because dehydration plays an increasingly significant role in heat cramps, heat exhaustion, and heatstroke, rehydration becomes increasingly pivotal to treatment success. Remember in milder forms of heat disorders, such as heat cramps, that the patient's perception of thirst is a poor indication of the degree of dehydration present. Fluid, whether it is administered orally or IV, is important in restoring the body's thermolytic abilities. In heat exhaustion and heatstroke, replacement of fluid (often by IV due to patient nausea, inability to swallow, or inability to take in fluids orally fast enough to be successful) is critical. Remember that an adult with moderate to severe dehydration can require 2–3 liters or more of replacement fluid.

11. Define hypothermia and list its common predisposing and preventive measures. p. 632

Hypothermia is a state of low body temperature, particularly low core body temperature. Important predisposing factors for hypothermia are the same: age, general health, and medications. Both the very young and the very old have less responsive heat generating systems to combat cold exposure and cannot tolerate cold environments. The elderly may become hypothermic in environments that are only somewhat cool to others. Persons with inadequately treated hypothyroidism have suppressed metabolisms, which prevents proper responsiveness to cold. In addition, malnutrition, hypoglycemia, Parkinson's disease, fatigue, and other medical conditions can interfere with the body's ability to combat cold exposure. Drugs that interfere with heat-generating mechanisms include narcotics, alcohol, phenothiazines, barbiturates, antiseizure medications, antihistamines and other allergy medications, antipsychotics, sedatives, antidepressants, and various analgesics such as aspirin, acetaminophen, and NSAIDs. Additional factors include prolonged or intense exposure, which directly affects both morbidity and mortality, and coexisting weather conditions (such as high humidity, brisk winds, or accompanying rain, all of which magnify the effect of cold). Preventive

©2008 Pearson Education, Inc.
Intermediate Emergency Care: 1985, 3rd ed.

measures can decrease the morbidity of cold-related injury, and these include dressing warmly, being rested, which maximizes the ability of the heat-generating mechanisms to replenish energy reserves, appropriate eating at proper intervals to support metabolism, and limitation of exposure to cold environments.

12. Identify differences between mild, moderate, and severe hypothermia. pp. 632–633

Mild hypothermia is defined by a core temperature greater than 93.2°F (34°C) in the presence of signs/symptoms of hypothermia, Moderate hypothermia is defined as a core temperature of 86 to 93.2°F with the signs/symptoms of hypothermia, whereas severe hypothermia is defined as core temperature less than 86°F in the presence of signs/symptoms of hypothermia. The mortality rate of someone with a core temperature of below 86°F is increased.

13. Identify signs, symptoms, and treatment for hypothermia. pp. 633–637

Signs and symptoms of hypothermia are given in Table 20-3 (text page 633). Your assessment of an individual with mild hypothermia will likely reveal lethargy, shivering, lack of coordination, pale, cold, dry skin, and an early rise in blood pressure, heart rate, and respiratory rates. In severe hypothermia, you may find no shivering, loss of voluntary muscle control, hypotension, and an unpredictable pulse and respiration. On the ECG, you may find dysrhythmias. The most common presenting dysrhythmia is atrial fibrillation. With progressive cooling of the body core, a variety of dysrhythmias may appear, with eventual bradycardia or asystole. Note: The severely hypothermic patient requires assessment of pulse and respirations for at least 30 seconds every 1–2 minutes. Management includes: (1) administration of oxygen, (2) CPR and defibrillation as needed, (3) removal of wet garments, (4) protection against further heat loss and wind chill (calling for passive external warming with blankets, moisture barriers, etc.), (5) monitor cardiac rhythm, (6) initiate IV access, administer warm fluids, (7) space cardiac arrest fluids out over longer intervals, (8) maintenance of patient in horizontal position. Persons with mild hypothermia may be rewarmed with active external techniques such as warmed blankets or heat packs. In contrast, active rewarming of the severely hypothermic patient is best carried out in the hospital because of the possibility of complications such as ventricular fibrillation. If transport to the hospital will require more than 15 minutes, you may need to begin active rewarming in the field. Beware of rewarming shock and cold diuresis. As a final aid in putting the pieces of hypothermia care together, review the algorithm on text page 635.

14. Discuss the impact of severe hypothermia on standard BCLS and ACLS algorithms and transport considerations. pp. 637–638

Severe hypothermia (core temperature less than 86°F or 30°C) mandates a switch from passive rewarming and some degree of active external rewarming to active internal rewarming, which may include use of warm IV fluids, warm, humid oxygen, peritoneal lavage, extracorporeal rewarming, and esophageal rewarming tubes. If pulse or breathing is absent, severe hypothermia mandates continuance of CPR but withholding of IV fluids and limitation of electrical conversion to three times maximum. There are also specific considerations for resuscitation when core temperature is 86°F or less (discussed on text pages 632–635). Drug metabolism in the severely hypothermic patient is significantly decreased, and levels may accumulate that will become toxic when the patient is rewarmed. In addition, it may not be possible to electrically defibrillate a heart that is at a temperature less than 86°F.

15. Define superficial and deep frostbite and discuss their treatment. pp. 637–638

Frostbite is an environmentally induced freezing of body tissues. As tissues freeze due to the excessive cold, ice crystals form within cells and water is drawn from cells into the extracellular space. As the ice crystals expand, cells are destroyed. Damage to blood vessels from ice-crystal formation causes loss of vascular integrity, which results in further tissue swelling and loss of distal blood flow. Peripheral tissues are more exposed to cold and thus more likely to be involved in frostbite. Thus, frostbite is largely seen in the extremities and in areas of the head and face.

©2008 Pearson Education, Inc.

Two types of frostbite are defined based on the extent of tissue freezing: superficial and deep frostbite. Superficial frostbite (also called frostnip) involves some freezing of epidermal tissue, resulting in initial redness followed by blanching and diminished sensation. Deep frostbite involves both the epidermal and subcutaneous layers; there is a white, hardened appearance. Sensation is lost. Subfreezing temperatures are necessary for frostbite (otherwise, cellular water wouldn't freeze) but are not necessary for hypothermia. You will find that many patients with frostbite also do have hypothermia. You will also find that there is tremendous variation in presentation of frostbite. Some patients will feel little pain at the outset, whereas other will complain of bitter pain. Physical exam is a better indicator of the extent of frostbite. In superficial frostbite, there will be some degree of compliance felt beneath the frozen layer upon palpation; in deep frostbite, the frozen part will be hard and noncompliant. Treatment involves the following steps. First, do not thaw the affected area if there is any possibility of refreezing and do not massage the frozen area or rub with snow. Both may result in more extensive damage. Do administer analgesia prior to thawing, and do transport to the hospital for rewarming by immersion. If transport will be delayed, thaw the frozen part in a 102–104°F water bath. Water will need to be changed frequently as it cools. Do cover the thawed part with loosely applied, dry, sterile dressings and elevate and immobilize the thawed part. Do not puncture or drain blisters, and do not rewarm frozen feet if they are required for walking out of a hazardous situation.

16. Define drowning, list its signs and symptoms, and discuss its treatment. **pp. 638–639**

Following submersion, a conscious person will have complete apnea for up to 3 minutes as an involuntary reflex as he struggles to keep his head above water, and during this period blood is shunted to the heart and brain. During apnea, $PaCO_2$ will rise to greater than 50 mmHg while PaO_2 falls to less than 50 mmHg. The hypoxic stimulus eventually overrides the sedative effects of the hypercarbia, resulting in CNS stimulation. While conscious, the panicky victim typically swallows a lot of water into the stomach, stimulating severe laryngospasm and bronchospasm. This effect prevents significant influx of water into the lungs (and is thus termed a dry drowning or near-drowning). Another effect of laryngospasm is worsening hypoxia, which causes a deepening coma. Morbidity or delayed mortality in drowning is primarily due to asphyxia from airway obstruction secondary to water in the airways (if a wet event) or laryngospasm and bronchospasm (if a dry near-drowning). Water in the lungs of a near-drowning survivor may cause lower-airway disease. A number of factors affect survival, and these include the cleanliness of the water, the duration of submersion, and the age and general health of the victim. Children have a longer survival time and a greater probability of successful resuscitation. Most significant is water temperature.

Field treatment for drowning in either saltwater or fresh water is similar: The first goal is to correct the profound hypoxia. Treatment includes the following steps: Remove the patient from the water. If possible, initiate ventilation while the victim is still in the water. Note that both steps require a trained, equipped rescue swimmer. Suspect head and neck injury if there was a fall or a dive involved; rapidly place victim on long backboard and use C-spine precautions. Then, protect from heat loss by removing wet clothing, laying the patient on a warm surface, and covering the body to the extent possible. The remaining steps are familiar to all resuscitations: Examine for airway patency, breathing, and pulse. If needed, begin CPR and defibrillation. Manage the airway as needed with suctioning and airway adjuncts. Administer 100% oxygen. Use respiratory rewarming, if available and if transport time will exceed 15 minutes. Establish an IV of lactated Ringer's or normal saline for venous access and run at 75 mL/hr. Follow ACLS protocols if the patient is normothermic. If hypothermic, the patient should be treated for hypothermia as discussed in the text. Note: Resuscitation is NOT indicated if immersion is known to have been extremely prolonged (unless hypothermia IS present) or if there is evidence of decomposition. All near-drowning victims should be admitted for observation for possible late complications including adult respiratory distress syndrome (ARDS).

17. Discuss the complications and protective role of hypothermia in the context of drowning. **pp. 638–639**

In general, the colder the water, the greater the patient's chance for survival. Usually, you expect brain death after 4–6 minutes without oxygen. However, some patients in cold water (below 68°F) may be resuscitated after 30 minutes or more in cardiac arrest. A possible physiologic factor in this phenomenon is the mammalian diving reflex. When a person dives into cold water, the

©2008 Pearson Education, Inc.
Intermediate Emergency Care: 1985, 3rd ed.

submersion of the face inhibits breathing, drops heart rate, and causes vasoconstriction in tissues relatively resistant to asphyxia even as blood flow to the heart and brain continues. The colder the water, the greater the shunting of blood to brain and heart. This is the origin of the saying "the cold water drowning victim is not dead until he is warm and dead."

18. Given several preprogrammed simulated environmental emergency patients, provide the appropriate assessment, management, and transportation. pp. 628–639

Attention to the ABCs is always important, and this doesn't change with environmental emergencies. The need to move the patient from the harmful environment to one conducive to recovery is special, although not unique (as with inhalation toxicological emergencies). Among the heat disorders, heatstroke is the most serious, and rapid transport is always required.

Hypothermia always requires transport to a hospital setting. The urgency in rewarming varies with the degree of hypothermia, as do some potential complications on rewarming such as cardiac dysrhythmias. Superficial and deep frostbite differ in the depth of tissue affected by freezing; care while en route to the hospital is similar. Early recognition is important to the EMS provider, but prevention is the most important of all steps.

Drownings require immediate care and rapid transport to the hospital. Although more than 90% of near-drowning patients survive without sequelae, ARDS can occur as a potentially deadly late complication. Emergencies related to air pressure (diving and altitude) can vary in severity and setting, but immediate care and removal to an appropriate environment as soon as possible are key to treatment. Again, these emergencies are better prevented than treated. Knowing what resources are available in the area is important to treating any of these types of emergencies.

Case Study Review

Reread the case study in Chapter 20 and then read the following discussion. This case study demonstrates how EMT-Is react to a wintertime emergency: a person through the ice. The case study demonstrates how resuscitation should proceed in a hypothermic environment and how that differs from normal arrest resuscitations.

Scene safety is the first concern for the arriving crew, both their own and that of bystanders. They will assure everyone stays off the ice while they assess the situation and plan their actions. Without proper training and equipment, Jenny and Catherine would risk becoming victims themselves if they tried a rescue. This is very hard for all of us because of the desire to help and the requests of the crowd.

Evaluating the scene, they have information the teenager just went under the water. They will try to verify this to determine just how long the submergence has lasted. They will also prepare to care for an arrest in a hypothermic environment. This crew frequently responds in an area of seasonal cold weather so they are prepared with training and IV fluid warmers. They also prepare for the arrival of the victim by warming the ambulance and preparing blankets.

Another 20 minutes pass before the teenager is recovered, and as expected, he is in cardiopulmonary arrest and CPR is initiated. They quickly dry the patient to reduce evaporative heat loss and prepare for defibrillation. They then do a dysrhythmia "quick look" and defibrillate. The team recognizes that low body temperature affects the action and blood concentration of drugs so they quickly determine the teenager's core temperature. Since it is above 86°, normal ACLS drugs can be used but the spacing between doses should be lengthened because they generally are less effective and take longer to leave the cardiovascular system. If the temperature was below 86, the team would withhold the administration of drugs. The team is also very careful in moving the teenager as sudden movement may cause ventricular fibrillation (which they already have) in the moderate to severely hypothermic patient. Note that the team intubates the patient carefully to minimize unnecessary patient movement. They are also careful to administer pre-warmed fluids to assure they contribute to the re-warming efforts.

The team provided the unfortunate teenager with the best chance for survival. The Emergency Department continued resuscitation until the patient's core temperature returned to close to normal, giving their resuscitation efforts (drugs and defibrillation) the best chance to work, before they terminated their efforts.

©2008 Pearson Education, Inc.

Content Self-Evaluation

Multiple Choice

______ 1. Homeostasis is the body's ability to maintain a steady, normal internal environment in the face of changing external conditions.
A. True
B. False

______ 2. Which process is NOT one that results in body heat loss into the environment?
A. evaporation
B. convection
C. respiration
D. radiation
E. diffusion

______ 3. Which group of medications does NOT predispose a person to hyperthermia?
A. psychotropics
B. antiepileptics
C. diuretics
D. beta blockers
E. antihistamines

______ 4. Dehydration is often intimately associated with heat disorders because it inhibits peripheral vasodilation and limits sweating.
A. True
B. False

______ 5. In situations where suspected heat exhaustion does not respond to fluids and patient position, treat for heat stroke.
A. True
B. False

______ 6. Medical conditions that may predispose to hypothermia include all of the following EXCEPT
A. hypothyroidism.
B. malnutrition.
C. Parkinson's disease.
D. thin body build.
E. hypoglycemia.

______ 7. Rewarming of the severely hypothermic patient is best affected by aggressive warming of the limbs and head.
A. True
B. False

______ 8. Which is appropriate as a rewarming measure for mild to moderate hypothermia?
A. warmed blankets
B. warmed IV fluids
C. warm water packs
D. warmed humidified oxygen
E. all of the above

______ 9. Management guidelines for frostbite include all of the following negatives EXCEPT:
A. Do not thaw affected area if possibility of refreezing exists.
B. Do not massage the frozen area or rub with snow.
C. Do not puncture or drain any blisters.
D. Do not warm frozen feet if patient will need to walk out of hostile environment.
E. Do not give analgesia prior to thawing.

______ 10. The physiology of dry versus wet drowning differs. In wet drowning you are likely to have which of the following?
A. surfactant washout
B. diminished gas exchange
C. ventilation-perfusion mismatch
D. atelectasis
E. all of the above

©2008 Pearson Education, Inc.
Intermediate Emergency Care: 1985, 3rd ed.

Chapter

21 Behavioral Emergencies

Review of Chapter Objectives

After reading this chapter, you should be able to do the following:

1. Distinguish between normal and abnormal behavior. **p. 644**

Behavior is a person's observable conduct and activity, while a behavioral emergency is a situation in which a patient's behavior becomes so unusual, bizarre, or threatening that it alarms the patient or another person and requires the intervention of EMS and/or mental health personnel. The differentiation between "normal" and "abnormal" behavior is largely subjective and widely variable based on culture, ethnic group, socioeconomic class, environment, and personal interpretation and opinion.

2. Discuss the pathophysiology of behavioral and psychiatric disorders. **pp. 644–645**

The general causes of behavioral and psychiatric disorders are biological (organic), psychosocial, and sociocultural. Biological (organic) causes are related to disease processes or structural changes in the brain. Psychosocial causes are related to the patient's personality, dynamics of unresolved conflict, or crisis management methods. Sociocultural causes are related to the patient's actions and interactions within society. It should be noted that many psychiatric disorders are due to altered brain chemistry.

3. Describe the medical-legal considerations for management of emotionally disturbed patients. **p. 656**

The laws of consent specify that any competent person has the right to refuse to consent to treatment. Further, no competent person may be transported against his/her will. Any person who is in imminent danger of harming him-/herself or others is not considered competent to refuse treatment and transport. Most states have laws that allow persons fitting this criterion to be transported against their will to a hospital or approved psychiatric facility for evaluation.

4. Describe the overt behaviors associated with behavioral and psychiatric disorders. **p. 644**

Overt behaviors that may be associated with behavioral emergencies include hand gestures (clenched fists, wringing hands, etc.) or postures (cowering, visible tension, etc.) that you may observe in your patient. The patient may display strange or threatening facial expressions. The patient's speech may reveal disorientation, fixations, unrealistic judgments, or unusual thought processes. Other behaviors you may observe include pacing, picking at one's skin, or appearing to pull things from the air. There are many different kinds of such overt behaviors, and they can differ or overlap depending on the specific disorder.

©2008 Pearson Education, Inc.

5. List the appropriate measures to ensure the safety of the EMT-Intermediate, the patient, and others. **pp. 645–646, 654–658**

As with any call, determining scene safety is critical. Many behavioral emergencies, for which you are dispatched, will also warrant mutual response by law enforcement personnel. Gain control of the scene. Remove anyone who agitates the patient or adds confusion to the scene. Examine the environment for signs of violence and potential weapons. Approach every situation cautiously and when feasible observe the patient from a distance first before approaching. Avoid invading the patient's personal space. Watch for signs of aggression. If a patient becomes violent, use of restraint may become necessary; in such cases, carefully follow your service's protocols for such circumstances and be sure to document your actions thoroughly.

6. Describe techniques to systematically gather information from the disturbed patient. **pp. 646–647, 654–655**

Your interpersonal skills are crucial to your success as an EMS professional but never more so than when you are caring for a patient who is having a behavioral emergency. Limit environmental distractions at the scene. Introduce yourself and note how the patient responds to you, altering your approach if the patient becomes agitated. Establish eye contact. Place yourself at the patient's level. Listen carefully. Take your time. Do not physically threaten the patient. Ask open-ended questions. Be truthful with the patient and never play along with hallucinations or delusions. Focus your questioning and assessment on the immediate problem.

7. Identify techniques for physical assessment in a patient with behavioral problems. **pp. 646, 654**

All of the interpersonal skills discussed above that allow you to effectively interview patients will need to be incorporated into your physical assessment activities. Generally, the examination of a behavioral emergency patient is largely conversational. If you need to perform hands-on assessment activities, defer their completion until you have had the opportunity to establish rapport and, even then, do not make any sudden moves that may startle the patient. If a patient is restrained, be sure to monitor him or her frequently and carefully to ensure that the airway is patent and that he or she is not experiencing positional asphyxia.

8. List situations in which you are expected to transport a patient forcibly and against his will. **pp. 655–656**

Any person who is in imminent danger of harming him-/herself or others is not considered competent to refuse treatment and transport. Patients who are suicidal or homicidal meet this criterion. Most states have laws that allow persons fitting this criterion to be transported against their will for evaluation. The authority to make this decision varies from state to state. Other situations are not so clear-cut and require you to use clinical judgment and follow your service's protocols.

9. Describe restraint methods necessary in managing the emotionally disturbed patient. **pp. 656–658**

The primary objective is to restrict the patient's movement to prevent him from harming himself or others. Your own agency's rules will dictate the appropriate technique and method for restraint. The following rules always apply: use minimum necessary force; use appropriate devices; remember that restraint is not punitive; and carefully monitor anyone who is restrained. Before initiating any restraint activities, make sure that you have sufficient help, as this minimizes the potential for injury to the patient or yourself.

10. List the risk factors and behaviors that indicate a patient is at risk for suicide. **pp. 653–654**

All of the following are considered to be risk factors for suicide: previously attempted suicide, depression, age (15 to 24 years of age or over 40), substance abuse, social isolation, major separation trauma, major physical stresses, loss of independence, suicide of a parent. Also significant is having possession of a mechanism for suicide and having a specific plan and/or expressing it.

©2008 Pearson Education, Inc.
Intermediate Emergency Care: 1985, 3rd ed.

11. Given several preprogrammed behavioral emergency patients, provide the appropriate scene size-up, initial assessment, focused assessment, and detailed assessment, then provide the appropriate care and patient transport. **pp. 645–658**

Throughout your training, you will encounter a variety of real and simulated patients with behavioral or psychiatric emergencies. Use the information in the text, as well as the application of this information as demonstrated by your instructors, preceptors, and mentors to enhance your ability to assess, manage, and transport patients with behavioral emergencies. Every emergency call has an element of behavioral emergency in it; your patience and professionalism will help minimize the emotional component for everyone involved.

Case Study Review

Reread the case study in Chapter 21 and then read the following discussion. This case study draws attention to the assessment and management of a commonly encountered patient presentation, in which an individual is exhibiting bizarre behavior in a public setting.

The EMT-Is arrive on-scene and obtain information about the situation from the store manager who has placed the 911 call. When the patient notices their arrival and becomes more agitated, they retreat to the ambulance and request assistance from law enforcement personnel.

As is often the case, the police officers recognize the patient from previous interactions with him. Before approaching the patient, the EMT-Is and police officers coordinate their plans and anticipate the potential need for restraint. Using a team approach to subdue and restrain the patient minimizes the risk of injury for all involved. Once the patient is safely restrained, a thorough assessment is performed to rule out possible medical or traumatic causes for the patient's altered mental status and agitation. This includes a glucose test to rule out hypoglycemia. Hypoglycemia can account for a patient's bizarre behavior and can rapidly become a life-threatening condition. En route to the hospital the patient is carefully monitored to ensure his well-being.

Content Self-Evaluation

Multiple Choice

_____ 1. Organic causes for behavioral emergencies include all of the following EXCEPT
A. tumor.
B. depression.
C. substance abuse.
D. infection.
E. hypoglycemia.

_____ 2. It is always safe to assume that a patient exhibiting bizarre behavior is suffering from a psychological problem or disease.
A. True
B. False

_____ 3. The term that describes the state of a patient's cerebral functioning is
A. affect.
B. mood.
C. mental status.
D. orientation.
E. sensorium.

_____ 4. The best approach for gaining information from a behavioral emergency patient is to
A. ask questions requiring yes or no answers.
B. talk loudly to establish control.
C. ask open-ended questions.
D. physically restrain the patient before questioning.
E. move quickly to expedite transport and then question.

©2008 Pearson Education, Inc.

______ 5. The most likely way to provoke violence or aggression in a behavioral emergency patient is to
A. listen carefully to his responses.
B. appear patient and unhurried.
C. ask open-ended questions.
D. invade his personal space.
E. avoid rapid or sudden movements.

______ 6. The structured exam designed to quickly evaluate a patient's level of mental functioning is the
A. neurologic exam.
B. mental status exam.
C. psychiatric evaluation.
D. Glasgow coma score.
E. stroke assessment scale.

______ 7. Common causes of dementia include all of the following EXCEPT
A. medical condition.
B. head trauma.
C. cardiac seizure.
D. intoxication.
E. substance withdrawal.

______ 8. Panic attack, phobias, and posttraumatic stress syndrome are classified as
A. types of schizophrenia.
B. personality disorders.
C. variants of depression.
D. bipolar disorders.
E. anxiety disorders.

______ 9. Hallucinations, delusions, and disorganized thought, speech, and behavior are commonly associated with
A. schizophrenia.
B. personality disorders.
C. depression.
D. bipolar disorders.
E. anxiety disorders.

______ 10. The most prevalent form of psychiatric problem is
A. schizophrenia.
B. personality disorder.
C. depression.
D. bipolar disorder.
E. anxiety disorder.

______ 11. Profound sadness, diminished ability to concentrate, and feelings of worthlessness are commonly associated with
A. schizophrenia.
B. personality disorders.
C. depression.
D. bipolar disorders.
E. anxiety disorders.

______ 12. Bipolar disorder is characterized by which of the following?
A. a manic episode
B. acute phobias
C. extreme guilt
D. prolonged depression
E. short-term depression

______ 13. The compelling desire to use a substance, inability to reduce use of a substance, and repeated unsuccessful efforts to quit using that substance are indicators of
A. psychological dependence.
B. physical dependence.
C. substance tolerance.
D. factitious disorder.
E. somatoform disorder.

______ 14. The primary objective in patient restraint is to
A. initiate punitive response.
B. stop dangerous behaviors.
C. limit patient strength.
D. reduce legal liability.
E. encourage patient cooperation.

______ 15. When a geriatric patient is experiencing a behavioral emergency, the EMT-I should always consider using physical restraints first.
A. True
B. False

©2008 Pearson Education, Inc.
Intermediate Emergency Care: 1985, 3rd ed.

Matching

Write the letter of the word or phrase in the space provided next to its definition.

A. delirium
B. dementia
C. schizophrenia
D. bipolar disorder
E. delusions
F. hallucinations

______ 16. Condition characterized by relatively rapid onset of widespread disorganized thought

______ 17. Fixed false beliefs

______ 18. Sensory perceptions with no basis in reality

______ 19. Condition characterized by one or more manic episodes, with or without subsequent or alternating periods of depression

______ 20. Common disorder involving significant behavioral changes and disorganized thought

______ 21. Condition involving gradual development of memory impairment and cognitive disturbance

©2008 Pearson Education, Inc.

Chapter 22 Gynecological Emergencies

Review of Chapter Objectives

After reading this chapter, you should be able to do the following:

1. Describe how to assess a patient with a gynecological complaint. **pp. 663–665**

The most common gynecological complaints are abdominal pain and vaginal bleeding. Complete your initial assessment in the usual manner and then proceed with a focused history and physical exam. Specific questions will need to be asked that are pertinent to reproductive function and dysfunction. If pertinent, be sure to gather information about her obstetrical history, including pregnancies and deliveries. It is important to document the date of the patient's last menstrual period (LMP). You should also ask what form of birth control, if any, she uses and, if pertinent, whether she uses it regularly. Pay particular attention to the physical exam, which will be limited to assessment of the abdomen and potentially (in the presence of serious bleeding) inspection of the patient's perineum. Gently auscultate and palpate the abdomen. Be sure to note the color, character, and volume of any blood lost. An internal vaginal exam should never be performed in the prehospital setting.

2. Explain how to recognize a gynecological emergency. **pp. 663–665**

As with any emergency situation, vital signs are useful clues as to your patient's status as well as its severity. Be alert for early signs of shock or a positive tilt test, both of which point to significant blood loss. If possible, estimate blood loss. The use of two sanitary pads per hour is considered significant bleeding.

3. Describe the general care for any patient experiencing a gynecological emergency. **pp. 667, 670**

Management of gynecological emergencies is focused on supportive care. Rely on your initial assessment guidance in your decision making about oxygen therapy, ventilatory support, and vascular access. In the presence of shock, follow your local protocols for fluid resuscitation and use of the PASG. In cases of heavy bleeding, do not pack dressings in the vagina. Continue to monitor the patient's status and bleeding en route to definitive care. Equally important is the psychological support that you give your patient. Protect her modesty and privacy.

4. Describe the pathophysiology, assessment, and management of the following gynecological emergencies.

a. Pelvic inflammatory disease **p. 666**

Pelvic inflammatory disease (PID), the most common cause of nontraumatic abdominal pain in women in the childbearing years, is an infection of the female reproductive tract that is most commonly caused by gonorrhea or chlamydia. Predisposing factors include multiple sexual partners, prior history of PID, recent gynecological procedure, or an IUD. The patient will look acutely ill and will often present with diffuse lower abdominal pain, and may also have fever,

©2008 Pearson Education, Inc.

chills, nausea, vomiting, and possibly a foul-smelling vaginal discharge. The patient may also walk with a shuffling gait due to pain. Blood pressure may be normal, and fever may or may not be present. Palpation of the lower abdomen usually elicits moderate to severe pain. The primary management in the field is supportive care and a position of comfort during transport. If the patient appears septic, then administer oxygen and initiate IV therapy.

b. Ruptured ovarian cyst **p. 666**

Cysts are fluid-filled pockets, and, when they develop in the ovary, they can rupture and be a source of abdominal pain. The rupture spills a small amount of blood into the abdomen, irritating the peritoneum and causing abdominal pain and rebound tenderness. Usually the patient complains of moderate to severe unilateral abdominal pain that may radiate to the back; it may be associated with vaginal bleeding. The patient may also report pain during intercourse or a delayed menstrual period. The primary management in the field is supportive care and a position of comfort during transport.

c. Cystitis **pp. 666–667**

A bacterial infection of the urinary bladder (cystitis) is a common cause of abdominal pain that may be accompanied by urinary frequency, dysuria, and a low-grade fever. The pain is generally located just above the symphysis pubis unless the infection has spread to the kidneys, in which case there is likely to be flank pain as well. The primary management in the field is supportive care and a position of comfort during transport.

d. Endometritis **p. 667**

Endometritis is an inflammation of the uterine lining that infrequently follows childbirth, miscarriage, or gynecologic procedures. The patient often complains of abdominal pain, foul-smelling discharge, and fever, 48 to 72 hours after the procedure. It may mimic PID and can be a serious life threat. Care usually involves antibiotics.

e. Endometriosis **p. 667**

Endometriosis is the growth of endometrial tissue found outside its normal location. It normally occurs in females between 30 and 40 and presents with dull pelvic cramping related to menstruation and abnormal uterine hemorrhage. Care involves antibiotics, analgesics, and possible surgery.

f. Ectopic pregnancy **p. 667**

Ectopic pregnancy is the implantation of a fetus outside of the uterus, most commonly in the fallopian tubes. Patients usually report severe unilateral abdominal pain that may radiate to the shoulder on the affected side, a late or missed menstrual period, and sometimes vaginal bleeding. As the fetus develops, the tube can rupture, triggering a massive, life-threatening hemorrhage. Absorb the bleeding but do not pack the vagina. Ectopic pregnancy is a surgical emergency, and the primary management in the field is supportive care and a position of comfort during transport, as well as oxygen administration and IV therapy for fluid resuscitation.

g. Vaginal hemorrhage **pp. 667–668**

Nontraumatic vaginal hemorrhage is rarely encountered in the prehospital setting unless it is severe. Do not presume that such bleeding is due to normal menstrual flow. Most commonly, it is due to a spontaneous abortion (miscarriage) and is associated with cramping abdominal pain and the passage of clots and tissue. Other possible causes include cancerous lesions, PID, or the onset of labor. Absorb bleeding but do not pack the vagina. The primary management in the field is supportive care and a position of comfort for the patient, as well as oxygen administration and IV therapy for fluid resuscitation. If the bleeding is due to miscarriage, this will likely be a significant emotional event for your patient, so your kind and considerate care is important.

h. Gynecological trauma **pp. 663–670**

Traumatic vaginal bleeding may result from sexual assault, blunt-force injuries to the lower abdomen, seat-belt injuries, objects inserted into the vagina, self-attempts at abortion, and lacerations following childbirth. Bleeding in such cases should be managed by direct pressure over a laceration or a cold pack applied to a hematoma. Never pack the vagina. Provide expedited transport to the hospital, with oxygen administration and IV access as necessary.

©2008 Pearson Education, Inc.
Intermediate Emergency Care: 1985, 3rd ed.

5. Describe the assessment, care, and emotional support of the sexual assault patient. **pp. 668–669**

Sexual assault victims are unique patients with unique needs. The psychological care of these patients is as important, if not more so, than the physical care they may need. Confine your questions to the physical injuries that the patient may have received. Unless your patient is unconscious, do not touch the patient, even to take vital signs, without her permission. Explain what's going to be done before initiating any treatment. Avoid touching the patient other than to take vital signs or to examine other physical injuries. Do not examine the external genitalia of the sexual assault victim unless there is life-threatening hemorrhage. Consider the patient to be a crime scene and protect that scene; handle clothing as little as possible, collect all bloody articles as potential evidence, do not allow the patient to change clothes or bathe, and do not clean wounds if possible. Be sure to document the treatment of the sexual assault victim carefully, thoroughly, and objectively.

6. Given several preprogrammed gynecological patients, provide the appropriate assessment, management, and transportation. **pp. 663–670**

Throughout your classroom, clinical, and field training, you will encounter a variety of real and simulated gynecologic patients. Use the information provided in this chapter of your text, as well as the application of this information as demonstrated by your instructors, preceptors, and mentors to enhance your ability to assess, manage, and transport these patients. Keep in mind that gynecological emergencies are likely to be very stressful situations for your patients, and they will appreciate your gentle, considerate care and professionalism.

Case Study Review

Reread the case study in Chapter 22 and then read the following discussion. This case study draws attention to the assessment and management of a sexual assault patient in the prehospital setting. Sexual assault continues to represent the most rapidly growing violent crime in the United States, so it is likely that you will encounter these patients in the course of your career.

In this scenario, the EMT-Is met their patient in the care of the park police officer that found her. Stephanie has been allowed to cover herself and afforded privacy prior to the arrival of the EMT-Is. Being mindful of the psychological aspects of her care, Erin explains every necessary procedure and asks her permission before any action is initiated. Recognizing the need to preserve potential evidence, Erin keeps the blanket around Stephanie. The initial and rapid trauma assessments revealed no significant injuries or immediate life threats and Stephanie's vital signs are normal. Erin consistently gives control to Stephanie and reassures her that she is safe now. She is transported to the hospital for evaluation by the Sexual Assault Nurse Examiner. The SANE nurse is specially trained to handle both chain of evidence and psychologically support the sexual assault victim.

Content Self-Evaluation

Multiple Choice

______ 1. Painful discomfort during menstrual periods is known as
- A. menarche.
- B. dyspareunia.
- C. cystitis.
- D. dysmenorrhea.
- E. pelvic inflammatory disease.

______ 2. The term used to describe the number of times a woman has been pregnant is parity.
- A. True
- B. False

©2008 Pearson Education, Inc.

______ 3. Which of the following questions is LEAST likely to get an accurate response from a female who is complaining of abdominal pain?
A. Are you currently menstruating?
B. Are you sexually active?
C. Could you be pregnant?
D. Have you ever experienced this pain before when menstruating?
E. Have you experienced dizziness?

______ 4. The term used to describe the number of deliveries a woman has had is
A. gravida.
B. gravity.
C. parity.
D. parita.
E. completa.

______ 5. A palpable abdominal mass found midway between the symphysis pubis and the umbilicus in the lower abdomen of a 25-year-old woman is most likely to be a(n)
A. tumor.
B. intrauterine pregnancy of 5 months gestation.
C. intrauterine pregnancy of 4 months gestation.
D. intrauterine pregnancy of 3 months gestation.
E. ovarian cyst.

______ 6. Pelvic inflammatory disease is most often caused by
A. gonorrhea and chlamydia.
B. streptococcus and staphylococcus.
C. gonorrhea and HIV.
D. chlamydia and streptococcus.
E. HIV and staphylococcus.

______ 7. Urinary infection is also called
A. endometriosis.
B. PID.
C. a miscarriage.
D. cystitis.
E. mittelschmerz.

______ 8. The most effective means to control vaginal hemorrhage is to pack the vaginal opening.
A. True
B. False

______ 9. All of the following signs and symptoms are associated with endometritis EXCEPT
A. history of gynecologic procedure.
B. severe abdominal pain.
C. fever.
D. bradycardia.
E. bloody, foul-smelling discharge.

______ 10. All of the following signs and symptoms are associated with endometriosis EXCEPT
A. history of gynecologic procedure.
B. dull cramping pain.
C. painful bowel movements.
D. women 30 to 40 years old.
E. bloody, foul-smelling discharge.

______ 11. All of the following signs and symptoms are associated with a ruptured ovarian cyst EXCEPT
A. dyspareunia.
B. severe abdominal pain.
C. fever.
D. delayed menstrual period.
E. irregular bleeding.

______ 12. If a female patient presents with severe unilateral abdominal pain that radiates to the shoulder on one side, a missed menstrual period, and vaginal bleeding, you should suspect
A. mittelschmerz.
B. ectopic pregnancy.
C. PID.
D. endometriosis.
E. cystitis.

©2008 Pearson Education, Inc.
Intermediate Emergency Care: 1985, 3rd ed.

______ 13. A female reports that during sexual assault she felt a sudden and sharp tearing sensation. She is now bleeding from the external genitalia, although the bleeding is minimal. Management should include

A. asking the woman to hold a dressing over the area and apply direct pressure.
B. establishing an IV and beginning fluid resuscitation regardless of blood loss.
C. packing the vagina with sterile dressings.
D. palpating the interior of the vagina to determine the extent of bleeding.
E. securing a hot pack over the vaginal opening with tape.

______ 14. The prehospital priorities for care of the sexual assault victim include all of the following EXCEPT

A. examining for perineal tears.
B. determining if life-threatening injuries exist.
C. providing emotional support.
D. preserving evidence.
E. protecting patient's privacy.

______ 15. The BEST prehospital management for a victim of a sexual assault is

A. aggressive questioning and internal examination.
B. discouraging the patient from dressing since this may taint evidence.
C. examining the genitalia.
D. psychological and emotional support.
E. prompt summoning of law enforcement officials.

Label the Diagram

In the spaces provided write the names of the organs of the female reproductive system marked A through E on the diagram below.

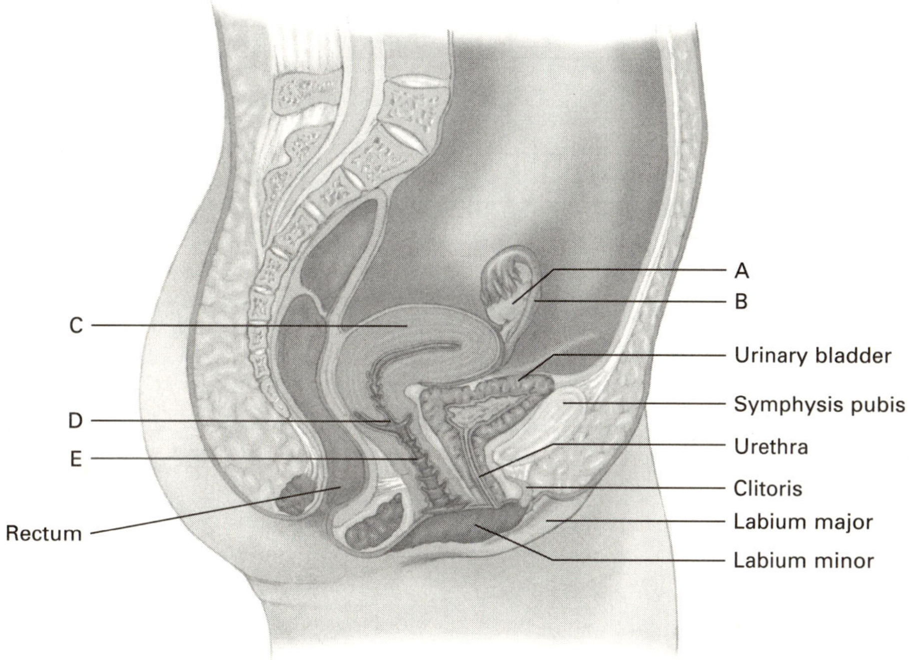

A. ______________________________

B. ______________________________

C. ______________________________

D. ______________________________

E. ______________________________

©2008 Pearson Education, Inc.

Special Project

Problem Solving—Abdominal Pain

You are dispatched for "woman with abdominal pain." Your patient is a 26-year-old female who looks acutely ill and complains of severe abdominal pain.

1. Given this information, what would you attempt to determine when gathering a focused history?

Having obtained the history, you perform a physical exam. Your findings include the following.

- tachypnea
- tachycardia
- pale, cool, diaphoretic skin
- narrowed pulse pressure
- vaginal bleeding or discharge
- abdominal exam: masses, distention, guarding, localized tenderness, rebound

2. Based on this information, provide a differential diagnosis for this patient.

©2008 Pearson Education, Inc.
Intermediate Emergency Care: 1985, 3rd ed.

Chapter

23 Trauma Emergencies

Review of Chapter Objectives

After reading this chapter, you should be able to do the following:

1. Identify, and explain by example, the laws of inertia and conservation of energy. **pp. 675–676**

- **Inertia** is the tendency for objects at rest or in motion to remain so unless acted upon by an outside force. In some cases, that force is the energy exchange that causes trauma. For example, a bullet will continue its travel until it exchanges all its energy with the tissue it strikes.
- **Conservation of energy** is the physical law explaining that energy is not lost but changes form in the auto or other impact. An example is the deformity in the auto when it impacts a tree.

2. Define kinetic energy and force as they relate to trauma. **pp. 675–678**

- **Kinetic energy** is the energy any moving object possesses. This energy is the potential to do harm if it is distributed to a victim.
- **Force** is the exchange of energy from one object to another. It is determined by an object's mass (weight) and the velocity of rate change (acceleration or deceleration). This force induces injury.

3. Explain the elements of trauma assessment. **pp. 678–690**

The assessment of the trauma patient follows the standard format for assessment including the special components that relate to trauma. The assessment progresses through the scene size-up, initial assessment, rapid trauma assessment (for the serious or critical patient) or the focused assessment and history, detailed physical exam (in rare cases), and finally, ongoing assessments.

During the scene size-up, you evaluate the scene to investigate and determine the mechanism of injury and, from that, identify an index of suspicion for specific injuries. You also analyze the potential hazards of the scene, including the need for body substance isolation procedures. You should search out and identify all patients. And, finally, you identify and summon all resources needed to manage the patients and scene.

In the initial assessment, you quickly apply spinal precautions and form a general patient impression and then determine the patient's mental status. Then, evaluate the patient's airway and breathing and perform any needed interventions (oxygen, oral or nasal airway or endotracheal intubation, and ventilation). Evaluate the circulation, control external hemorrhage, and, if hypovolemia and shock are possible, then initiate a large-bore IV. At the conclusion of the initial assessment, the patient is categorized as needing the rapid trauma assessment (emergency patients) or the focused trauma assessment.

During the rapid trauma assessment, you examine areas where significant injury is expected either from the mechanism of injury analysis or the initial assessment. It is also a time to examine

©2008 Pearson Education, Inc.

the patient's chief and minor complaints, as time and priority permit. In general, during this assessment you should look in detail at the head, neck, chest, abdomen, and pelvis, as these are the areas likely to produce life-threatening injury. Take a quick set of vital signs and an abbreviated patient history. At the end of the rapid trauma assessment, decide the priority of the patient for transport. That decision is made by comparing the assessment findings against the trauma triage criteria used in your system.

The focused trauma assessment is used for the patient with limited mechanism of injury and expected, isolated, and moderate to minor injuries. During the focused assessment, you direct consideration to the likely injuries and the specific patient complaints. It usually concludes with slow transport to a nearby emergency department, or in some cases, treatment and release.

The detailed physical exam is a head-to-toe assessment of the patient while you search for signs and symptoms of injury. This procedure is useful for the unconscious patient for whom all other known or suspected life threats have been attended to, and it is then provided only during transport. However, portions of the techniques and process of the detailed assessment are used for elements of the initial and focused assessments.

During the ongoing assessment, you retake the vital signs, make a mental status assessment, reevaluate chief or serious patient complaints and significant signs of injury, and recheck any intervention you have performed. Perform an ongoing assessment every 5 minutes with seriously injured patients and every 15 minutes with other patients. Also perform the ongoing assessment after every major intervention or any sign that the patient's condition has changed or is changing.

4. Explain the management of soft-tissue injury patients. **pp. 691–694**

Soft-tissue injury care is generally a lower priority in trauma patient management and is often deferred until you care for serious injury. The management of soft-tissue injuries is directed at three objectives: stop any hemorrhage, keep the wound clean, and immobilize the wound site. As needed, employ direct pressure, elevation (where indicated), arterial pressure points and, only as a last resort, a tourniquet to control any serious blood loss. Then apply a sterile, properly sized dressing, secured firmly in place, with bandaging material. Assure that the wound site is properly immobilized to assist the coagulation and wound repair processes are unimpeded.

5. Explain the management of head, facial, and neck injury patients. **pp. 702–711**

Direct management of the patient with injury to the head, face, and neck focuses first on the potential for brain injury, airway compromise, injury to the sense organs, and hemorrhage control. Assure the airway with proper patient positioning while employing the proper spinal precautions. Use suctioning and intubation as needed. Control any hemorrhage with direct pressure but be careful of any unstable fracture of the skull. If instability is possible, apply gentle pressure around the wound to help control hemorrhage. Hemorrhage can be especially severe from neck wounds, and circumferential pressure is not indicated. Also be aware that some neck wounds may aspirate air and cause life-threatening air emboli. Cover any open neck wound with an occlusive dressing held in place with gentle direct pressure. Allow blood and possibly cerebral spinal fluid to drain from the ears and protect an injured eye with a paper cup and cover the uninjured eye. Monitor and record any changes in the patient's vital signs and level of consciousness.

6. Explain the management of spinal injury patients. **pp. 711–721**

Whenever you encounter a patient who could be a spinal injury patient, treat him as though he has an injury. Gently bring the spine into alignment by bringing the nose, belly button, and toes into one plane, the shoulders and buttocks against a firm flat surface, the knees bent, and the head (of the adult) $1^1/_2$ to 2 inches above the flat surface. Assure that all movement and immobilization maintains this position and does not cause either axial loading or distraction. Once a potential for injury is recognized, have a rescuer apply manual immobilization of the head and neck. Once the neck is assessed during the initial assessment, apply a properly sized cervical collar. Frequently, the short spine board, KED, or other similar device is needed to bring the patient from a seated position to a full supine position. In an emergency (clear need for rapid extrication) you (and two other rescuers) may manually support the patient as he or she is brought from a seated or other position

©2008 Pearson Education, Inc.
Intermediate Emergency Care: 1985, 3rd ed.

to the supine position. If the patient is found supine or prone, logroll him or her, using spinal precautions, to the long spine board. Once the patient is supine on a spine board, secure the shoulders, hips, legs, and head to the board.

7. Discuss the epidemiology, pathophysiology, assessment findings, and management—including the need for rapid intervention and transport—of the patient with chest wall injuries, including:

a. Chest wall contusion **p. 722**
Chest wall contusion is the most common of chest injuries and presents with pain, made worse by deep breathing. The area may discolor (presenting the shape of the object struck or the underlying ribs), and the pain may limit air movement. Care is directed to assuring good respiratory volume and assessing for pulmonary injuries beneath the contusion.

b. Rib fracture **pp. 722–723, 732**
Blunt or penetrating trauma induces a fracture and possible associated injury underneath. The fracture itself is of only limited concern; however, the pain from such an injury may limit chest excursion and suggests more serious injury beneath. Care is directed to administering oxygen, considering the possibility of underlying injury, and supplying pain medication to ensure respirations are not limited by pain. These injuries do not by themselves require immediate intervention or transport.

c. Flail segment **pp. 723–725, 732–733**
A flail segment is the result of several ribs (three or more) broken in numerous (two or more) places. This creates a rib segment that is free to move independently from the rest of the thorax. This paradoxical motion greatly decreases the efficiency of respiration as air that would be exhaled moves to the region under the flail segment and then returns to the unaffected lung with inspiration. Care includes seeing that the section is stabilized, the patient is given oxygen, possibly using overdrive ventilation. Consider the flail chest patient a candidate for rapid transport. Because of the severity of forces required to compromise the chest wall with this injury and the likelihood of serious underlying injury, this patient is given a high priority for care and transport.

8. Discuss the pathophysiology, assessment findings, and management—including the need for rapid intervention and transport—of the patient with injury to the lung, including:

a. Simple pneumothorax **pp. 725–726**
A simple or closed pneumothorax is an injury caused by either blunt or penetrating trauma that opens the airway to the pleural space. Air accumulates within the space and displaces the lung, resulting in less effective respirations and reduced oxygenation of the blood. This patient has a history of trauma and progressive dyspnea. Oxygen is administered and the patient is observed for progression to tension pneumothorax.

b. Open pneumothorax **pp. 726–727, 733**
Open pneumothorax is like simple pneumothorax, though in this case the injury penetrates the thoracic wall. The injury must be significantly large in order for air to move preferentially through the wound. The patient will have an open chest wound and dyspnea. Care includes sealing the wound on three sides to prevent further progress of the pneumothorax, provision of oxygen, and monitoring the patient for the development of tension pneumothorax.

c. Tension pneumothorax **pp. 727, 734**
Tension pneumothorax is a pneumothorax created under the mechanisms associated with simple or open pneumothorax that progresses because of a valve-like injury site. The valve permits air to enter the pleural space but not exit. This results in a progressive lung collapse, followed by increasing pressure that displaces the mediastinum and restricts venous return to the heart. The patient has a trauma history and progressive dyspnea that becomes very severe. The patient may also display subcutaneous emphysema and distended jugular veins. Care is directed at decompressing the thorax with the insertion of a catheter into the 2nd intercostal space, providing oxygen, and monitoring the patient for a recurring tension pneumothorax.

©2008 Pearson Education, Inc.

d. Hemothorax **pp. 727–728, 734**

A hemothorax is a collection of blood in the pleural space. It may occur with or without pneumothorax. Hemothorax will generally become a hypovolemic problem before it seriously endangers respiration because the amount of fluid loss necessary to restrict respiration is great. The patient may experience dyspnea and the signs and symptoms of hypovolemic compensation (shock). Provide the patient with shock care, oxygen, fluid replacement, and rapid transport.

e. Hemopneumothorax **p. 727**

A hemopneumothorax is simply the existence of blood loss into the pleura and an accumulation of air there. Its presentation includes the signs and symptoms associated with both these pathologies. Care is directed at oxygen administration and rapid transport.

f. Pulmonary contusion **p. 728**

Pulmonary contusion is a blunt trauma injury to the tissue of the lung resulting in edema and stiffening of the lung tissue. This reduces the efficiency of air exchange and causes an increased workload associated with respiration. If the region involved is limited, the patient may only experience very mild dyspnea. If the area is extensive, the patient may experience severe dyspnea. Care is centered around ensuring good oxygenation, including overdrive ventilation when indicated, and rapid transport.

9. Discuss the pathophysiology, findings of assessment, and management—including the need for rapid intervention and transport—of the patient with myocardial injuries, including:

a. Myocardial contusion **pp. 729–730, 735**

Myocardial contusion is simply a contusion to the myocardium, usually related to blunt anterior chest trauma. The patient will present with myocardial-infarction-like pain and possible dysrhythmias. Care is directed at oxygen therapy, cardiac medications as indicated, and rapid transport.

b. Pericardial tamponade **pp. 730–731, 735–736**

Pericardial tamponade is usually related to penetrating trauma in which a wound permits blood from within the heart to enter the pericardium. It progressively fills the pericardium and restricts ventricular filling. The cardiac output drops and circulation is severely restricted. The patient will present with a penetrating trauma mechanism and will move quickly into shock, and possibly, sudden death. Care is insertion of a needle into the pericardial sac and the withdrawal of fluid. Any patient suspected of this injury requires immediate transport to the closest hospital.

c. Traumatic aortic aneurysm or rupture **pp. 731–732, 736**

Traumatic aortic aneurysm and rupture are associated with blunt chest trauma and occur as the heart and aorta are twisted with impact. The aorta is attached as it leaves the heart, where it exits the diaphragm, and at the ligamentum arteriosum. These forces may separate the layers of the vessel, permit blood to flow between them, and cause the aorta to bulge. This damage to the vessel may cause it to rupture. Aneurysm is most commonly related to severe lateral impact or falls and presents with a tearing chest pain and may have a pulse deficit between extremities.

10. Explain the management of abdominal injury patients. **pp. 736–738**

The care for a patient with abdominal injuries is for the most part supportive. If you suspect serious internal hemorrhage, then provide fluid therapy and rapid transport. Give high-flow, high-concentration oxygen, keep the patient warm, and monitor vital signs and level of consciousness. Immobilize objects impaled within the abdomen in place and dress open wounds and cover eviscerations with occlusive dressings.

11. Identify and describe the depth classifications of burn injuries, including superficial burns, partial-thickness burns, and full-thickness burns. **pp. 738–740**

- **Superficial (first-degree) burns** involve only the upper layers of the epidermis and dermis. The effects are limited to an irritation of the upper sensory tissues with some pain, minor edema, and erythema.

©2008 Pearson Education, Inc.
Intermediate Emergency Care: 1985, 3rd ed.

- **Partial-thickness (second-degree) burns** penetrate slightly deeper than first-degree burns and cause blistering, erythema, swelling, and pain. Since the cells that reproduce the skin's upper layers are still alive, complete regeneration is expected.
- **Full-thickness (third-degree) burns** penetrate the entire dermis, causing extensive destruction. The burned area may display a variety of appearances and colors, the site is anesthetic, and healing is prolonged. Third-degree burns may involve not only the skin, but also underlying tissues and organs. (Organ and other tissue involvement is sometimes called fourth-degree burn.)

12. Describe and apply the "rule of nines," and the "rule of palms" methods for determining body surface area percentage of a burn injury. **p. 741**

The "rule of nines" approximates the body surface area burned by assigning each body region nine percent of the total. These regions include each upper extremity, the anterior of each lower extremity, the posterior of each lower extremity, the anterior of the abdomen, the anterior thorax, the upper back, the lower back, and the entire head and neck. The remaining one percent is assigned to the genitalia. For children, the head is given 18 percent, and the lower extremities are assigned $13^1/_2$ percent.

The "rule of palms" method of approximating burn surface area assumes the victim's palm surface is equivalent to one percent of the total body surface area. The care provider then estimates the burn surface area by determining the number of palmar surfaces it would take to cover the wound.

13. Describe burn management including considerations for airway and ventilation, circulation, pharmacological and nonpharmacological measures, transport decisions, and psychological support/communication strategies. **pp. 744–746**

The management of the burn patient is a rather complicated, multifaceted process. The first consideration is to extinguish the fire to ensure the burn does not continue. If necessary, use water from a low-pressure hose and remove all jewelry, leather, nylon, or other material that may continue to smolder or hold heat and continue to burn the patient. Also consider removing any restrictive jewelry or clothing, as such an item may act as a tourniquet, restricting distal blood flow as the burn region swells.

Then assess and ensure that the airway remains adequate. With any history suggestive of an inhalation burn or injury, carefully assess and monitor the airway for any signs of restriction. If they are found, move to protect the airway with rapid sequence intubation early, before the progressive airway swelling prevents intubation or significantly restricts the size of the endotracheal tube you can introduce. Small and painful burns may be covered with wet dressings to occlude airflow and reduce the pain; however, any extensive burn should be covered with a sterile dry dressing to prevent body cooling and the introduction of pathogens through the dressing.

Resuscitation for extensive burns must include large volumes of prehospital fluid (0.5 mL/kg × BSA) as burns often account for massive fluid loss into and through the burn. The patient must also be kept warm because by their nature burns account for rapid heat loss.

Any burns on opposing tissue, such as between the fingers and toes, should be separated by nonadherent dressings, as the burned surfaces are likely to adhere firmly together and cause further damage as they are pulled apart. In painful burns consider morphine, in 2 mg increments, for pain relief as long as there is no evidence of hypotension or respiratory depression.

Watch for any constriction from eschar formation that may reduce or halt distal circulation or restrict respiration. Medical direction may request a surgical incision to relieve the pressure (an escharotomy).

Any burn patient with serious injury should be transported to the burn center where he or she can receive the specialized treatment needed. Also ensure that the burn patient receives therapeutic communication while you are at the scene and during transport. The burn injury is very painful and the appearance can be very frightening. Constantly talk with the patient. Try to distract him or her from the injury, and monitor level of consciousness and anxiety level throughout your care and transport.

©2008 Pearson Education, Inc.

14. Explain the management of musculoskeletal injury patients. **pp. 747–760**

Musculoskeletal injuries are usually a lower priority for the seriously injured trauma patient and are attended to only after the patient's serious injuries are stabilized, and then, only during transport. The first priority in caring for the patient with a musculoskeletal injury is to assure distal circulation and innervation. Then immobilize the injury using a splinting device. Assure that the device firmly immobilizes the joint above and the joint below the injury (be it a sprain, strain, dislocation, or fracture). There are many splinting devices to choose from including the traction splint (for the femur fracture), padded board splints, air splints, vacuum splints, ladder splints, and specialized splints. Choose one that is easy to apply and will firmly stabilize the wound site. Be sure to assess the distal pulse and nervous function distal to the injury before, during, and after the splinting process. If the pulse is absent after splinting, move the splint and limb around slightly to re-establish circulation or innervation.

Case Study Review

Reread the case study in Chapter 23 and then read the following discussion. This scenario represents a typical serious auto collision in which knowledge of the kinetics of trauma assists in analyzing the mechanism of injury and helps guide assessment and care. Using this approach results in a better understanding of the potential injuries. It also provides for an orderly scene approach in which the patients are quickly assessed, prioritized, immediately stabilized, and then quickly transported. The incident is evaluated carefully, using an analysis of the mechanism of injury to anticipate both the nature and severity of patient injuries. This information is then used in combination with the data gathered through the patient assessments to develop a clear picture of what happened to the auto passengers and to determine what resources will be distributed to each patient.

The information given by the dispatcher allows Kris and Bob to begin planning for arrival at the scene. The dispatch information describes a severe accident with the potential for several seriously injured patients. While still en route, Kris and Bob locate equipment in the ambulance and set it out on the stretcher for quick transport to their patients' side. Lactated Ringer's solution in 1,000 mL bags might be readied in the ambulance with trauma tubing, pressure infusers, and large-bore catheters readied, just in case the decision is made to rapidly transport the patient. Kris and Bob may also use this time to review their responsibilities, which begin with arrival at the scene.

Given the police update, the team begins thinking about the kinetic energy associated with the collision and the injuries that it is likely to cause. One auto was stopped and was hit from behind by a vehicle at "highway speed." In the auto hit, the suspected injuries should include cervical spine injury, with the rest of the body well protected except for secondary impacts. Kris and Bob should anticipate the need for spinal precautions and ready a collar, vest-type immobilization device, and long spine board.

The auto traveling at highway speed most likely impacted the other frontally. If the occupants were unrestrained, they may have traveled either through the down-and-under or up-and-over pathway. If they were restrained, the lap, lap and shoulder, or airbag restraint systems may have protected them. (Remember that the airbag restraint system is beneficial only for the initial frontal impact.) Internal head injuries, chest trauma, and shock are the leading trauma killers. The team will anticipate these types of injuries and treat their patients accordingly.

Kris and Bob gain a great deal of information quickly during the scene size-up. Potential hazards, the number of patients, the resources needed, and the mechanism of injury all are identified. From analysis of the mechanism of injury, they anticipate the nature and extent of injuries for each of the three expected patients. By examining what happened, how badly the autos are damaged, and from what direction the impacts came, the team can garner enough information to anticipate which patient is likely to be the most seriously injured.

In this collision, the green car struck the red one from behind. The red car sustained severe rear-end damage, reflecting a strong impact. The passenger would have been pushed forward with great acceleration by the auto seat, while the unsupported head rotated backward, extending the cervical spine. An important observation was that the headrest was in the "up" position. This positioning probably limited the forceful hyperextension of the head and neck and reduced the potential for injury. The

©2008 Pearson Education, Inc.
Intermediate Emergency Care: 1985, 3rd ed.

seatbelt also limited the danger of secondary impact, assuring the driver came to rest with the vehicle, not afterward.

The second car (the green one) sustained front-end damage and two spiderweb cracks in the windshield. This suggests an unrestrained driver and passenger, the up-and-over pathway, and a potential for severe head, neck, thoracic, and abdominal injuries. The deformed steering wheel also provides evidence that the driver may have sustained a chest injury. Using the analysis of the mechanism of injury, Kris and Bob have a good preliminary picture of the collision process and the likely injuries it produced. As they leave their vehicle and approach the scene, they don gloves and assure the scene is safe for them, their patients, fellow rescuers, and bystanders. They also request anticipated resources (another ambulance) to handle the multiple patients they expect. Because the mechanism of injury analysis suggests the most serious patients will be found in the green car, Kris and Bob head there first.

Assessment confirms the injuries anticipated by review of the impact and the degree of auto damage. As reported by the police officer, the driver of the red car appears only shaken up with a possible spine injury. His vitals are within normal limits, given the circumstances. The choice is made to leave him with a first responder while Kris and Bob remain with the patients in the green car. While it would be more preferable to have an ALS provider by the side of each patient, this decision is justified based upon the findings at the scene. Bob and Kris will have another First Responder hold spinal immobilization for the driver of the green car as they attend to the unconscious passenger.

The initial assessment reveals that the occupants of the green auto are in serious condition. The driver has sustained chest trauma and is experiencing dyspnea, though her breath sounds are clear at this time. She is stable for now. However, she has the potential to deteriorate rapidly at any time. Her passenger is moving rapidly into hypovolemic shock, presumably due to pelvic and femur fractures and internal hemorrhage. She is also unconscious either due to the hypovolemia or the head injury from striking the windshield. The passenger is critical and a candidate for immediate transport. The driver, though more stable, is a candidate for immediate transport also.

This case study demonstrates the value a good scene analysis can have in triaging, in anticipating the findings of assessment, and in determining the care needed by the patient or patients. While the mechanism of injury analysis does not give definitive information regarding the nature and extent of patient injuries, it can complement the overall assessment of both the scene and each individual patient.

Content Self-Evaluation

MULTIPLE CHOICE

______ 1. The study of trauma is related to a branch of physics called
- A. kinetics.
- B. velocity.
- C. ballistics.
- D. inertia.
- E. heuristics.

______ 2. The anticipation of injuries based upon the analysis of the collision mechanism is referred to as the
- A. mechanism of injury.
- B. index of suspicion.
- C. trauma triage criteria.
- D. mortality potential.
- E. RTS.

______ 3. The tendency of an object to remain at rest or remain in motion unless acted upon by an external force is
- A. kinetics.
- B. velocity.
- C. ballistics.
- D. inertia.
- E. deceleration.

©2008 Pearson Education, Inc.

_____ 4. Two autos accelerate from a stop sign to a speed of 30 mph, the first one by normal acceleration and the second when it was struck from behind by another vehicle. Assuming that both vehicles have the same weight, which vehicle gained the most kinetic energy?
A. the vehicle in normal acceleration
B. the vehicle struck from behind
C. both vehicles gained the same kinetic energy
D. cannot be determined since the kinetic energy is not known
E. cannot be determined since the force is not known

_____ 5. Which of the following is an example of energy dissipation from an auto accident?
A. sound of the impact
B. bending of the structural steel
C. heating of the compressed steel
D. internal injury to the occupant
E. all of the above

_____ 6. Which of the following increases the kinetic energy of a collision most quickly?
A. the temperature of the object
B. increasing object speed
C. decreasing object speed
D. increasing object mass
E. decreasing object mass

_____ 7. Blunt trauma may cause
A. rupture of the bowel.
B. bursting of the alveoli.
C. crushing of blood vessels.
D. contusion of the liver or kidneys.
E. all of the above

_____ 8. The scene size-up includes four elements. They include all of the following EXCEPT
A. analysis of the mechanism of injury.
B. identifying scene hazards.
C. locating all patients.
D. evaluating the ABCs.
E. requesting additional resources.

_____ 9. Employ spinal precautions when you note the patient has experienced extremes of
A. flexion.
B. axial loading.
C. rotation.
D. distraction.
E. all of the above

_____ 10. A person who does not recognize friends and family is NOT
A. oriented to time.
B. oriented to place.
C. oriented to persons.
D. oriented to one's own person.
E. none of the above

_____ 11. Which examination technique should be performed first?
A. inspection
B. palpation
C. percussion
D. auscultation
E. questioning

_____ 12. At what angle should the normo-tensive patient display jugular vein distention?
A. 10 degrees
B. 15 degrees
C. 25 degrees
D. 35 degrees
E. 45 degrees

_____ 13. Which of the following is NOT a part of the ongoing assessment?
A. mental status check
B. vital sign assessment
C. rapid trauma assessment
D. circulation check
E. breathing check

_____ 14. Which of the following types of hemorrhage is characterized by bright red blood?
A. capillary bleeding
B. venous bleeding
C. arterial bleeding
D. A and C
E. A and B

©2008 Pearson Education, Inc.
Intermediate Emergency Care: 1985, 3rd ed.

______ 15. Which of the following types of hemorrhage is characterized by dark red blood?
A. capillary bleeding
B. venous bleeding
C. arterial bleeding
D. A and C
E. none of the above

______ 16. Bleeding from capillary or venous wounds is easy to halt because the pressure driving the hemorrhage is limited.
A. True
B. False

______ 17. Fractures of the femur can account for a blood loss
A. from 500 to 750 mL.
B. up to 1,500 mL.
C. in excess of 2,000 mL.
D. less than 500 mL.
E. in excess of 2,500 mL.

______ 18. Which list places the stages of shock in the order of their occurrence?
A. irreversible, decompensated, compensated
B. compensated, decompensated, irreversible
C. compensated, irreversible, decompensated
D. decompensated, irreversible, compensated
E. decompensated, compensated, irreversible

______ 19. Which stage of shock begins with a precipitous drop in blood pressure?
A. compensatory
B. decompensatory
C. irreversible
D. hypovolemic
E. none of the above

______ 20. Which of the following does NOT occur during the compensated stage of shock?
A. increasing pulse rate
B. decreasing pulse strength
C. decreasing systolic blood pressure
D. skin becomes cool and clammy
E. the patient experiences thirst and weakness

______ 21. The first line drug for the patient with a head injury is
A. oxygen.
B. epinephrine.
C. mannitol.
D. furosemide.
E. thiamine.

______ 22. A protective helmet must be removed from the patient when the helmet
A. does not immobilize the head within.
B. cannot be securely immobilized to the spine board.
C. obstructs airway care.
D. prevents assessment of anticipated injuries.
E. all of the above

______ 23. The vest-type device for the movement of the spinal injured patient is well suited for lifting the patient.
A. True
B. False

______ 24. Which of the following is an appropriate reason to employ rapid extrication instead of normal spinal precautions?
A. the needed procedure is time consuming
B. the needed procedure is complicated
C. scene safety requires immediate movement
D. the patient condition requires immediate transport
E. C and D

©2008 Pearson Education, Inc.

______ 25. Rib fracture is found in slightly more than what percent of significant chest trauma?
A. 10 percent
B. 25 percent
C. 35 percent
D. 50 percent
E. 65 percent

______ 26. Which rib group results in mortality up to 30 percent when they are fractured?
A. ribs 1 and 3
B. ribs 4 through 8
C. ribs 7 through 9
D. ribs 8 through 11
E. ribs 9 through 12

______ 27. Which of the following is a sign or symptom of rib fracture?
A. local pain
B. crepitus
C. limited chest excursion
D. hemothorax
E. all of the above

______ 28. Air from under the flail segment in flail chest does which of the following?
A. moves out from under the segment during expiration
B. moves toward the segment during expiration
C. does not move with the segment
D. moves toward the segment during inspiration
E. none of the above

______ 29. As the pain of the flail chest increases with time, the amount of paradoxical movement will decrease due to muscular splinting.
A. True
B. False

______ 30. The condition in which a part of the chest wall moves in opposition to the rest of the chest due to numerous rib fractures is called
A. pneumothorax.
B. tension pneumothorax.
C. hemothorax.
D. atelectasis.
E. none of the above

______ 31. The chest injury that causes the patient to experience increasing dyspnea because of an open or closed pneumothorax that has a valve-like function and allows intrathoracic pressure to increase is referred to as
A. subcutaneous emphysema.
B. traumatic asphyxia.
C. hyperbaric mediastinal displacement.
D. tension pneumothorax.
E. flail chest.

______ 32. Which of the following is a very late sign of tension pneumothorax?
A. head and neck petechiae
B. intercostal bulging
C. a narrowing pulse pressure
D. tracheal deviation away from the injury
E. distended jugular veins

______ 33. Each hemithorax can hold up to what volume of blood from a hemothorax?
A. 500 mL
B. 750 mL
C. 1,500 mL
D. 3,000 mL
E. 4,500 mL

______ 34. Distant or absent breath sounds heard during auscultation of the chest and the signs of shock are suggestive of which pathology?
A. pneumothorax
B. tension pneumothorax
C. aortic aneurysm
D. pulmonary contusion
E. hemothorax

______ 35. Which of the following problems would most likely result in a chest area that was dull to percussion?
A. pneumothorax
B. tension pneumothorax
C. hemothorax
D. subcutaneous pneumothorax
E. pericardial tamponade

©2008 Pearson Education, Inc.
Intermediate Emergency Care: 1985, 3rd ed.

______ 36. Your patient has received chest trauma yet did not initially present with crackles. However, as the assessment continues, they are heard in both the lower lung fields. This condition is most likely a result of which of the following?
A. pulmonary contusion
B. hemothorax
C. pneumothorax
D. aortic aneurysm
E. pericardial tamponade

______ 37. The most common cause of myocardial contusion is
A. blunt anterior chest trauma.
B. blunt lateral chest trauma.
C. penetrating anterior chest trauma.
D. blunt posterior chest trauma.
E. the pressure wave of an explosion.

______ 38. A patient presents with the signs of shock, jugular vein distention, distant heart sounds, and a narrowing pulse pressure. The lung fields are clear. Which condition is most likely the cause?
A. tension pneumothorax
B. hemothorax
C. traumatic asphyxia
D. pericardial tamponade
E. atelectasis

______ 39. Which of the following is a sign of pericardial tamponade?
A. pulsus paradoxus
B. a narrowing pulse pressure
C. distended jugular veins
D. hypotension
E. all of the above

______ 40. A decrease in jugular vein distention during inspiration is known as
A. Beck's triad.
B. pulsus paradoxus.
C. Cushing's reflex.
D. Kussmaul's sign.
E. electrical alternans.

______ 41. Your patient was involved in a lateral impact auto accident. The car is greatly deformed, though the patient does not have many signs of injury. During your assessment, he complains of a tearing sensation in his central chest and numbness in his left upper extremity. Your highest index of suspicion of injury is for
A. traumatic asphyxia.
B. pulmonary contusion.
C. aortic aneurysm.
D. myocardial contusion.
E. pericardial tamponade.

______ 42. In a patient with a history of blunt lateral trauma and a suspected traumatic aortic aneurysm, which signs or symptoms would you expect to find?
A. severe tearing chest pain
B. pulse deficit between extremities
C. reduced pulse strength in the lower extremities
D. hypertension
E. all of the above

______ 43. A harsh systolic murmur is heard over the central chest. This is suggestive of which pathology?
A. pneumothorax
B. tension pneumothorax
C. traumatic aortic aneurysm
D. pulmonary contusion
E. hemothorax

______ 44. Overdrive ventilation (bag-valve masking) of the patient with flail chest will cause the flail segment to move with, rather than in opposition to, the chest wall.
A. True
B. False

______ 45. Meperidine, diazepam, or morphine sulfate may be given to the minor rib fracture patient to reduce pain and increase respiratory excursion.
A. True
B. False

©2008 Pearson Education, Inc.

______ 46. The patient who is suspected of a flail chest or other thoracic cage injury, without suspected spine injury, should be positioned
A. on the uninjured side.
B. on the injured side.
C. supine with legs elevated.
D. on the left lateral side.
E. on the right lateral side.

______ 47. The open pneumothorax should be cared for using which of the following techniques?
A. Pack the wound with a sterile dressing.
B. Cover the wound with an occlusive dressing and tape securely.
C. Cover the wound with an occlusive dressing, taped on three sides.
D. Attempt to close the wound with a hemostat and then cover with a sterile dressing.
E. Cover the wound loosely with a sterile dressing.

______ 48. Which location is recommended for prehospital pleural decompression?
A. 2nd intercostal space, midclavicular line
B. 5th intercostal space, midclavicular line
C. 5th intercostal space, midaxillary line
D. A and B
E. A and C

______ 49. A few minutes after you have inserted a needle and decompressed a tension pneumothorax, you notice that a patient's dyspnea is getting worse and breath sounds on the injured side are becoming diminished. Which action would you take?
A. Insert a second needle.
B. Remove the dressing.
C. Provide overdrive ventilation.
D. Consider nitrous oxide administration.
E. all of the above

______ 50. The major emphasis of abdominal injury care in the prehospital setting is
A. stopping internal hemorrhage.
B. assuring patient comfort.
C. bringing the patient to surgery as rapidly as possible.
D. identifying the exact injuries and providing essential care.
E. none of the above

______ 51. The burn characterized by erythema, pain, and blistering is the
A. superficial burn.
B. partial-thickness burn.
C. full-thickness burn.
D. electrical burn.
E. chemical burn.

______ 52. The burn characterized by discoloration and lack of pain is the
A. superficial burn.
B. partial-thickness burn.
C. full-thickness burn.
D. electrical burn.
E. chemical burn.

______ 53. An adult has received burns to the entire anterior chest and to the entire left upper extremity, circumferentially. Using the rule of nines, the percentage of body surface (BSA) area involved is
A. 9 percent.
B. 18 percent.
C. 27 percent.
D. 36 percent.
E. 48 percent.

______ 54. A child has received burns to the entire left lower extremity and the genitals. Using the rule of nines, the percentage of the body surface area involved is:
A. 9 percent.
B. 10 percent.
C. 14½ percent.
D. 19 percent.
E. 22½ percent.

©2008 Pearson Education, Inc.
Intermediate Emergency Care: 1985, 3rd ed.

______ 55. An adult has received burns to the entire left lower extremity and the genitals. Using the rule of nines, the percentage of the body surface area involved is
A. 9 percent.
B. 10 percent.
C. 18 percent.
D. 19 percent.
E. 21 percent.

______ 56. A child receives burns to his entire head and neck and upper back. What percentage of body surface area is involved?
A. 9 percent
B. 10 percent
C. 18 percent
D. 19 percent
E. 27 percent

______ 57. Which of the following systemic complications should you suspect with all serious burns?
A. hypothermia
B. hypovolemia
C. infection
D. eschar formation
E. all of the above

______ 58. Which of the following conditions would increase the impact a burn has on a patient?
A. being very young
B. being very old
C. having the flu
D. emphysema
E. all of the above

______ 59. In general, moderate to severe burns should be covered with
A. moist occlusive dressings.
B. dry sterile dressings.
C. cool water immersion.
D. plastic wrap covered by a soft dressing.
E. warm water immersion.

______ 60. Adjacent full-thickness burns, such as those affecting the fingers and toes, should be held together without dressings to ensure rapid healing.
A. True
B. False

______ 61. The Parkland formula for fluid administration calls for administration of 4 mL of fluid to a patient multiplied by the patient's BSA involved. What other factor(s) determines the total fluid administered in the first 24 hours?
A. patient's age
B. patient's weight
C. depth of burns
D. age of the patient
E. all of the above

______ 62. Which of the following drugs may be given to the patient with severe burns in the prehospital setting?
A. ipratropium
B. morphine
C. epinephrine
D. furosemide
E. haloperidol

______ 63. Which of the following is an objective of musculoskeletal injury care?
A. reduce the possibility of further injury during transport
B. protect open wounds
C. immobilize the injured extremity
D. reduce patient discomfort
E. all of the above

______ 64. Proper limb positioning is important for maintaining distal circulation, sensation, and increasing patient comfort.
A. True
B. False

©2008 Pearson Education, Inc.

______ 65. Which of the following should halt the movement of an angulated limb to an aligned position?
A. a significant increase in patient discomfort
B. a strong distal pulse
C. regaining distal sensation
D. significant resistance to movement
E. A and D

Special Project

Drip Math Worksheet 2

Formulas

Rate = Volume/Time		mL/min = drops per min/drop per mL	
Volume = Rate × Time		drops/min = mL per min × drop per mL	
Time = Volume/Rate		mL = drops/drops per mL	

Please complete the following drug and drip math problems:

1. Upon arriving at the emergency department the physician asks how much fluid you infused into your trauma patient. Your on-scene and transport time was 35 minutes, and you ran normal saline at a rate of 120 drops/minute through a 10 drops/mL administration set. What would you report?
2. Protocol calls for a drug to be hung and administered by drip at 45 drops per minute based upon a 60 drops/mL administration set. You find that the set you have administers 45 drops/mL. How many drops per second should you set your chamber for?
3. The transferring physician requests that you infuse 100 mL of a drug during your transport. Anticipated transport time is 1 hour and 55 minutes. At what rate would you set a 60 drops/mL administration set?
4. You are allowed to administer a drug by IV drip at a rate of between 45 and 100 mL per hour. What drip rate range can you use with a

   60 drops/mL set?

   45 drops/mL set?

   10 drops/mL set?
5. After a call, you can't remember at what rate you ran a fluid. You do know that 350 mL is left in the 500 mL bag and that the IV was running for 1 hour and 5 minutes. What would you record?

©2008 Pearson Education, Inc.
Intermediate Emergency Care: 1985, 3rd ed.

Chapter 24

Obstetrical Emergencies

Review of Chapter Objectives

After reading this chapter, you should be able to do the following:

1. Describe the anatomic structures and physiology of the reproductive system during pregnancy. **pp. 766–769**

The primary "organ of pregnancy" is the placenta, which arises from the site on the uterine wall where the blastocyst (fertilized egg) implants itself. This temporary, blood-rich structure serves as a lifeline for the developing fetus via the umbilical cord. Its functions include the transfer of heat while exchanging oxygen and carbon dioxide, delivering nutrients, and removing waste. The placenta also serves as an endocrine gland throughout the pregnancy, secreting hormones necessary for fetal survival as well as the estrogen and progesterone required to maintain the pregnancy. The placenta is also a protective barrier against harmful substances that might cross the placental barrier to the fetus.

The fetus develops within the amniotic sac, a thin-walled membranous covering containing amniotic fluid that surrounds and protects the fetus during intrauterine life.

2. Describe how to assess an obstetrical patient. **pp. 769–772**

The initial assessment for an obstetric patient is the same as for any other patient. Utilization of the SAMPLE history will allow you to obtain specific information about the pregnancy. Ask about gravidity, parity, length of gestation, and EDC (estimated date of confinement or due date). You should also obtain information about past OB/GYN history (e.g., C-section) or complications as well as prenatal care. Determine current medications and any drug allergies as well. It is important to obtain the past medical history because pregnancy may aggravate preexisting medical problems or trigger new ones such as gestational diabetes. It is possible to estimate the due date by measuring fundal height above the symphysis pubis. Continue the physical exam, which is essentially the same for any patient, while being mindful of the need for modesty and privacy.

3. Identify the stages of labor and the EMT-Intermediate's role in each stage. **pp. 779–785**

Labor is the physiologic and mechanical process by which the baby, placenta, and amniotic sac are expelled through the birth canal. The three stages of labor are dilatation, expulsion, and placental. The first stage (dilatation stage) begins with the onset of true labor and ends with the complete dilatation and effacement of the cervix. The second stage (expulsion stage) begins with the complete dilatation of the cervix and ends with the delivery of the baby. The third and final stage of labor (placental stage) begins immediately after the birth of the baby and ends with the delivery of the placenta. The role of the EMT-I during labor is to assist in the delivery and to recognize and treat life-threatening problems for the mother or baby.

©2008 Pearson Education, Inc.

4. Differentiate between normal and abnormal delivery. **pp. 780–789**

Normally, most infants present from the birth canal in a headfirst, face-down position (vertex presentation), which allows the infant to be delivered vaginally. Abnormal delivery situations generally preclude vaginal delivery and are likely to require cesarean section, so transport must be expedited. These situations include breech presentation (buttocks present first), prolapsed cord (umbilical cord protrudes from the birth canal), limb presentation (baby's arm or leg protrudes from the birth canal) or occiput posterior presentation (baby's brow is facing forward).

5. Identify and describe complications associated with pregnancy and delivery. **pp. 773–778, 790–791**

Medical complications of pregnancy include ectopic pregnancy, bleeding problems, supine hypotensive syndrome, gestational diabetes, and hypertensive disorders. Ectopic pregnancy refers to the implantation of the fertilized egg outside of the uterus. Abdominal pain and evidence of intra-abdominal and/or vaginal bleeding usually herald this event. Bleeding is generally differentiated as painful or painless. Vaginal bleeding, accompanied by cramping abdominal pain, prior to the 20th week of gestation is almost always associated with a spontaneous abortion. Painless bleeding is most commonly associated with *placenta previa* where, due to abnormal implantation of the placenta on the uterine wall, labor is accompanied by bleeding. Painful bleeding is the hallmark of *abruptio placenta* or the premature separation of the placenta from the uterine wall. It poses an immediate life threat to mother and child.

Supine hypotensive syndrome occurs most commonly in the third trimester as a result of compression of the inferior vena cava by the gravid uterus. Insulin resistance and decreased glucose tolerance characterize gestational diabetes, occurring in the last 20 weeks of pregnancy. Hypertensive disorders of pregnancy (formerly called toxemia) include preeclampsia or eclampsia and chronic and transient hypertension. Major motor seizures are the hallmark of eclampsia, which is the most serious of the hypertensive disorders, posing a life threat to the mother and child.

Some complications associated with delivery are discussed in objective 5. Other problems can occur after delivery. One of these is postpartum hemorrhage, which is the loss of 500 cc or more of blood immediately following delivery. A common cause of the condition is lack of uterine muscle tone, and it occurs most frequently in the multigravida, with multiple births, and with the births of large infants. Uterine rupture is another complication of delivery. It can result from blunt abdominal trauma, prolonged uterine contractions, or a surgically scarred uterus. Uterine rupture presents with a patient in excruciating abdominal pain and often in shock. Blood loss from 800 to 1,800 cc occurs, and the patient often experiences profound shock. Pulmonary embolism can also occur after pregnancy as a result of venous thromboembolism. It often presents with sudden dyspnea accompanied by sharp chest pain and a sense of impending doom.

6. Identify predelivery emergencies. **pp. 773–778**

Recognition of a predelivery emergency is based on information obtained from the focused history and physical exam that relates to the reported abnormality, such as pain, discomfort, or bleeding. While any of the complications listed above has potential to be an emergency, the most likely are *abruptio placenta* and eclampsia, both of which pose potential life threats to mother and child and require prompt and appropriate intervention.

7. State indications of an imminent delivery. **pp. 771, 779**

Increasing frequency and duration of contractions and the sensation of needing to move one's bowels (urge to push) are all signs of impending delivery. However, crowning is the definitive sign that birth is imminent.

8. Differentiate the management of a patient with predelivery emergencies from a normal delivery. **pp. 773–778**

Management of predelivery emergencies requires that EMT-Is correctly recognize their presence based on information obtained from the focused history and physical exam and then expedite transport while anticipating the development of shock and maintaining adequate oxygenation,

©2008 Pearson Education, Inc.
Intermediate Emergency Care: 1985, 3rd ed.

fluid resuscitation as necessary, and, if appropriate, pharmacological intervention. Most of the time, the mother will be transported in the left lateral recumbent position.

9. State the steps in the predelivery preparation of the mother. pp. 780–781

The first priority is to provide the mother with privacy. Then, time permitting, administer oxygen via a nasal cannula and establish vascular access. Position the mother on her back with knees and hips flexed and buttocks slightly elevated, or the mother may prefer squatting or to be in a semi-Fowler position with knees and hips flexed. Drape the mother's perineum to minimize contamination of the infant during delivery.

Normally, preparation for childbirth in the prehospital setting would entail thoroughly washing hands and forearms before donning a gown, in addition to sterile gloves and goggles. Body substance isolation for childbirth generally includes draping the mother to minimize contamination of the baby during delivery.

10. State the steps to assist in the delivery of a newborn, including cutting the umbilical cord and delivery of placenta. pp. 780–785

Key EMS actions during a routine (normal) delivery are primarily supportive, but you should remain vigilant to signs of impending problems. Providing gentle support to thc perineum as the delivery progresses decreases the likelihood of an explosive delivery causing vaginal tears and the potential for neonatal head trauma. While supporting the head, gently slide your finger along the head and neck to ensure that the cord is not wrapped around the baby's head and neck. As the head emerges from the vaginal opening, suction the airway (mouth first, then nose) to insure that the airway is clear prior to the neonate taking his first breath. It may be necessary to tear the amniotic sac to release the amniotic fluid and permit the baby to breathe.

Gently guide the baby's head downward to allow delivery of the upper shoulder. Do not pull! Then gently guide the baby's body upward to allow delivery of the lower shoulder. Once the shoulders are delivered, the rest of the body will be quickly delivered. Keep the baby at the level of the mother's hips until the cord has been clamped and cut. Once the body has fully emerged from the birth canal, the baby should again be suctioned until the airway is clear. Once the baby's body has been delivered, suction the airway until clear while keeping the baby at the level of the mother's hips until the cord has been clamped and cut. Do not "milk" the cord. Supporting the baby's body, place the first umbilical clamp approximately 10 cm from the baby and the second clamp at 15 cm and carefully cut in between.

Following delivery of the baby, the vaginal opening will continue to ooze blood. Do not pull on the umbilical cord! Eventually, the cord will appear to lengthen indicating separation of the placenta from the uterine wall. Once the placenta is expelled through the vaginal opening, it should be placed in a biohazard bag and be transported to the hospital for examination.

11. Describe how to care for the newborn, including routine care and neonatal resuscitation. pp. 785–786

The essential emergency care of the newborn includes the establishment and maintenance of adequate airway and breathing status and the prevention of heat loss. Support the infant's head and torso, using both hands. Maintain warmth, repeat suctioning of the mouth and nose as needed until the airway is clear, and then assess using the APGAR score. Do not delay resuscitation or transport to perform APGAR scoring.

If the infant's respirations are below 30 per minute and tactile stimulation does not increase the rate to a normal range (30–60), immediately assist ventilations using a pediatric bag-valve mask with high-flow oxygen. If the heart rate is below 80 and does not increase in response to ventilations, initiate chest compressions. Transport to a facility with neonatal intensive care capabilities.

12. Describe the management of the mother post-delivery. pp. 781, 784–785, 790

The mother should receive fundal massage to control postpartum bleeding and the perineum should be inspected for tears. Continuously monitor vital signs. If not accomplished prior to delivery, vascular access should be established should fluid resuscitation become necessary.

©2008 Pearson Education, Inc.

13. Describe the procedures for handling abnormal deliveries, complications of pregnancy, and maternal complications of labor. **pp. 773–778, 780–791**

Management of abnormal deliveries or complications of pregnancy and labor require that the EMT-I correctly recognize the problem and expedite transport while anticipating the development of shock and maintaining adequate oxygenation, fluid resuscitation as necessary and, if appropriate, pharmacological intervention. Most of the time, the mother will be transported in the left lateral recumbent position. When the baby's position (breech presentation, prolapsed cord, or limb presentation) dictates, the mother should be placed on oxygen and then assisted in assuming the knee-chest position. Additionally, in the management of prolapsed cord, two gloved fingers should be placed inside the vagina to prevent the baby's weight from compressing the cord and inhibiting oxygen delivery to the baby.

14. Given several simulated delivery situations, provide the appropriate assessment, management, and transport for the mother and child. **pp. 769–791**

Throughout your training, you will encounter a variety of real and simulated obstetric patients. Use the information provided in this chapter, as well as the application of this information as demonstrated by your instructors, preceptors, and mentors to enhance your ability to assess, manage, and transport these patients. Keep in mind that this is likely to be a stressful situation for your patient, and she will appreciate your kind, considerate care and professionalism.

Case Study Review

Reread the case study in Chapter 24 and then read the following discussion. This case study draws attention to the management of childbirth in the prehospital setting. In most cases, the role of the EMS provider in a childbirth situation is merely supportive, as often no "emergency" care is needed.

In this scenario, you are presented with a woman, well along in the second stage of delivery. Her cervix has fully dilated and the infant is moving down the birth canal. The infant is now pushing the tissue surrounding the vaginal opening outward and you can see the infant's head during a forceful contraction. This is called crowning and clearly identifies that the delivery is imminent and you don't have much time to prepare.

The history of three previous deliveries suggests this delivery will progress quickly (the first is usually the slowest). The prenatal care suggests the mother has been well monitored and cared for, preparing just for this moment. Her vital signs are normal given the stress of delivery. As the mother again begins to push crowning is again visible. The head slowly progresses out of the opening as you cradle it and prevent an explosive delivery. This slight pressure prevents rapid decompression of the infant's head and possible brain injury. You are careful to assure you do not put any pressure on the fontenalles.

As the head delivers, you break the amniotic sac and are ready with a bulb syringe to suction the airway. It will only be a few seconds before the infant takes his first breath and you would like to remove as much of the amniotic fluid as you can. The fluid is free of meconium, suggesting there was no fetal distress and the umbilical cord is not wrapped around the neck which would indicate another delivery problem. You guide the rest of the delivery and dry the infant, cover him with a blanket and prepare to cut the cord. You also monitor the mother for excessive post partum hemorrhage, the delivery of the placenta, and any respiratory problems (that might indicate pulmonary emboli). All goes well, and you can't stop smiling.

©2008 Pearson Education, Inc.
Intermediate Emergency Care: 1985, 3rd ed.

Content Self-Evaluation

MULTIPLE CHOICE

______ 1. The structure that supplies circulation to the developing fetus is the
A. uterus.
B. placenta.
C. amniotic fluid.
D. umbilical cord.
E. amniotic sac.

______ 2. All of the following are placental functions EXCEPT
A. acting as the "organ of pregnancy."
B. production of hormones.
C. serving as a protective barrier.
D. providing fertilization.
E. providing a means of heat transfer.

______ 3. Blood volume increases by what percentage during pregnancy?
A. 10%
B. 25%
C. 30%
D. 45%
E. 60%

______ 4. When performing a focused history on a pregnant patient, which of the following questions would be appropriate?
A. Are you experiencing any pain or discomfort?
B. Have you had any vaginal discharge or bleeding?
C. When is your due date?
D. Have you ever been pregnant before?
E. all of the above

______ 5. All of the following are common signs or symptoms of a predelivery emergency EXCEPT
A. abdominal pain or trauma.
B. vaginal bleeding or discharge.
C. painful deformed extremities.
D. altered mental status or seizures.
E. hypertension or hypotension.

______ 6. All of the following are causes of bleeding during pregnancy EXCEPT
A. abortion.
B. ovarian cyst.
C. ectopic pregnancy.
D. placenta previa.
E. abruptio placenta.

______ 7. Treatment of a female patient who is 16 weeks pregnant, is complaining of cramping abdominal pain, and has bright red vaginal bleeding should include all of the following EXCEPT
A. packing the vagina to control bleeding.
B. treating for shock if indicated.
C. maintaining oxygenation.
D. providing emotional support.
E. saving any tissue and clots for evaluation.

______ 8. You suspect the patient in the situation described in question 7 is having a(n)
A. abortion.
B. ovarian cyst.
C. ectopic pregnancy.
D. placenta previa.
E. abruptio placenta.

______ 9. Pelvic inflammatory disease, endometriosis, and tubal ligation are predisposing factors for
A. abortion.
B. ovarian cyst.
C. ectopic pregnancy.
D. placenta previa.
E. abruptio placenta.

©2008 Pearson Education, Inc.

______ 10. You find that your patient is 36 weeks pregnant, has an altered mental status, and is reported to have had a major motor seizure, which you suspect is due to

A. placenta previa.
B. eclampsia.
C. epilepsy.
D. abruptio placenta.
E. supine hypotensive syndrome.

______ 11. Care of the patient in question 10 should include all of the following EXCEPT

A. administering high-flow oxygen via a nonrebreather mask.
B. protecting the patient from injury if seizures recur.
C. minimizing noise and light to prevent seizure activity.
D. administering magnesium sulfate per protocol.
E. transporting on right side to protect airway.

______ 12. There is a significant risk of infection if labor does not begin within 24 hours of the rupture of the membranes.

A. True
B. False

______ 13. All of the following are signs and symptoms of an imminent delivery EXCEPT

A. the presence of crowning.
B. contractions occurring every 1–2 minutes.
C. passage of "bloody show."
D. sensation of an urge for bowel movement.
E. rupture of membranes.

______ 14. The stage of labor that begins with complete cervical dilatation and ends with the delivery of the fetus is called the dilatation stage.

A. True
B. False

______ 15. During delivery the fetal heart rate must be monitored. If it falls below what value should immediate transport of the mother occur?

A. 120
B. 100
C. 90
D. 80
E. 65

______ 16. Elements of the APGAR assessment include appearance, pulse, grimace, activity and respirations.

A. True
B. False

______ 17. Acrocyanosis in the neonate is always a sign of inadequate oxygenation.

A. True
B. False

______ 18. Management of a limb presentation should include all of the following EXCEPT

A. administration of high-flow oxygen to the mother.
B. immediate transport to the hospital.
C. attempting to push the limb back into the vagina.
D. positioning the mother with her head down and pelvis elevated.
E. providing reassurance to the mother.

______ 19. During a breech delivery there is a significant pause between the delivery of the torso and the delivery of the head. During this time you should do which of the following?

A. Clamp and cut the umbilical cord.
B. Insert two fingers into the vagina to open an airway.
C. Pull gently on the feet.
D. Place the mother in the knee-chest position and transport.
E. Wait for up to 10 minutes.

©2008 Pearson Education, Inc.
Intermediate Emergency Care: 1985, 3rd ed.

______ 20. Your patient has just delivered a healthy baby boy. Following the delivery of the placenta, her vaginal bleeding seems to increase. Which of the following best describes what you should do to provide emergency care for this patient?
A. Massage the uterus and position your patient on her right side.
B. Administer oxygen and firmly massage the uterus.
C. Massage the uterus and pack the vagina to control bleeding.
D. Administer oxygen and pack the vagina with sanitary napkins.
E. Provide fluid resuscitation and position patient on her right side.

MATCHING

Write the letter of the definition in the space provided next to the term it describes.

______ 21. amniotic sac

______ 22. ovulation

______ 23. fetus

______ 24. placenta

______ 25. umbilical cord

______ 26. effacement

______ 27. parity

______ 28. placenta and membranes

______ 29. puerperium

A. newborn infant from the third month of pregnancy to birth

B. fetal lifeline, a placental extension through which the child is nourished

C. organ of pregnancy for the exchange of oxygen and waste products

D. transparent membrane forming the sac that holds the fetus

E. release of an egg from the ovary

F. the time period surrounding the birth of the fetus

G. thinning and shortening of the cervix during labor

H. number of pregnancies carried to term

I. afterbirth

©2008 Pearson Education, Inc.

Chapter

25 Neonatal Resuscitation

Review of Chapter Objectives

After reading this chapter, you should be able to do the following:

1. Define newborn and neonate. **p. 795**

A newborn is a baby in the first few hours of its life, also called a *newly born infant*. A neonate is a baby less than one month old.

2. Identify the primary signs utilized for evaluating a newborn during resuscitation. **pp. 796–797**

The newborn should be assessed immediately after birth. The primary signs used for evaluating a newborn during resuscitation include respiratory rate, heart rate, and skin color. The newborn's respiratory rate should average 40–60 breaths per minute. The normal heart rate is between 150 and 180 beats per minute at birth, slowing to 130–140 beats per minute thereafter. A pulse less than 100 beats per minute indicates distress and requires emergency intervention. Some cyanosis of the extremities is common immediately after birth. However, if the newborn is cyanotic in the central part of the body or if peripheral cyanosis persists, the newborn must be treated with 100% oxygen.

3. Identify the appropriate use of the APGAR scale and calculate the APGAR score given various newborn situations. **pp. 796–797**

The APGAR scale—designed for use at 1 and 5 minutes after birth—helps distinguish between newborns who need only routine care and those who need greater assistance. The system also predicts long-term survival. A severely distressed newborn (one with an APGAR score of less than 4) requires immediate resuscitation.

To calculate the APGAR score, a value of 0, 1, or 2 is given for each of the following categories: pulse rate (heart rate), grimace (irritability), activity (muscle tone), and respiratory rate.

4. Discuss the initial steps in resuscitation of a newborn. **pp. 798–807**

Resuscitation of the newborn follows an inverted pyramid. In chronological order, initial steps include drying, warming, positioning, suctioning, and tactical stimulation; administration of supplemental oxygen; bag-valve ventilation; and chest compressions. If these steps fail, advanced measures include intubation and administration of medications.

5. Describe the indications, equipment needed, application, and evaluation of the following management techniques for the newborn in distress.

a. Blow-by oxygen **pp. 800, 804**

Blow-by oxygen—the process of blowing oxygen across a newborn's face—is applied if central cyanosis is present or if the adequacy of ventilations is uncertain. If possible, the oxygen should be warmed and humidified.

©2008 Pearson Education, Inc.

b. Ventilatory assistance **pp. 800–801, 804**

Positive-pressure ventilation should be applied to a newborn if any of the following conditions exist: heart rate less than 100 beats per minute, apnea, or persistence of central cyanosis after administration of supplemental oxygen. A bag-valve-mask unit is the device of choice. A self-inflating bag of appropriate size should be used (450 mL is optimal). If prolonged ventilation is required, it may be necessary to disable the pop-off valve.

c. Chest compressions **pp. 805–806**

Chest compressions should be applied to newborns with heart rates of less than 60 beats per minute or with heart rates between 60 and 80 beats per minute *that do not increase* with 30 seconds of positive-pressure ventilation and supplemental oxygen. Begin chest compressions by encircling the newborn's chest, placing both thumbs on the lower one-third of the sternum. Compress the sternum 1.5 to 2.0 cm (1/2 to 3/4 inch) at a rate of 120 times per minute. Maintain a ratio of 3 compressions to 1 ventilation. Reassess the newborn after 20 cycles of compressions (1-minute intervals). Discontinue compressions if the spontaneous heart rate exceeds 80 beats per minute.

6. Describe the epidemiology, including the incidence, morbidity/mortality, risk factors and prevention strategies, pathophysiology, assessment findings, and management for the following neonatal problems.

a. Meconium aspiration **pp. 808–809**

Meconium-stained amniotic fluid occurs in approximately 10–15 percent of deliveries, mostly in post-term or small-for-gestational-age newborns. Meconium aspiration accounts for a significant proportion of neonatal deaths. Fetal distress and hypoxia can cause meconium to be passed into the amniotic fluid. Either *in utero* or more often with the first breath, thick meconium is aspirated into the lungs, resulting in small airway obstruction and aspiration pneumonia. The infant may have respiratory distress within the first hours, or even the first minutes, of life as evidenced by tachypnea, retraction, grunting, and cyanosis in severely affected newborns. The partial obstruction of some airways may lead to a pneumothorax.

An infant born through thin meconium may not require treatment, but depressed infants born through thick, particulate (pea-soup) meconium-stained fluid should be intubated immediately, prior to the first ventilation. Before stimulating such infants to breathe, apply suction with a meconium aspirator attached to an endotracheal tube. Connect to suction at 100 cc/H_2O or less to remove meconium from the airway. Withdraw the ET tube as suction is applied. It may be necessary to repeat this procedure to clear the airway. The patient should then be taken to a facility that can manage a high-risk neonate.

b. Bradycardia **p. 809**

Bradycardia is most commonly caused by hypoxia in newborns. However, the bradycardia may also be due to several other factors, including increased intracranial pressure, hypothyroidism, or acidosis. In cases of hypoxia, the infant experiences minimal risk if the hypoxia is corrected quickly. In providing treatment, follow the procedures in the inverted pyramid. Resist the inclination to treat the bradycardia with pharmacological measures alone. Keep the newborn warm and transport to the nearest facility.

7. Given several neonatal emergencies, provide the appropriate procedures for assessment, management, and transport. **pp. 796–809**

During your classroom, clinical, and field training, you will assess and develop a management plan for the real and simulated patients you attend. Use the information presented in this chapter, the information on neonatal emergencies in the field provided by your instructors, and the guidance given by your clinical and field preceptors to develop the skills needed to assess, manage, and transport the newborn and neonate patient. Continue to refine these skills once your training ends and you begin your career as an EMT-I.

©2008 Pearson Education, Inc.
Intermediate Emergency Care: 1985, 3rd ed.

Case Study Review

Reread the case study in Chapter 25 and then read the following discussion. This case study draws attention to one of the complications that may occur at an out-of-hospital delivery of a newborn.

In this case, you arrive on scene to attend one patient, a woman who has just gone into labor, and quickly find yourself managing a second patient—a newly born infant who remains blue and limp, even after suctioning. The situation can be highly stressful, especially with the two parents nearby. You recall the steps in the inverted pyramid for resuscitating a distressed newborn. You quickly dry the infant and wrap her in a dry blanket, reducing the life-threatening risk of hypothermia. As you prepare to suction, you remember that you will also need to apply tactile stimulation, either by flicking the soles of the newborn's feet or by gently rubbing her back.

When the baby does not "pink up," many thoughts probably run through your mind. You know, for example, that a prolonged lack of oxygen can cause permanent brain damage—and death. You must immediately provide the patient with oxygen. Again following the inverted pyramid, you administer supplemental oxygen (preferably warmed and humidified) using the "blow-by" method. When the patient's heart rate remains below 100 beats per minute, you begin positive-pressure ventilation with a bag-valve-mask unit.

Because the baby starts breathing spontaneously, you do not have to initiate endotracheal intubation or chest compressions. You might consider using the pulse oximeter to evaluate the neonate's oxygenation. When the baby responds to ventilation with vigorous crying you breathe a sigh of relief and present the new mother with her new daughter. Your calm, professional conduct throughout the call helped reassure the parents—the two other people in your care—of their daughter's safety.

Content Self-Evaluation

Multiple Choice

_____ 1. The APGAR score should be assigned at 1 and 10 minutes after the infant's birth.
A. True
B. False

_____ 2. The most important indicator of neonatal distress is the fetal respiratory rate.
A. True
B. False

_____ 3. EMS units should contain all of the following equipment in their neonatal resuscitation kit EXCEPT a(n)
A. meconium aspirator.
B. laryngoscope with size 3 and 4 blades.
C. device to secure the endotracheal tube.
D. umbilical catheter and 10 mL syringe.
E. DeLee suction trap.

_____ 4. Following the inverted pyramid of neonatal resuscitation, which would be done first?
A. intubation
B. bag-valve-mask ventilations
C. chest compressions
D. drying and warming
E. administration of medications

_____ 5. Which of the following are indications to ventilate the neonate?
A. apnea
B. heart rate less than 100
C. central cyanosis
D. meconium stained amniotic fluid
E. all but D

______ 6. The danger of deep suctioning a newborn is that it can cause a(n)
A. vagal response.
B. increased heart rate.
C. decreased respiratory rate.
D. allergic reaction.
E. tachypnea.

______ 7. Suctioning of a newborn should last no longer than 10 seconds.
A. True
B. False

______ 8. Initiate chest compressions in the neonate who has which of the following conditions?
A. weak cry
B. heart rate of 50
C. blue extremities
D. blue trunk
E. bleeding from the umbilical cord

______ 9. Insertion of an endotracheal tube is recommended when prolonged ventilation of a newborn will be required.
A. True
B. False

______ 10. A dark green material found in the intestine of the full-term newborn is called
A. bile.
B. meconium.
C. mucus.
D. vomitus.
E. hyperbilirubinemia.

Special Project

The APGAR Scale

The APGAR scoring system will help you distinguish between newborns who need only routine care and those who need greater assistance. To gain practice in using this system, complete the following exercises.

Part I

You have just assisted in the delivery of a newborn. Your quick assessment reveals a blue baby with very slow movement of the extremities. Your initial vital signs indicate a slow respiratory rate and a heart rate around 80–90 beats per minute. The infant seems distressed but does not cry when touched. Complete the first 1-minute APGAR score for this infant using the following chart.

©2008 Pearson Education, Inc.
Intermediate Emergency Care: 1985, 3rd ed.

The APGAR Score					
				Score	
Sign	0	1	2	1 min	5 min
Appearance (Skin color)	Blue, pale	Body pink, extremities blue	Completely pink		
Pulse Rate (Heart rate)	Absent	Below 100	Above 100		
Grimace (Irritability)	No response	Grimace	Cries		
Activity (Muscle tone)	Limp	Some flexion of extremities	Active motion		
Respiratory Effort	Absent	Slow and irregular	Strong cry		
			TOTAL SCORE =		

Part II

You have begun to follow the inverted pyramid by drying, warming, positioning, suctioning, and providing tactile stimulation to the newborn. Based upon the inverted pyramid, what would be the next steps if the infant does not "perk up"? Indicate these steps, in the correct order, on the following incomplete diagram.

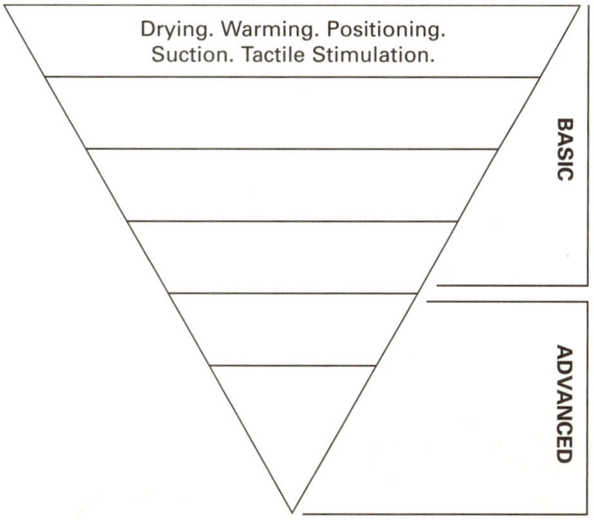

Part III

Fortunately, the stimulation that you provided has been helpful. At this time, both the family and your crew feel immense relief as the infant begins to cry and thrash about. A quick assessment of the vitals reveals a pulse rate well over 100 beats per minute. The infant's body is now pink, but the extremities are still a bit blue. Recalculate the APGAR score, using the chart in Part I, now that 5 minutes have quickly gone by.

Special Considerations

Drying.

Warming.

Positioning.

Suction.

Tactile stimulation.

©2008 Pearson Education, Inc.
Intermediate Emergency Care: 1985, 3rd ed.

Chapter

26 Pediatric Emergencies

Review of Chapter Objectives

After reading this chapter, you should be able to do the following:

1. **Identify the common family responses to acute illness and injury of an infant or child. p. 819**

   As you might expect, the reaction of parents or caregivers to a pediatric emergency will vary. Initial responses by parents or caregivers might include shock, grief, denial, anger, guilt, fear, or complete loss of control. Their behavior may change during the course of the emergency.

2. **Identify key anatomical, physiological, growth, and developmental characteristics of infants and children and their implications. pp. 813–818, 819–823**

   Children are broken into age groups because they differ in terms of anatomical, physiological, growth, and developmental characteristics. The following are some of the differences:

   - **Newborns (first hours after birth).** The term "newborn" refers to a baby in the first hours of extrauterine life. These patients are assessed using the APGAR scoring system, which was described in Chapter 25. Resuscitation of the newborn generally follows the inverted pyramid and the guidelines established in the Neonatal Advanced Life Support (NALS) curriculum.
   - **Neonates (ages birth to 1 month).** The neonate typically loses up to 10 percent of its birth weight as it adjusts to extrauterine life. This lost weight, however, is ordinarily recovered within 10 days. Gestational age affects early growth. Children born at term (40 weeks) should follow accepted developmental guidelines. Infants born prematurely will not be as developed, either neurologically or physically, as their term counterparts.

     The neonatal stage of development centers on reflexes. The neonate's personality also begins to form. Obviously, the history must be obtained from the parents or caregivers. However, it is also important to observe the child. Common illnesses in this age group include jaundice, vomiting, and respiratory distress. The approach to this age group should include several factors. First, the child should always be kept warm. Observe skin color, tone, and respiratory activity. The absence of tears when crying may indicate dehydration. The lungs should be auscultated early during this exam, while the infant is quiet.
   - **Infants (ages 1 to 5 months).** Infants should have doubled their birth weight by 5 to 6 months of age and can follow the movement of others with their eyes. Muscle control develops in a cephalo-caudal ("head-to-tail") progression, with control spreading from the trunk toward the extremities. Although the infant's personality continues to form, it still centers strongly on the parents or caregivers. Concentrate on keeping these patients warm and comfortable, allowing them to remain on the parent's or caregiver's lap, if possible. A pacifier or bottle can be used to help keep the baby quiet during the examination.
   - **Infants (ages 6 to 12 months).** Patients in this age group are active and enjoy exploring the world with their mouths. In this stage of development, the risk of foreign body airway obstruction (FBAO) becomes a serious concern. Infants 6 months and older have more fully formed

©2008 Pearson Education, Inc.

personalities and express themselves more readily than younger babies. They have a considerable anxiety toward strangers. They don't like lying on their backs, and they tend to cling to their mother, though the father "will do." Common illnesses and accidents include febrile seizures, vomiting, diarrhea, dehydration, bronchiolitis, car accidents, croup, child abuse, poisonings, falls, airway obstructions, and meningitis. These children should be examined while sitting in the lap of the parent or caregiver. The exam should progress in a toe-to-head order, since starting at the face may upset the child. If time and conditions permit, allow the child to become familiar with you before beginning the examination.

- **Toddlers (ages 1 to 3 years).** Great strides in gross motor development occur during this stage. Children tend to run underneath or stand on almost anything. As they grow older, toddlers become braver and more curious or stubborn. They begin to stray away from the parents or caregivers more frequently. Yet these remain the only people who can comfort them quickly, and most children will cling to a parent or caregiver if frightened. At ages 1 to 3, language development begins. Although the majority of the history comes from interaction with the parent or caregiver, it is possible to ask the toddler simple questions.

  Be cautious when treating toddlers. Approach toddlers slowly and try to gain their confidence. Conduct the exam in a toe-to-head order. The child may be difficult to examine and may resist being touched. Be sure to tell the child if something will hurt. If at all possible, avoid procedures on the dominant arm/hand, which the child will try to pull away.
- **Preschoolers (ages 3 to 5 years).** Children in this age group show a tremendous increase in fine and gross motor development. Language skills increase greatly. However, if frightened, these children often refuse to speak. They usually have vivid imaginations and may see monsters as part of their world. Preschoolers may have tempers and will express them. During this stage of development, children fear mutilation and may feel threatened by treatment. Avoid frightening or misleading comments. When evaluating a child in this age group, question the child first, keeping in mind that imagination may interfere with the facts. The child often has a distorted sense of time, and thus you must rely on the parents or caregivers to fill in the gaps. Common illnesses and accidents in this age group include croup, asthma, poisonings, auto accidents, burns, child abuse, ingestion of foreign bodies, drownings, epiglottitis, febrile seizures, and meningitis.

  Start the examination with the chest and evaluate the head last. Do not lie or try to trick the patient. Avoid baby talk. If time and situation permit, give the preschooler health care choices.
- **School-age children (ages 6 to 12 years).** School-age children are active and carefree. Growth spurts sometimes lead to clumsiness. The personality continues to develop, and these children are proud and protective of their parents and caregivers. Common illnesses and injuries for this age group include drownings, auto accidents, bicycle accidents, falls, fractures, sports injuries, child abuse, and burns.

  When examining school-age children, give them responsibility for providing the history. However, remember that children may be reluctant to provide information if they sustained an injury while doing something forbidden. The parents or caregivers can fill in the pertinent details. During assessment, respect the modesty of school-age children. Also, remember to be honest and tell the child what is wrong.
- **Adolescents (ages 13 to 18).** Adolescence covers the period from the end of childhood to the start of adulthood (age 18). It begins with puberty, roughly at age 13 for males and 11 for females. Puberty is highly child specific and can begin at various ages. Adolescents vary significantly in their development. Those over age 15 are physically nearer to adults in terms of their vital signs but emotionally may still be children. Regardless of physical maturity, remember that teenagers as a group are "body conscious." The slightest possibility of a lasting scar may be a tremendous issue to the adolescent patient. Common illnesses and injuries in this age group include mononucleosis, asthma, auto collisions, sports injuries, drug and alcohol problems, suicide gestures, and sexual abuse. Remember that pregnancy is also possible in female adolescents.

  In examining an adolescent patient, it may be wise to conduct the interview away from the parents or caregivers. If you must perform a detailed physical exam, respect the teenager's sense of privacy. If the patient exhibits modesty or bodily shame, have an EMT-I of the same sex as the teenager conduct the exam. Although patients in this age group are not legally adults, keep in mind that most of them see themselves as grown up and will take offense at the use of the word "child."

©2008 Pearson Education, Inc.
Intermediate Emergency Care: 1985, 3rd ed.

3. Outline differences in adult and childhood anatomy, physiology, and "normal" age-group-related vital signs. **pp. 819–823, 827**

Anatomical or physiological differences in infants and children as compared with adults include:

- A proportionally larger tongue
- Smaller airway structures
- Abundant secretions
- Deciduous (baby) teeth
- Flatter nose and face
- Head heavier relative to body and less-developed neck structures and muscles
- Fontanelle and open sutures (soft spots) palpable on top of a young infant's head
- Thinner, softer brain tissue
- Head larger in proportion to the body
- Shorter, narrower, more elastic (flexible) trachea
- Shorter neck
- Abdominal breathers with a faster respiratory rate
- In the case of newborns, breathe primarily through the nose (obligate nose breathers)
- Larger body surface relative to their body mass
- Softer bones
- More exposed spleen and liver
- More easily dehydrated
- Less blood and in greater danger of developing severe shock or bleeding to death from a relatively minor wound
- Immature temperature control mechanism (unstable in babies)

Age-related differences in vital signs include:

- Pulse rates (average) by age group:
  —Newborn: 100–180
  —Infant 0–5 months: 100–160
  —Infant 6–12 months: 100–160
  —Toddler 1–3 years: 80–110
  —Preschooler 3–5 years: 80–110
  —School-age child 6–10 years: 65–110
  —Early adolescent 11–14 years: 60–90

- Respiratory rates (average) by age group:
  —Newborn: 30–60
  —Infant 0–5 months: 30–60
  —Infant 6–12 months: 30–60
  —Preschooler 3–5 years: 22–34
  —School-age child 6–10 years: 18–30
  —Early adolescent 11–14 years: 12–26

- Blood pressure (average/mmHg at rest) by age group:

	Systolic Approx. 90 plus 2 × age	*Diastolic Approx. 2/3 systolic*
—Preschooler 3–5 years:	average 98 (78–116)	average 65
—School-age child 6–10 years:	average 105 (80–122)	average 69
—Early adolescent 11–14 years:	average 114 (88–140)	average 76

©2008 Pearson Education, Inc.

4. Describe techniques for successful assessment and treatment of infants and children. pp. 823–848

Many of the components of the initial patient assessment can be done during a visual examination of the scene ("assessment from the doorway"). Whenever possible, involve the parent or caregiver in efforts to calm or comfort the child. Depending on the situation, you may decide to allow the parent or caregiver to remain with the child during treatment and transport. The developmental stage of the patient and the coping skills of the parents or guardians will be key factors in making this decision.

When interacting with parents or other responsible adults, pay attention to the way in which parents or caregivers interact with the child. Are the interactions appropriate to the emergency? Are family members concerned? Are they angry? Are they overly emotional or entirely indifferent?

From the time of dispatch, you will continually acquire information relative to the patient's condition. As with all patients, personal safety must be your first priority. In treating pediatric patients, follow the same guidelines in approaching the scene as you would with any other patient. Observe for potentially hazardous situations, and make sure you take appropriate BSI precautions. Remember that infants and young children are at especially high risk of an infectious process.

5. Discuss normal age-group vital signs and the appropriate equipment used to obtain pediatric vital signs. pp. 824–827

Remember that poorly taken vital signs are of less value than no vital signs at all. Therefore, you must have the correct equipment to obtain pediatric vital signs. Items include appropriate-sized BP cuffs, a pediatric stethoscope, and so on. Modern noninvasive monitoring devices all have their application to emergency care. These devices may include pulse oximeter, capnography, automated blood pressure devices, self-registering thermometers, and ECGs. However, these devices may frighten a child. Before applying any monitoring device, explain what you are going to do and then demonstrate the device.

6. Determine appropriate airway adjuncts, ventilation devices, and endotracheal intubation equipment; their proper use; and complications of use for infants and children. pp. 833–840

As a general rule, use airway adjuncts in pediatric patients only if prolonged artificial ventilations are required. There are two reasons for this. First, infants and children often improve quickly through the administration of 100% oxygen. Second, airway adjuncts may create greater complications in children than in adults.

Keeping this in mind, be sure to have available the appropriate-sized airway adjuncts for each pediatric age group. Basic equipment includes oral and nasal airways, a pediatric BVM, smaller-sized suction catheters, smaller-sized masks for the BVM, age-appropriate nasogastric tubes, and a pediatric laryngoscope, blades, and endotracheal tubes. It is also a good idea to carry a Broselow® tape, which, after measuring the child's height, displays the appropriate sizes of tubes.

The biggest complication of airway management for the pediatric patient is the possibility of overinflation, which allows air to gather in the stomach. Gastric distention can cause pressure on the diaphragm, making full expansion of the lungs difficult. For specific techniques in airway management in the pediatric patient, review the steps and scans in the textbook, especially those dealing with advanced airway and ventilatory management.

7. List the indications and methods of gastric decompression for infants and children. pp. 840, 841

If gastric distention is present in a pediatric patient, you may consider placing a nasogastric tube (NG tube). In infants and children, gastric distention may result from overly aggressive artificial ventilations or from air swallowing. Placement of an NG tube will allow you to decompress the stomach and the proximal bowel of air. An NG tube can also be used to empty the stomach of blood or other substances. Indications for use of nasogastric intubation include an inability to achieve adequate tidal volumes during ventilation due to gastric distention and the presence of gastric distention in an unresponsive patient.

©2008 Pearson Education, Inc.
Intermediate Emergency Care: 1985, 3rd ed.

As with nasopharyngeal airways, an NG tube is contraindicated in pediatric patients who have sustained head or facial trauma. Because the NG tube might migrate into the cranial sinuses, consider the use of an orogastric tube instead. Other contraindications include possible soft-tissue damage in the nose and inducement of vomiting.

In determining the correct length of NG tube, measure the tube from the top of the nose, over the ear, to the tip of the xiphoid process. To insert an NG tube, you should:

- Oxygenate and continue to ventilate, if possible.
- Measure the NG tube from the tip of the nose, over the ear, to the tip of the xiphoid process.
- Lubricate the end of the tube. Then pass it gently downward along the nasal floor to the stomach.
- Auscultate over the epigastrium to confirm correct placement. Listen for bubbling while injecting 10–20 cc of air into the tube.
- Use suction to aspirate stomach contents.
- Secure the tube in place.

8. Define and discuss the pathophysiology and assessment findings associated with pediatric respiratory distress, failure, and arrest. pp. 848–849

The severity of respiratory compromise can be quickly classified into the following categories:

- **Respiratory distress.** The mildest form of respiratory impairment is classified as respiratory distress. The most noticeable finding is the increased work of breathing. The signs and symptoms of respiratory distress include a normal mental status deteriorating to irritability or anxiety, tachypnea, retractions, nasal flaring (in infants), good muscle tone, head bobbing, grunting, and cyanosis that improves with supplemental oxygen. If not corrected immediately, respiratory distress will lead to respiratory failure.
- **Respiratory failure.** Respiratory failure occurs when the respiratory system is not able to meet the demands of the body for oxygen intake and for carbon dioxide removal. It is characterized by inadequate ventilation and oxygenation. During respiratory failure, the carbon dioxide level begins to rise as the body is not able to remove it. This ultimately leads to respiratory acidosis. The signs and symptoms of respiratory failure include irritability or anxiety deteriorating to lethargy, marked tachypnea later deteriorating to bradypnea, marked retractions later deteriorating to agonal respirations, poor muscle tone, marked tachycardia later deteriorating to bradycardia, and central cyanosis. Respiratory failure is a very ominous sign. If immediate intervention is not provided, the child will deteriorate to full respiratory arrest.
- **Respiratory arrest.** The end result of respiratory impairment, if untreated, is respiratory arrest. The cessation of breathing typically follows a period of bradypnea and agonal respirations. The signs and symptoms of respiratory arrest include unresponsiveness deteriorating to coma, bradypnea deteriorating to apnea, absent chest wall movement, bradycardia deteriorating to asystole, and profound cyanosis. Respiratory arrest will quickly deteriorate to full cardiopulmonary arrest if appropriate interventions are not made. The child's chances of survival markedly decrease when cardiopulmonary arrest occurs.

9. Describe the general approach to the treatment of children with respiratory distress, failure, or arrest from upper or lower airway disease. pp. 848–854

The general approach to the child with respiratory distress or failure from an upper or lower airway problem is to assess the child in the least stressful way possible and to administer oxygen. If the child has a complete upper airway obstruction, the appropriate FBAO maneuvers will need to be quickly done. If the child is in respiratory arrest, begin BVM resuscitation and consider the need for ET tube insertion. An NG tube may be useful to minimize gastric distention. If the child is in respiratory failure, assisted ventilations should also be considered.

When treating lower airway diseases, the primary goal is to support ventilations through the use of supplemental, humidified oxygen and appropriate pharmacological therapy such as bronchodilator medications (asthma and bronchiolitis). If prolonged ventilation will be required, perform endotracheal intubation.

©2008 Pearson Education, Inc.

10. Describe the epidemiology, including the incidence, morbidity/mortality risk factors, preventive strategies, pathophysiology, assessment, and treatment of infants and children with:

a. Croup **pp. 849–851**

Croup (or laryngotracheobronchitis) is a viral infection of the upper airway affecting children of 6 months to 4 years of age, most commonly in the fall and winter months. The child will have a barking cough secondary to inflammation and swelling of the tissues just beneath the glottis and larynx. In the evening the child develops a harsh barking cough with inspiratory stridor, nasal flaring, and tracheal tugging. Management is supportive with calming and reassurance to both the child and parents. Administer oxygen, preferably with a cool water mist and racemic epinephrine or albuterol, as per physician order.

b. Epiglottitis **pp. 851–852**

Epiglottitis presents similarly to croup and occurs usually at night. The child awakens with a high fever and brassy cough. There is often pain on swallowing, sore throat, dyspnea, inspiratory stridor, and drooling. Do not attempt to visualize the airway as the procedure may result in complete airway obstruction. Management includes reduction of the child's anxiety and blow-by oxygen, humidified if possible. Do not attempt intubation unless absolutely necessary and then be prepared to use a tube somewhat smaller than otherwise indicated. The airway will be restricted by the glottic swelling.

c. Bronchiolitis **p. 852**

Bronchiolitis is a contagious viral infection affecting the medium-sized airways and most often occurs in early childhood. It resembles asthma and presents with an expiratory wheeze in children under 2 years of age. Management is much the same as with asthma: reassurance, blow-by, humidified oxygen, and albuterol.

d. Pneumonia **pp. 852–853**

Pneumonia is an infectious disease affecting the lower airways and lungs of pediatric patients between 1 and 5 years old. The child will often present with a history of respiratory infection, low-grade fever, decreased breath sounds, crackles, and chest pain. Management is basically supportive with emphasis on patient comfort and reassurance, oxygen, and bag-valve-masking as necessary.

e. Asthma **pp. 853–854**

Asthma is a chronic inflammation of the lower respiratory tract and is usually associated with allergies. It is associated with bronchospasm and excessive mucus production that obstructs airflow. The lungs become progressively hyperinflated, which reduces vital capacity and gas exchange in the alveoli. Asthma is often recognized by patient history, though it can be difficult to differentiate from other pediatric respiratory disease. The patient is often sitting bolt upright and using the accessory muscles of respiration. Wheezing is often present, though in a severe attack, air exchange may be so compromised that it and respiratory sounds may be absent. Management includes calming and reassurance, the administration of high-flow/high-concentration oxygen, and an inhaled beta agonist. Status asthmaticus is a serious and prolonged asthma attack that cannot be broken by pharmacologic means. It is a serious event that often precedes respiratory arrest.

f. Shock (hypoperfusion) **pp. 854–856**

The second major cause of pediatric cardiopulmonary arrest—after respiratory impairment—is shock. Shock can most simply be defined as inadequate perfusion of the tissues with oxygen and other essential nutrients and inadequate removal of metabolic waste products.

When compared with the incidence of shock in adults, shock is an unusual occurrence in children because their blood vessels constrict so efficiently. However, when the blood pressure does drop, it drops so far and so fast that the child may quickly develop cardiopulmonary arrest. A number of factors place infants and young children at risk for shock. Newborns and neonates will develop shock as a result of a loss of body heat. Other causes include dehydration (from vomiting and/or diarrhea), infection (particularly septicemia), trauma, and blood loss. Less common causes of shock in infants and children include allergic reactions, poisoning, and cardiac events.

As in adults, the severity of shock in a pediatric patient is classified as compensated shock, decompensated shock, and irreversible shock. It can also be categorized as *cardiogenic* or

©2008 Pearson Education, Inc.
Intermediate Emergency Care: 1985, 3rd ed.

noncardiogenic. Cardiogenic shock results from an inability of the heart to maintain an adequate cardiac output to the circulatory tissues. Cardiogenic shock in a pediatric patient is ominous and often fatal. Noncardiogenic shock—types of shock that result from causes other than inadequate cardiac output—is more frequently encountered in pediatric patients, because they have a much lower incidence of cardiac problems than adults. Causes of noncardiogenic shock may include hemorrhage, abdominal trauma, systemic bacterial infection, spinal cord injury, and others.

The definitive care of shock takes place in the emergency department of a hospital. Because shock is a life-threatening condition in pediatric patients, it is important to recognize early signs and symptoms—or even the possibility of shock in a situation where the signs and symptoms may not have yet developed. In a situation in which you suspect a possibility of shock, provide oxygen to boost tissue perfusion and transport as quickly as possible. Also, keep the patient in a supine position and take steps to protect the child from hypothermia and agitation that might worsen the condition. In some cases (compensated shock), fluid therapy as ordered by medical direction can buy time until the patient arrives at an appropriate treatment center.

g. Dysrhythmias including tachydysrhythmias, bradydysrhythmias, and arrest **pp. 856–858, 859–860**

Dysrhythmias in children are uncommon. When dysrhythmias occur, bradydysrhythmias are the most common. Supraventricular tachydysrhythmias are very uncommon. Dysrhythmias can cause pump failure, ultimately leading to cardiogenic shock. Children have a very limited capacity to increase stroke volume. The primary mechanism through which they increase cardiac output is through changes in the heart rate. The treatment of dysrhythmias is specific for the dysrhythmia in question.

h. Seizures **pp. 861–862**

The etiology for seizures is often unknown. However, several risk factors have been identified. They include fever, hypoxia, infections, idiopathic epilepsy (epilepsy of unknown origin), electrolyte disturbances, head trauma, hypoglycemia, toxic ingestions or exposure, tumor, or CNS malformations. Management of pediatric seizure is essentially the same as for the seizing adult. Place patients on the floor or on the bed. Be sure to lay them on their side, away from furniture. Do not restrain patients, but take steps to protect them from injury. Maintain the airway, but do not force anything, such as a bite stick, between the teeth. Administer supplemental oxygen. Then take and record all vital signs. If the patient is febrile, remove excess layers of clothing, while avoiding extreme cooling. If status epilepticus is present, institute the following steps:

- Start an IV of normal saline or lactated Ringer's and perform a glucometer evaluation.

Administer dextrose if the patient is hypoglycemic

- Administer diazepam as follows:
  —*Children 1 month to 5 years:* 0.2–0.5 mg slow IV push every 2–5 minutes up to a maximum of 2.5 milligrams.
  —*Children 5 years and older:* 1 mg slow IV push every 2–5 minutes to a maximum of 5 milligrams.
- Contact medical direction for additional dosing. Diazepam can be administered rectally if an IV cannot be established.
- If the seizure appears to be due to a fever and a long transport time is anticipated, medical direction may request the administration of acetaminophen to lower the fever. Acetaminophen is supplied as an elixir or as suppositories. The dose should be 15 mg/kg body weight.

i. Meningitis **pp. 862–863**

Meningitis is a bacterial or viral infection of the covering of the brain and spinal cord. It is more common in children than adults. The child or infant will appear very ill and will show discomfort with any movement as well as headache or stiff neck (not in infants), recent ear or respiratory infection, and high fever. Care is supportive with standard precautions.

j. Gastrointestinal conditions **p. 863**

Childhood gastrointestinal problems most commonly present with nausea, vomiting, and diarrhea. They represent fluid loss and dehydration. Care is supportive and fluid resuscitation (20 mL/kg) as needed.

©2008 Pearson Education, Inc.

k. Poisoning and toxic exposure **pp. 864–865**

Children account for the majority of poisonings (usually toddlers and preschoolers). Signs and symptoms vary though a thorough history may be helpful. General steps of care include maintaining the airways and oxygen, ventilating, as necessary activated charcoal, and transport with any evidence available.

l. Trauma emergencies, including injuries to the head, neck, chest, abdomen, and extremities and burns **pp. 865–873**

Trauma is the number one cause of death in infants and children. Most pediatric injuries result from blunt trauma. Children have thinner body walls that allow forces to be more readily transmitted to body contents, increasing the possibility of injury to internal tissues and organs. If you serve in an urban area, you can expect to see a higher incidence of penetrating trauma, mostly intentional and mostly from gunfire or knife wounds. There is also a significant incidence of penetrating trauma outside the cities (mostly unintentional) from hunting accidents and agricultural accidents.

Although pediatric patients can be injured in the same way as adults, children tend to be more susceptible to certain types of injuries than grownups. Falls, for example, are the single most common cause of injury in children. Other mechanisms of injury include motor vehicle collisions, car vs. pedestrian collisions, drownings and near drownings, penetrating injuries, burns, and physical abuse.

The treatment of trauma is injury specific. It involves management of the ABCS, management of the injury (e.g., spinal immobilization, splinting of fractures, control of bleeding), and treatment for possible shock.

Burn injuries are the leading cause of death in the home for children under 14 years of age. Burns in children are assessed as for adults except that the child's surface area to body weight is increased and the child's fluid reserves are decreased. Therefore, the burn injuries are more serious in children than adults due to this factor.

m. Abuse or neglect **pp. 874–877**

Child abuse is the second leading cause of death in infants less than 6 months of age. An estimated 1,200 children die each year as a result of abuse or neglect. There are several characteristics common among abused children. Often the child is seen as "special" and different from others. Premature infants and twins stand a higher risk of abuse than other children. Many abused children are less than 5 years of age. Physically and mentally handicapped children as well as those with special needs are at greater risk. So are uncommunicative children. Boys are more often abused than girls. A child who is not what the parents wanted (e.g., the "wrong" gender) is at increased risk of abuse, too.

Signs of abuse or neglect can be startling. As a guide, the following findings should trigger a high index of suspicion:

- Any obvious or suspected fractures in a child under 2 years of age
- Injuries in various stages of healing, especially burns and bruises
- More injuries than usually seen in children of the same age or size
- Injuries scattered on many areas of the body
- Bruises or burns in patterns that suggest intentional infliction
- Increased intracranial pressure in an infant
- Suspected intra-abdominal trauma in a young child
- Any injury that does not fit with the description of the cause given

Information in the medical history may also raise the index of suspicion. Examples include:

- A history that does not match the nature or severity of the injury
- Vague parental accounts or accounts that change during the interview
- Accusations that the child injured himself or herself intentionally
- Delay in seeking help
- Child dressed inappropriately for the situation
- Revealing comment by bystanders, especially siblings

Suspect child neglect if you spot any of the following conditions:

- Extreme malnutrition
- Multiple insect bites

©2008 Pearson Education, Inc.
Intermediate Emergency Care: 1985, 3rd ed.

- Long-standing skin infections
- Extreme lack of cleanliness
- Verbal or social skills far below those you would expect for a child of similar age and background
- Lack of appropriate medical care

In cases of child abuse or neglect, the goals of management include appropriate treatment of injuries, protection of the child from further abuse, and notification of proper authorities.

n. Children with special needs, including children dependent on various technological devices **pp. 877–881**

For most of human history, infants and children with devastating congenital conditions or diseases died or remained confined to a hospital. In recent decades, however, medical technology has lowered infant mortality rates and allowed a greater number of children with special needs to live at home. Some of these infants and children include:

- Premature babies
- Infants and children with lung disease, heart disease, or neurological disorders
- Infants and children with chronic diseases, such as cystic fibrosis, asthma, childhood cancers, cerebral palsy, and others
- Infants and children with altered functions from birth (e.g., spina bifida, congenital birth defects, and cerebral palsy)

On some calls, you may be asked to treat technology-assisted children who depend, in varying degrees, upon special equipment. Commonly found devices include tracheostomy tubes, apnea monitors, home artificial ventilators, central intravenous lines, gastric feeding tubes, gastrostomy tubes, and shunts.

In treating pediatric patients with special needs, remember that they require the same assessment as other patients. (Recall that in the initial assessment, "disability" refers to a patient's neurological status—not to the child's special need.) Keep in mind that the child's special need is often an ongoing process, which may make the parent or caregiver an excellent source of information. In most cases, you should concentrate on the acute problem—the reason for the call. In managing patients with special needs, try to keep several thoughts in mind.

- Avoid using the term "disability" (in reference to the child's special need). Instead, think of the patient's many abilities.
- Never assume that the patient cannot understand what you are saying.
- Involve the parents, caregivers, or the patient, if appropriate, in treatment. They manage the illness or congenital condition on a daily basis.
- Treat the patient with a special need with the same respect as any other patient.

11. Discuss the primary etiologies of cardiopulmonary arrest in infants and children. **pp. 824, 849, 858**

The primary causes of cardiopulmonary arrest in infants and children include untreated respiratory failure, immaturity of the cardiac conductive system, bradycardia, hypoxia, vagal stimulation (rare), drug overdose, drowning, multiple system trauma, electrocution, pericardial tamponade, tension pneumothorax, acidosis, hypothermia, hypoglycemia, and FBAO.

12. Discuss basic cardiac life support (CPR) guidelines for infants and children. **pp. 831–836**

See the current CPR guidelines for infants and children at the Brady website at: www.bradybooks.com will provide a link to the most up-to-date information on these standards.

13. Discuss age-appropriate sites, equipment, techniques, and complications of vascular access and fluid therapy for infants and children. **pp. 846, 870**

Intravenous techniques for children are basically the same as for adults. (See Chapter 10, "Fluids and Shock.") However, additional veins may be accessed in an infant. These include veins of the neck and scalp, as well as of the arms, hands, and feet. The external jugular vein, however, should only be used in life-threatening situations.

©2008 Pearson Education, Inc.

The use of intraosseous (IO) infusion has become popular in the pediatric patient. This is especially true when large volumes of fluid must be administered, as occurs in hypovolemic shock, and when other means of venous access are unavailable. The indications for IO include the existence of shock or cardiac arrest, an unresponsive patient, or an unsuccessful attempt at a peripheral IV insertion. The contraindications for IO infusion include the presence of a fracture in the bone chosen for infusion and a fracture of the pelvis or extremity fracture in the bone proximal to the chosen site.

In performing IO perfusion, you can use a standard 16- or 18-gauge needle (either hypodermic or spinal). However, an intraosseous needle is preferred and significantly better. Basic steps are as follows: Prep the anterior surface of the leg below the knee with antiseptic solution (povidone iodine), and insert the needle in twisting fashion 1–3 centimeters below the tuberosity. Insertion should be slightly inferior in direction (to avoid the growth plate) and perpendicular to the skin. Signs of correct placement of the needle into the marrow cavity include a lack of resistance as the needle passes through the bony cortex, the ability of the needle to stand upright without support, the ability to aspirate bone marrow into a syringe, or free flow of the infusion without infiltration into the subcutaneous tissues.

14. Identify common lethal mechanisms of injury in infants and children. **pp. 865–868**

The most common pediatric mechanisms of injury (MOI) include falls, motor vehicle crashes, car vs. pedestrian collisions, drownings and near drownings, penetrating injuries, burns, and physical abuse.

15. Discuss anatomical features of children that predispose or protect them from certain injuries. **pp. 871–872**

Head. Small children have larger heads in proportion to the rest of their bodies. For this reason, when they fall or are thrown through the air, they often land head first, predisposing them to serious head injury. The larger relative mass of the head and lack of neck muscle strength also provide increased momentum in acceleration-deceleration injuries and a greater stress on the cervical spine. Because the skull is softer and more compliant in infants and young children than in adults, brain injuries occur more readily.

Chest and abdomen. Infants and young children lack the rigid rib cages of adults. Therefore, they suffer fewer rib fractures and more intrathoracic injuries. Remember that chest injuries are the second most common cause of pediatric trauma death. Because of the compliance of the chest wall, severe intrathoracic injury can be present without signs of external injury. Likewise, their relatively underdeveloped abdominal musculature affords minimal protection to the viscera, particularly the spleen.

Extremities. Because children have more flexible bones than adults, they tend to have incomplete fractures such as bend fractures, buckle fractures, and greenstick fractures. Therefore, you should treat "sprains" and "strains" as fractures and immobilize accordingly. In younger children, the bone growth plates have not yet closed. Some growth plate fractures can lead to permanent disability if not managed correctly.

Body surface area. There are three distinguishing features of the pediatric patient's skin and BSA. First, the skin of an infant or child is thinner than that of an adult. Second, infants and children generally have less subcutaneous fat. Finally, they have a larger body-surface-area-to-weight ratio. As a result of these features, children risk greater injury from extremes in temperature or thermal exposure. They lose fluids and heat more quickly than adults and have a greater likelihood of dehydration and hypothermia. They also burn more easily and deeper than adults, which explains why burns are one of the leading causes of death among pediatric trauma patients.

16. Describe aspects of infant and child airway management that are affected by potential cervical spine injury. **pp. 868–870**

An infant's open airway is in the neutral or extended position but not in the hyperextended position. This needs to be kept in mind when positioning the infant who may have sustained a neck injury where there can be little to no movement of the neck for fear of worsening the potential neck injury. Children under the age of 6 usually have large heads in proportion to the rest of their bodies. Therefore, it is often necessary to pad behind the shoulders when a cervical collar is applied as a part of the spinal immobilization. Keep infants, toddlers, and preschoolers with the cervical spine in a neutral in-line position by placing padding from the shoulders to the hips.

©2008 Pearson Education, Inc.
Intermediate Emergency Care: 1985, 3rd ed.

Always make sure that you use appropriate-sized pediatric immobilization equipment. These supplies may include rigid cervical collars, towel or blanket rolls, foam head blocks, commercial pediatric immobilization devices, vest-type or short wooden backboards, and long boards with the appropriate padding.

17. Given several preprogrammed simulated pediatric patients, provide the appropriate assessment, treatment, and transport. **pp. 823–881**

During your classroom, clinical, and field training, you will be presented with real and simulated pediatric patients and assess and treat them. Use the information provided in this chapter and the information and skills you gain from your instructors and clinical and field preceptors to develop your skill for caring for these patients. Continue to refine newly learned skills once your training ends and you begin your EMT-I career.

Case Study Review

Reread the case study in Chapter 26 and then read the following discussion. This case study examines the treatment of a severely dehydrated pediatric patient—a common condition encountered on calls involving infants and young children.

This case involves an infant who has been unable to hold down any food for three days. In just a short time, she has developed signs and symptoms that point to possible severe dehydration, which the EMT-Is immediately notice. Their initial assessment starts as soon they observe the quality of the baby's skin (pale, cool, clammy) and the noticeably sunken anterior fontanelle. As the EMT-Is take vital signs and assess the level of consciousness, they note that the baby cries but does not produce tears. After taking appropriate standard precautions, they wisely check the infant's diaper to see if it is dry or wet. (If it had been wet, they would have checked the quality of the urine. Dehydrated patients, when they do urinate, have very dark yellow urine because it is a concentrated solute with less solvent [water] than usual.) The dry diaper and the mother's comment confirms a suspicion of dehydration, giving the crew enough information to develop a treatment plan.

The EMT-Is take this patient very seriously and begin transport before starting fluid therapy. En route to the hospital, they start an IV, which is not always an easy task in a patient this small. They keep in mind the use of an intraosseous needle in case an IV cannot be placed. For a patient this dehydrated, it would not be surprising that she might have needed a second bolus of 20 mL/kg of the normal saline. Of course, as is always the case, a parent should be nearby to assist in comforting the patient.

During your EMT-I career, you can expect to take part in a call similar to this one. Dehydration in infants and small children is a common condition, and you should be prepared to respond, assess, and manage the patient accordingly. Remember that dehydration is one of the causes of hypoperfusion (shock) in pediatric patients.

Content Self-Evaluation

Multiple Choice

______ 1. The leading cause of death in pediatric patients in the United States is
- A. AIDS
- B. asthma.
- C. trauma.
- D. neglect.
- E. cardiac arrest.

______ 2. The term neonate describes a baby that is
- A. newly born.
- B. 10 days or less in age.
- C. up to 1 month in age.
- D. 1 to 5 months in age.
- E. 6 months or more in age.

©2008 Pearson Education, Inc.

______ 3. The age group for which foreign body airway obstruction (FBAO) becomes a concern is
A. infants ages 1–5 months.
B. infants ages 6–12 months.
C. toddlers.
D. preschoolers.
E. school-age children.

______ 4. The pediatric airway differs from that of an adult in all of the following ways EXCEPT that it
A. is narrower at all levels.
B. has a softer and more flexible trachea.
C. is less likely to be blocked by secretions.
D. has a greater likelihood of soft-tissue injury.
E. is more prone to obstruction by the tongue.

______ 5. In comparing pediatric heart and respiratory rates with those of an adult, infants and young children have
A. about the same heart and respiratory rates as an adult.
B. slower heart rates and slower respiratory rates.
C. slower heart rates and faster respiratory rates.
D. faster heart rates and slower respiratory rates.
E. faster heart rates and faster respiratory rates.

______ 6. Unlike an adult, the trachea of a child can collapse if the neck and head are hyperextended because
A. the trachea is softer and more flexible.
B. a child's tongue takes up more space proportionately.
C. the cricoid rings are firmer.
D. a child's larynx is higher.
E. the airway is wider at all levels.

______ 7. The two abdominal organs that are most likely to suffer traumatic injury in a pediatric patient are the
A. kidney and gallbladder.
B. liver and spleen.
C. stomach and small intestine.
D. colon and appendix.
E. bladder and pancreas.

______ 8. A child's larger body-surface-area-to-weight ratio causes a pediatric patient to be
A. resilient to temperature changes.
B. prone to hypothermia.
C. difficult to assess.
D. prone to excess subcutaneous fat.
E. less likely to lose fluids quickly.

______ 9. Although infants and children have a circulating blood volume proportionately larger than adults, their absolute blood volume is
A. about the same.
B. smaller.
C. even larger.
D. rate dependent.
E. variable.

______ 10. The pediatric assessment triangle focuses on airway, breathing, and circulation.
A. True
B. False

______ 11. In an infant or small child, tachypnea, an abnormally rapid rate of breathing, may indicate
A. fear.
B. pain.
C. inadequate oxygenation.
D. exposure to cold (neonate).
E. all of the above

______ 12. A respiratory rate of 18–30 breaths per minute would be considered normal for a(n)
A. newborn.
B. 6-month-old infant.
C. toddler.
D. preschooler.
E. school-age child.

©2008 Pearson Education, Inc.
Intermediate Emergency Care: 1985, 3rd ed.

______ 13. Which of the following approaches is the correct method for conducting the physical examination of a younger child?
A. toe-to-head
B. head-to-chest
C. head-to-toe
D. chest-to-head
E. A and B

______ 14. To obtain the blood pressure of a pediatric patient, the cuff should be ______ the width of the patient's arm.
A. one-fourth
B. one-third
C. one-half
D. two-thirds
E. three-fourths

______ 15. The hallmark of pediatric management is
A. frequent pulse checks.
B. prompt transport.
C. administration of fluids.
D. adequate oxygenation.
E. diagnosis of medical conditions.

______ 16. As a rule, an oropharyngeal airway should only be used on pediatric patients who
A. have sustained head or facial trauma.
B. are known to suffer from seizures.
C. show signs of cardiac arrest.
D. exhibit a vagal response.
E. lack a gag reflex.

______ 17. An indication to perform abdominal thrusts in the pediatric patient is
A. conscious patient.
B. desire to suction the airway.
C. a severe airway obstruction.
D. desire to ventilate by a BVM.
E. both A and C

______ 18. Indications for performing an endotracheal intubation in a pediatric patient include all of the following EXCEPT the
A. need to relieve gastric distension.
B. necessity of providing a route for drug administration.
C. need for prolonged artificial ventilations.
D. failure to provide adequate ventilations with a BVM.
E. cardiac or respiratory arrest.

______ 19. The optimal positioning of the head for pediatric intubation in the absence of a spinal injury is
A. neutral.
B. hyperextended.
C. sniffing.
D. head-tilt.
E. spine.

______ 20. If gastric distention is present in a non-responsive pediatric patient, an EMT-I might consider placing a(n)
A. oropharyngeal airway.
B. nasopharyngeal airway.
C. needle cricothyrotomy.
D. nasogastric tube.
E. endotracheal tube.

______ 21. In obtaining vascular access in a pediatric patient, the external jugular vein should only be used in life-threatening situations.
A. True
B. False

______ 22. The indications for use of intraosseous infusion include all of the following EXCEPT
A. a patient less than 5 years old.
B. existence of shock or cardiac arrest.
C. presence of a pelvic fracture.
D. an unresponsive patient.
E. failure to place a peripheral IV.

©2008 Pearson Education, Inc.

______ 23. You are more likely to use electrical therapy on pediatric patients than adult patients.
A. True
B. False

______ 24. All of the following are symptoms of epiglottitis EXCEPT
A. a rapid onset.
B. occasional stridor.
C. a barking cough.
D. drooling.
E. a fever of approximately 102–104°F.

______ 25. In treating a patient with epiglottitis, an EMT-I should
A. take blood pressure regularly.
B. attempt to visualize the oropharynx.
C. take the child's temperature orally.
D. place the child in a supine position.
E. none of the above

______ 26. Common causes of lower airway distress include all of the following EXCEPT
A. pneumonia.
B. asthma.
C. croup.
D. bronchiolitis.
E. status asthmaticus.

______ 27. When a child experiences a severe asthma attack without wheezing, this is
A. an ominous sign.
B. because of a lack of expectorant.
C. a sign of improvement.
D. because of an inability to cough.
E. common, and should not alarm the EMT-I.

______ 28. All of the following are signs and symptoms of shock in a child EXCEPT
A. pale, cool, clammy skin.
B. impaired mental status.
C. absence of tears when crying.
D. increased urination.
E. a rapid respiratory rate.

______ 29. Cardiogenic shock is more frequently encountered in prehospital pediatric care than hypovolemic shock.
A. True
B. False

______ 30. When dysrhythmias do occur in children, the most common form is a(n)
A. bradydysrhythmia.
B. supraventricular tachydysrhythmia.
C. ventricular tachydysrhythmia.
D. asystole.
E. ventricular fibrillation.

______ 31. A pediatric patient is seen by an EMT-I for a seizure. Assessment and history reveal that the child has a fever of 103°F, with a headache, was very sleepy and irritable before the seizure, and has had no similar episodes. The child complained of a stiff neck and headache earlier in the day. You suspect that the episode may have been caused by
A. febrile convulsions.
B. meningitis.
C. hypoglycemia.
D. hypoxia.
E. hyperglycemia.

______ 32. The single most common cause of trauma-related injuries in children is:
A. motor-vehicle collisions.
B. burns.
C. falls.
D. physical abuse.
E. drownings.

______ 33. Appropriate-sized pediatric immobilization equipment includes all of the following EXCEPT
A. towel or blanket roll.
B. vest-type device (KED).
C. sandbag.
D. straps and cravats.
E. padding.

©2008 Pearson Education, Inc.
Intermediate Emergency Care: 1985, 3rd ed.

______ 34. The normal first bolus of fluid for a pediatric patient is
A. 5 mL/kg.
B. 10 mL/kg.
C. 20 mL/kg.
D. 30 mL/kg.
E. 250 mL.

______ 35. A moderate brain injury in a pediatric patient would likely have a Glasgow coma score of:
A. 15.
B. 10.
C. 3.
D. 8.
E. none of the above

______ 36. When intubating the pediatric patient with head injury, consider the use of lidocaine to reduce the rise in intracranial pressure associated with the procedure.
A. True
B. False

______ 37. If a pediatric patient suffer burns that involve an area equal to about three of their palms, the approximate body surface involved is
A. 1%.
B. 2%.
C. 10%.
D. 3%.
E. 15%.

______ 38. Child abuse can take the form of
A. psychological abuse.
B. physical abuse.
C. sexual abuse.
D. neglect.
E. all of the above

______ 39. In cases of suspected child abuse, management goals include all of the following EXCEPT
A. protection of the child from further injury.
B. notification of proper authorities.
C. appropriate treatment of injuries.
D. cross-examination of the parents or caregivers.
E. documentation of all findings and statements.

______ 40. A surgical connection that runs from the brain to the abdomen in a pediatric patient is called a(n)
A. central IV.
B. tracheostomy.
C. shunt.
D. inner cannula.
E. epigastric tube.

Special Project

Burn Injuries

Burn injuries are the leading cause of accidental death in the home for children under 14 years of age. As with other assessment tools, you must modify the "rule of nines" to estimate the extent of a burn in a pediatric patient. Read the following short patient description and complete the diagram on the following page. Then answer the questions that follow.

You have been called to the scene of a fire at a single-family residence. The dispatcher tells you that a two-year-old female patient has been critically burned. Upon arrival at the scene, first responders with the fire department lead you to the little girl. They report that the patient has full-thickness burns on the entire right arm, entire right leg, and the anterior trunk.

©2008 Pearson Education, Inc.

THE RULE OF NINES

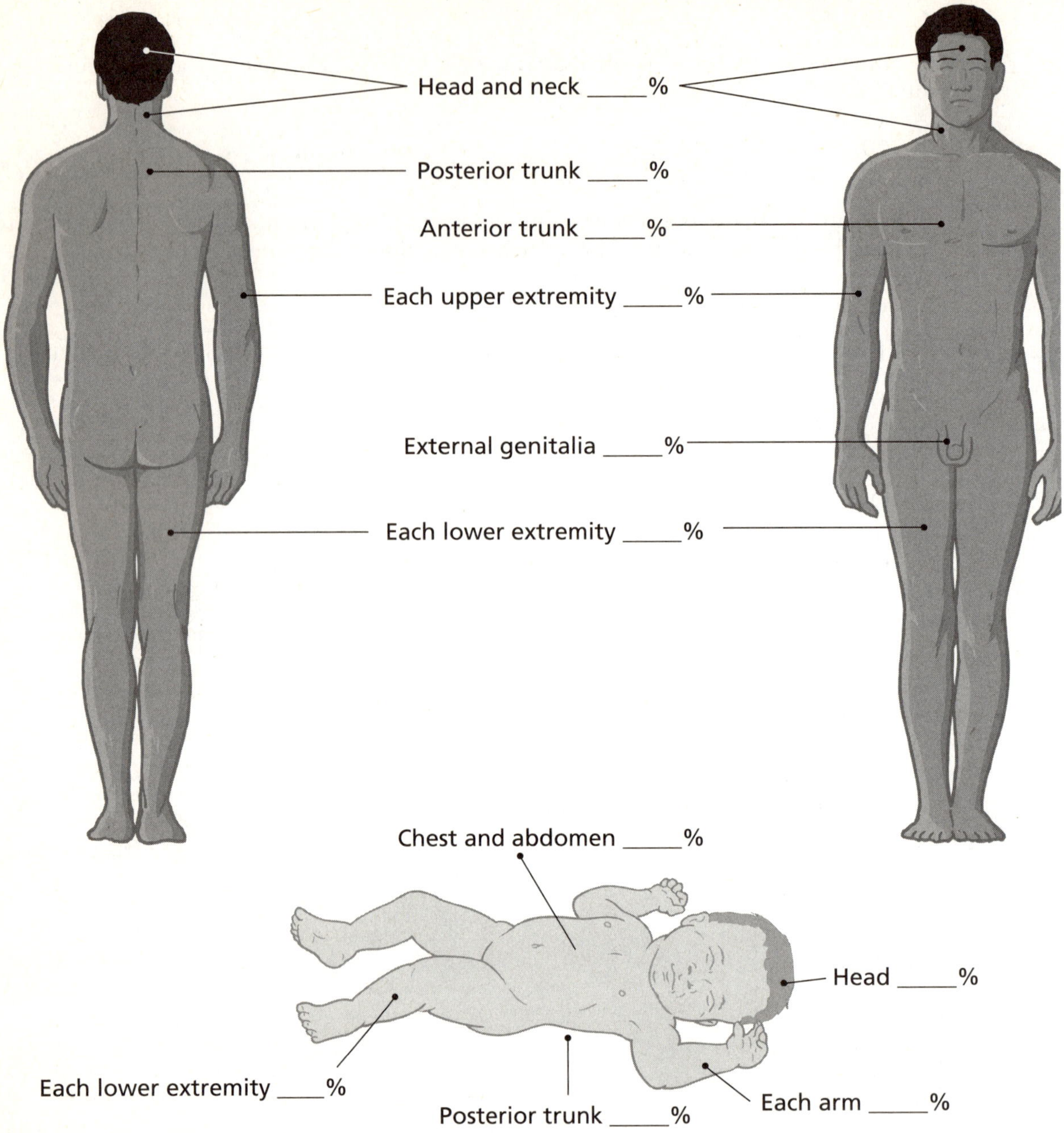

1. If the patient had been an adult, what would the rule of nines add up to? ____________________
2. What does the rule of nines add up to for this toddler? ____________________
3. Why do the percentages differ? ____________________
4. Suppose the burns had been less extensive. What alternative method for calculating the burn area might be used? ____________________

©2008 Pearson Education, Inc.
Intermediate Emergency Care: 1985, 3rd ed.

Chapter

27 Geriatric Emergencies

Review of Chapter Objectives

After reading this chapter, you should be able to do the following:

1. Discuss pathophysiology changes associated with the elderly in regard to drug distribution, metabolism, and elimination—including polypharmacy, dosing errors, increased drug sensitivity, and medication noncompliance. **p. 889**

In general, a person's sensitivity to drugs increases with age. When compared with younger patients, the elderly experience more adverse drug reactions, more drug–drug interactions, and more drug–disease interactions. Because of age-related pharmacokinetic changes such as a loss of body fluids and atrophy of organs, drugs concentrate more readily in the plasma and tissues of elderly patients. As a result, drug dosages often must be adjusted to prevent toxicity. Additionally, due to differences in the GI tract, medications are metabolized and excreted at a slower rate in the elderly patient.

If medications are not correctly monitored, polypharmacy can cause a number of problems among the elderly. In taking a medical history of an elderly patient, remember to ask questions to determine if the patient is taking a prescribed medication as directed. Noncompliance with drug therapy, usually underadherence, is common among the elderly. Up to 40% do not take medications as prescribed. Of these individuals, 35% experience some type of medical problem.

Factors that can decrease compliance in the elderly include limited income, memory loss (due to decreased or diseased neural activity), limited mobility, sensory impairment (cannot hear/read/understand directions), multiple or complicated drug therapies, fear of toxicity, child-proof containers (especially difficult for arthritic patients), and lengthy drug therapy plans.

2. Discuss the use and effects of commonly prescribed drugs for the elderly patient. **pp. 889, 907**

Functional changes in the kidneys, liver, and gastrointestinal system slow the absorption and elimination of many medications in the elderly. In addition, the various compensatory mechanisms that help buffer against medication side effects are less effective in the elderly than in younger patients.

Approximately 30% of all hospital admissions are related to drug-induced illness. About 50% of all drug-related deaths occur in people over the age of 60. Accidental overdoses may occur more frequently in the aged due to confusion, vision impairment, self-selection of medications, forgetfulness, and concurrent drug use. Intentional drug overdose also occurs in attempts at self-destruction. Another complicating factor is the abuse of alcohol among the elderly.

3. Discuss the problem of mobility in the elderly, and develop strategies to prevent falls. **pp. 889–890**

Regular exercise and a good diet are two of the most effective prevention measures for ensuring mobility among the elderly. Some elderly may suffer from a severe medical problem, such as crippling arthritis. They may fear for their personal safety, either from accidental injury or intentional

©2008 Pearson Education, Inc.

injury, such as robbery. Certain medications also may increase their lethargy. Whatever the cause, a lack of mobility can have detrimental physical and emotional effects. Some of these include poor nutrition, difficulty with elimination, poor skin integrity, a greater predisposition for falls, loss of independence and/or confidence, depression from "feeling old," and isolation.

Falls present an especially serious problem for the elderly. Fall-related injuries represent the leading cause of accidental death among the elderly and the seventh highest cause of death overall. As a result, the EMT-I should consider strategies for making a home safe for the elderly and point these out to the elderly patient or family of the elderly patient, whichever may be appropriate. Examples of hazards that can easily be corrected include torn or slippery rugs, chairs without armrests, chairs with low backs, chairs with wheels, obstructing furniture, slippery bathtubs, dim lighting, high cabinet shelves, missing handrails on stairways, and high steps on stairways.

4. Discuss age-related changes in sensations in the elderly, and describe the implications of these changes for communication and patient assessment. p. 890

Most elderly patients suffer from some form of age-related sensory changes. Normal physiological changes may include impaired vision or blindness, impaired or loss of hearing, an altered sense of taste or smell, and/or a lower sensitivity to pain or touch. Any of these conditions can affect your ability to communicate with the patient. In general, be prepared to spend more time obtaining histories from elderly patients.

5. Discuss the problems with continence and elimination in the elderly patient. p. 891

The elderly often find it embarrassing to talk about problems with continence and elimination. They may feel stigmatized, isolated, and/or helpless. When confronted with these problems, DO NOT make a big deal out of them. Respect the patient's dignity, and assure the person that, in many cases, the problem is treatable.

Remember, too, that problems with continence and elimination are not necessarily caused by aging. They may be the result of drug therapy or medical conditions such as diabetes. As a result, in assessing a patient with incontinence or constipation, inquire about their medications and any chronic medical disorders. Also keep in mind the variety of other conditions that can result from problems with continence or elimination. In the case of incontinence, for example, a patient may experience rashes, skin infections, skin breakdown (ulcers), urinary tract infections, sepsis, and falls or fractures (caused by a frequent need to eliminate). In elderly people with cerebrovascular disease or impaired baroreceptor reflexes, efforts to force a bowel movement can lead to a transient ischemic attack (TIA) or syncope.

6. Discuss factors that may complicate the assessment of the elderly patient. pp. 891–895

In assessing an elderly patient, keep in mind the variety of causes of functional impairment. If identified early, an environmental or disease-related condition can often be reversed. Your success depends upon a thorough understanding of age-related changes and the implications of these changes for patient assessment and management. You will need to recall at all times the complications that can arise from comorbidity (having more than one disease at a time) and polypharmacy (concurrent use of a number of drugs).

Communications challenges may also complicate the assessment. Patients may be blind, have speech difficulties, or have some kind of hearing loss that can make assessment more difficult. They also often have a lower sensitivity to pain or touch.

In general, assessment of the elderly patient follows the same basic approach used with any other patient. However, you should keep in mind these points:

- Set a context for illness, taking into account the patient's living situation, level of activity, network of social support, level of dependence, medication history (both prescriptive and nonprescriptive), and sleep patterns.
- Pay close attention to an elderly person's nutrition, noting conditions that may complicate or discourage eating.
- Keep in mind that elderly patients may minimize or fail to report important symptoms. Therefore, try to distinguish the patient's chief complaint from the patient's primary problem.

©2008 Pearson Education, Inc.
Intermediate Emergency Care: 1985, 3rd ed.

- Because of presence of multiple chronic diseases, treat the patient on a "threat-to-life" basis.
- Recall at all times that alterations in the temperature-regulating mechanism can result in a lack of fever, or a minimal fever, even in the presence of a severe infection.
- When confronted with a confused patient, try to determine whether the patient's mental status represents a significant change from normal for them. DO NOT assume that a confused, disoriented patient is "just senile," thus failing to assess for a serious underlying problem.
- Remember that some patients are often easily fatigued and cannot tolerate a long physical examination. Also, because of problems with temperature regulation, the patient may be wearing several layers of clothing.
- Be aware that the elderly patient may minimize or deny symptoms because of a fear of institutionalization or a loss of self-sufficiency.
- Try to distinguish signs of chronic disease from acute problems. For example:
  — Peripheral pulses may be difficult to evaluate because of peripheral vascular disease and arthritis.
  — The elderly may have nonpathological crackles (rales) upon lung auscultation.
  — The elderly often exhibit an increase in mouth breathing and a loss of skin elasticity, which may be confused with dehydration.
  — Dependent edema may be caused by inactivity, not congestive heart failure.

7. Discuss common complaints of elderly patients. **pp. 896–908**

Common complaints of elderly patients include fatigue and weakness, dizziness, vertigo or syncope, falls, headaches, insomnia, dysphagia, loss of appetite, inability to void, and constipation or diarrhea. Many of these complaints in and of themselves would not be too serious. However, given the context of complicated medical histories of the elderly, each of these complaints are important and should be followed up and taken very seriously.

8. Discuss the assessment and management of the elderly patient with complaints related to the following body systems:

a. Respiratory **pp. 896–899**

Respiratory emergencies are some of the most common reasons elderly persons summon EMS or seek emergency care. Most elderly patients with a respiratory disorder present with a chief complaint of dyspnea. However, coughing, congestion, and wheezing are also common chief complaints

- *Pneumonia* occurs more frequently in the elderly than younger patients due to the following reasons found in an elderly population: decreased immune response, reduced pulmonary function, increased colonization of the pharynx by gram-negative bacteria, abnormal or ineffective cough reflex, and decreased effectiveness of mucociliary cells of the upper respiratory system. Common signs and symptoms of pneumonia include increasing dyspnea, congestion, fever, chills, tachypnea, sputum production, and altered mental status. Occasionally, abdominal pain may be the only symptom, and a fever may be absent in the elderly patient. In treating an elderly patient with pneumonia, manage the life-threats, maintain ABCs, and transport to the hospital for diagnosis.
- *Chronic obstructive pulmonary disease (COPD)* is a collection of diseases characterized by chronic airflow obstruction with reversible and/or irreversible components. COPD patients often have a combination of emphysema, chronic bronchitis, and asthma. The usual signs and symptoms include cough, increased sputum production, dyspnea, accessory muscle use, pursed-lip breathing, tripod positioning, exercise intolerance, wheezing, pleuritic chest pain, and tachypnea. When confronted by an elderly patient with COPD, treatment is essentially the same as for all age groups. Administer supplemental oxygen and drug therapy, most frequently bronchodilators, according to your local medical direction to reduce the patient's dyspnea.
- *Pulmonary embolism* (PE) should always be considered as a possible cause of respiratory distress in the elderly patient. Blood clots are the most frequent cause of PE, yet they may also be caused by fat, air, bone marrow, tumor cells, or foreign bodies. Risk factors for

©2008 Pearson Education, Inc.

developing a PE include deep venous thrombosis, prolonged immobility, malignancy, paralysis, fractures of the pelvis, hip, or leg, obesity, trauma to the leg vessels, major surgery, presence of a venous catheter, use of estrogen (in women), and atrial fibrillation. Treatment goals involve delivery of high-flow, high-concentration oxygen via mask, maintaining oxygen levels above SaO_2 or 90%. An IV should be established but vigorous fluid therapy avoided. Pain medications should be discussed with medical direction.

- *Pulmonary edema* is an escape of serous fluids into the alveoli and interstitial tissues of the lungs. Pulmonary edema can develop very rapidly in the elderly patient having an acute myocardial infarction. It can also be caused by pulmonary factors such as infections, inhaled toxins, narcotic overdose, pulmonary embolism, and decreased atmospheric pressure. The treatment is directed at altering the cause of the condition through actively positioning the patient in the Fowler's position, administering high-flow, high-concentration oxygen, assessing the need for ventilatory assistance, obtaining IV access, ECG monitoring, and providing appropriate drug therapy including morphine, nitrates, Lasix, or other medications as ordered by medical direction.

b. Cardiovascular **pp. 899–901**

The leading cause of death in the elderly is cardiovascular disease. When conducting a patient history, determine the patient's level of cardiovascular fitness, changes in exercise tolerance, recent diet history, use of medications, and use of cigarettes and/or alcohol. Ask questions about breathing difficulty, especially at night, and evidence of palpitations, flutter, or skipped beats. In performing the physical exam watch for hypertension, orthostatic hypotension, and consider checking both arms for BP differences from side-to-side. Look for signs of dehydration or dependent edema. In evaluating the problem, recall the cardiovascular disorders commonly found in elderly patients. They include angina pectoris, myocardial infarction, heart failure, dysrhythmias, aortic dissection, aneurysm, hypertension, and syncope.

- *Angina pectoris* literally means "pain in the chest." However, the pain of angina is actually felt in only about 10% to 20% of elderly patients. The changes in sensory nerves, combined with the myocardial changes of aging, make dyspnea a more likely symptom of angina than pain. In the elderly patient, exercise intolerance is a key symptom of angina. In obtaining a history, you should ask the patient about sudden changes in routine. In addition, inquire about any increased stresses on the heart, such as anemia, infection, dysrhythmias, and thyroid changes.
- *Myocardial infarction* (MI) involves actual death of muscle tissue due to a partial or complete occlusion of one or more of the coronary arteries. The greatest number of patients hospitalized for acute MI are older than 65. The elderly patient with MI is less likely to present with the classic symptoms such as chest pain that a younger patient would have. These "atypical" presentations seen in the elderly may also include absence of pain, exercise intolerance, confusion and dizziness, syncope, dyspnea (especially >85 years old), neck, dental, and/or epigastric pain, fatigue, and weakness. The mortality rate associated with MI and/or resulting complications doubles after age 70. Unlike younger patients, the elderly are more likely to suffer a silent MI. They also tend to have larger MIs. The majority of the deaths that occur in the first few hours following a MI are due to dysrhythmias.
- *Heart failure* takes place when cardiac output cannot meet the body's metabolic demands. The incidence rises exponentially after age 60. The causes of heart failure fall in one of four categories: impairment to flow, inadequate cardiac filling, volume overload, and myocardial failure. Typical age-related factors, such as prolonged myocardial contractions, make the elderly vulnerable to heart failure. Assessment findings specific to the elderly include fatigue from left heart failure; two-pillow orthopnea; dyspnea on exertion; dry, hacking cough progressing to a productive cough; dependent edema from right heart failure; nocturia; anorexia; hepatomegaly; and ascites.
- *Dysrhythmias* usually develop with age, and atrial fibrillation is the most common of the rhythms. Dysrhythmias occur primarily as a result of degeneration of the patient's conductive system. Anything that decreases myocardial blood flow can produce a dysrhythmia. They may also be caused by electrolyte abnormalities. To complicate matters further, the elderly do not tolerate extremes in heart rate as well as a younger person would. Treatment considerations depend upon the type of dysrhythmia. Patients who may already

©2008 Pearson Education, Inc.
Intermediate Emergency Care: 1985, 3rd ed.

have a pacemaker have a low but significant rate of complications such as a failed battery, fibrosis around the catheter site, lead fracture, or electrode dislodgement. Drug therapy may be indicated. Whenever you discover a dysrhythmia remember the irregular heart rhythm may be the only clinical finding in an elderly patient suffering an acute MI.

- *Aortic dissection* is the degeneration of the wall of the aorta, either in the thoracic or abdominal cavity. It can result in an aneurysm or in the rupture of the vessel. Approximately 80% of thoracic aneurysms are due to atherosclerosis combined with hypertension. The remaining cases occur secondary to other factors like Marfan's syndrome or blunt trauma to the chest. These patients often present with tearing chest pain radiating to the back or if ruptured, cardiac arrest. The distal portion of the aorta is the most common site for abdominal aneurysms. The aneurysm may appear as a pulsatile mass in a patient with a normal girth, but lack of identifiable mass does not eliminate this condition. The patient may have a tearing abdominal pain or unexplained low back pain. Pulses in the legs are diminished or absent and the lower extremities feel cold to the touch. The treatment of an aneurysm depends on its size, location, and the severity of the condition. Rapid transportation is in order, and many of these patients will need a surgical procedure.
- Today over 50% of the people in the U.S. over the age of 65 have clinically diagnosed *hypertension*—defined as blood pressure greater than 140/90 mmHg. Prolonged elevated blood pressure will eventually damage the heart, brain, or kidneys. As a result of hypertension, the elderly are at greater risk for heart failure, stroke, blindness, renal failure, coronary heart disease, and peripheral vascular disease. Management of hypertension depends upon its severity and the existence of other conditions. Hypertension is often treated chronically with beta blockers which are contraindicated in patients who have COPD, asthma, or heart blocks greater than a first degree. Diuretics are another common drug used to treat hypertension but should be used cautiously in patients who are also taking digitalis.
- *Syncope* is a common presenting complaint in the elderly. The condition results when blood flow to the brain is temporarily interrupted or decreased. It is usually caused by problems with either the nervous system or the cardiovascular system. Common presentations of syncope would include the following:
  - — Vasodepressor syncope or common fainting may occur following an emotional distress, pain, prolonged bed rest, mild blood loss, prolonged standing in warm crowded rooms, anemia, or fever.
  - — Orthostatic syncope occurs when a person rises from a seated or supine position. This is due to pooling of the blood in the legs reducing the flow of blood to the brain. This is common in hypovolemia, venous varicosities, prolonged bed rest, and autonomic dysfunction. It can also be drug induced by blood pressure medications.
  - — Vasavagal syncope occurs as a result of a valsalva maneuver during defecation, coughing, or similar maneuvers. This slows the heart rate and cardiac output, thus decreasing the blood flow to the brain.
  - — Cardiac syncope results from transient reduction in cerebral blood flow due to a sudden decrease in cardiac output. It can result from a silent MI or a dysrhythmia, such as a bradycardia, Stokes-Adam syndrome, heart block, tachydysrhythmia, and sick sinus syndrome.
  - — Seizures may result from a seizure disorder or syncope may cause seizure activity. Syncope due to seizures tends to occur without warning. It is associated with muscular jerking or convulsions, incontinence, and tongue-biting.
  - — Transient ischemic attacks occur more frequently in the elderly and may cause syncope.

c. Nervous **pp. 901–904**

Elderly patients are at risk for several neurological emergencies. Many of these disorders involve an altered mental status and are discussed below:

- *Cerebrovascular disease (stroke/brain attack).* Strokes are the third leading cause of death in the U.S. Older patients are at higher risk than younger patients because of atherosclerosis, hypertension, immobility, limb paralysis, congestive heart failure, and atrial fibrillation. Transient ischemic attacks (TIAs) are also more common in older patients. Strokes usually fall in one of two major categories: (1) brain ischemia injuries caused by inadequate supply of oxygen and nutrients, which accounts for 80% of the strokes, and (2) subarachnoid

©2008 Pearson Education, Inc.

hemorrhage or intracerebral hemorrhages which account for the rest. Due to the different types of strokes, signs and symptoms can present in many ways including altered mental status, coma, paralysis, slurred speech, a change in mood, and seizures. When assessing a stroke, complete a GCS for later comparison in the ED. Many EMS systems also use the Cincinnati Prehospital Stroke Scale which assesses the smile, pronator drift, and speech to predict the potential for a stroke. Stroke patients need to be assessed and removed to the most appropriate facility quickly so that fibrinolytics (thrombolytics) can be utilized if the patient is an appropriate candidate and it is within three hours of the onset of the symptoms. By far the most preferred treatment for a stroke is prevention. Strategies for stroke prevention include control of hypertension, treatment of cardiac disorders and blood disorders, cessation of smoking, cessation of recreational drug use, moderate use of alcohol, regular exercise, improving eating habits.

- *Seizures* may be mistaken for stroke in the elderly patient. Some seizures are subtle in the elderly, and the common causes include seizure disorders (epilepsy), syncope, recent or past head trauma, mass lesion (tumor or bleed), alcohol withdrawal, hypoglycemia, or stroke. If the patient has fallen during a seizure, always remember to check for evidence of trauma and treat accordingly.
- *Dizziness* is a frequent complaint of the elderly. It may indicate the patient has suffered syncope, pre-syncope, lightheadedness, or true vertigo. Vertigo is a specific sensation of motion perceived by the patient as spinning or whirling. Vertigo is often accompanied by sweating, pallor, nausea, and vomiting. Meniere's disease can cause severe, intractable vertigo as well as a "roaring" sound in the ears. Any factor that impairs visual input, inner-ear function, peripheral sensory input, or the central nervous system can cause dizziness, including alcohol and many prescription drugs. Therefore, it is virtually impossible to distinguish dizziness, syncope, and pre-syncope in the prehospital setting.
- *Delirium* can be caused by organic brain disease or disorders that occur elsewhere in the body. Delirium in the elderly is a serious condition leading to death in approximately 18% of hospitalized patients. Delirium is a global mental impairment of sudden onset and self-limited duration. Common signs and symptoms include the acute onset of anxiety, an inability to focus, disordered thinking, irritability, inappropriate behavior, fearfulness, excessive energy, or psychotic behavior such as hallucinations or paranoia. Aphasic or speaking errors and/or prominent slurring may be present. In distinguishing between delirium and dementia, err on the side of delirium.
- *Dementia* is more prevalent in the elderly than delirium. Over 50% of all nursing home patients have some form of dementia. Dementia is a chronic global cognitive impairment, often progressive or irreversible. This mental deterioration is often called "organic brain syndrome," "senile dementia," or "senility." Causes of dementia include small strokes, atherosclerosis, age-related neurological changes, neurological diseases, certain hereditary diseases (e.g., Huntington's disease), and Alzheimer's disease. The signs and symptoms of dementia include progressive disorientation, shortened attention span, aphasia or nonsense talking, and hallucinations. Stay alert for signs of abuse or neglect which occurs in a disproportionate number of elderly suffering from dementia.
- *Alzheimer's disease* is a specific type of dementia that affects 4 million people in the United States. It is a chronic degenerative disorder that attacks the brain and results in impaired memory, thinking, and behavior. The disease generally occurs in three stages: early, intermediate and terminal stages. The early stage is characterized by loss of recent memory, inability to learn new material, mood swings, and personality changes. Patients may believe someone is plotting against them when they lose items or forget things. Aggression or hostility is common and poor judgment is evident. In the intermediate stage, the patient has a complete inability to learn new material. They wander, particularly at night, have increased falls, lose the ability for self-care, including bathing and use of the toilet. In the terminal stage, the patient is unable to walk and regresses to an infant stage including the loss of bowel and bladder function. Eventually the patient loses the ability to eat and swallow. Remember that the families of these patients also have need for support. If they show signs of stress, you may want to alert the emergency department so additional assistance in caring for their loved ones can be provided.

©2008 Pearson Education, Inc.
Intermediate Emergency Care: 1985, 3rd ed.

- *Parkinson's disease* is a degenerative disorder characterized by changes in muscle response, including tremors, loss of facial expression, and gait disturbances. It mainly appears in people over age 50 and peaks at age 70. Primary Parkinson's disease still has an unknown cause. Secondary Parkinson's disease has one of a number of potential causes such as viral encephalitis, atherosclerosis of cerebral vessels, reaction to certain drugs or toxins (such as antipsychotic or carbon monoxide), metabolic disorders (such as anoxia), tumors, head trauma, and degenerative disorders (such as Shy-Drager syndrome). Patients have a resting tremor and a pill rolling motion. As the disease progresses, muscles become more rigid and movements become slower and/or jerkier. Their feet may feel "frozen to the ground." Gaits become shuffled with short steps and unexpected bursts of speed, often used to avoid falling. Kyphotic deformity is a hallmark of the disease. They also develop a mask-like face devoid of all expression and speak in a slow, monotone voice. Difficulties in communication, coupled with a loss of mobility, often lead to anxiety and depression. In treating the patient with Parkinson's, observe for conditions that may indicate a fall or the inability to move. Manage treatable conditions and transport as needed.

d. Endocrine **p. 904**

The endocrine system undergoes a number of age-related changes, which affect hormone levels. The most common endocrine disorders include diabetes mellitus and thyroid gland disorders.

- *Diabetes mellitus* (primarily Type II) is estimated to be present in 20% of older adults, and almost 40% of the elderly have a form of glucose intolerance. The reasons the elderly develop these disorders include poor diet, decreased physical activity, loss of lean body mass, impaired insulin production, and resistance by body cells to the actions of insulin. Left unchecked, over time vague constitutional symptoms like fatigue or weakness may actually be indications of diabetes and ultimately lead to high glucose levels, neuropathy, and visual impairment. The acute management of an elderly diabetic and/or hypoglycemic patient is generally the same as for any other patient. Do not rule out alcohol as a complicating factor, especially in cases of hypoglycemia. In addition, remember that diabetes places the elderly at increased risk of other complications, including atherosclerosis delayed healing, retinopathy, blindness, altered renal function, and severe peripheral vascular disease, leading to foot ulcers and even amputations.
- *Thyroid disorders* occur due to the moderate atrophy and changes in hormone production that come with aging of the thyroid gland. Often when an elderly patient presents with complaints of typical signs and symptoms of hypothyroidism, they are attributed to aging. Common nonspecific complaints in the elderly include mental confusion, anorexia, falls, incontinence, and decreased mobility. Some patients may also experience an increase in muscle or joint pain. Hyperthyroidism is less common among the elderly but may result from medication errors such as an overdose of thyroid hormone replacement. The typical symptom of heat intolerance is often present in the elderly patient. Common nonspecific features or complaints include atrial fibrillation, failure to thrive, abdominal distress, diarrhea, exhaustion, and depression. Since thyroid disorders are not diagnosed in the field, these patients should always be encouraged to go to the hospital for further evaluation.

e. Gastrointestinal **pp. 904–905**

The most frequent GI emergency is bleeding; however, the elderly will describe a variety of other GI complaints such as nausea, poor appetite, diarrhea, and constipation. Remember these conditions may be symptomatic of more serious diseases and should not be downplayed. Keep in mind that older patients are far more intolerant of hypotension and anoxia than younger patients. Treatment should include airway management, support of breathing and circulation, high-flow, high-concentration oxygen therapy, IV fluid replacement with a crystalloid solution, PASG placement (if indicated), and rapid transport. The following are the most serious of the GI problems found in the elderly patient in the field:

- *GI hemorrhage* falls into two general categories of upper GI and lower GI bleeds. The upper GI bleeds include peptic ulcer disease, gastritis, esophageal varices, and Mallory-Weiss tears. Lower GI bleeds include diverticulosis, tumors, ischemic colitis, and arterio-venous malformations. Signs of significant GI blood loss include the presence of "coffee ground" emesis, black tar-like stool (melena), obvious blood in the emesis or stool, orthostatic hypotension,

©2008 Pearson Education, Inc.

pulse greater than 100 (unless the patient is on beta blockers), and confusion. GI bleeding in the elderly may result in such complications as a recent increase in angina symptoms, congestive heart failure, weakness, or dyspnea.

- *Bowel obstruction* in the elderly typically involves the small bowel. Causes include tumors, prior abdominal surgery, use of certain medications, and occasionally the presence of vertebral compression fractures. The patient will typically complain of diffuse abdominal pain, bloating, nausea, and vomiting. The abdomen may feel distended when palpated and the bowel sounds may be hypoactive or absent. If the obstruction has been present for a prolonged period of time, the patient may have a fever, weakness, shock, and various electrolyte disturbances.
- *Mesenteric infarct* involves the vessels arising from the superior or inferior mesenteric arteries which serve the bowel. An infarct occurs when a portion of the bowel does not receive enough blood to survive. The primary symptom of a bowel infarct is pain out of proportion to the physical exam. Signs include bloody diarrhea (but usually not a massive hemorrhage), some tachycardia (although there may be a vagal effect masking the sign), and abdominal distention. The patient is at great risk for shock as the dead bowel attracts interstitial and intravascular fluids, thus removing them from use. Necrotic products are released to the peritoneal cavity, leading to a massive infection.

9. Describe the assessment and management of the elderly patient with an environmental emergency. pp. 905–907

Hypothermia. Thermoregulatory emergencies represent some of the most common EMS calls involving the elderly. As a group, the elderly are vulnerable to low temperatures, suffering about 750,000 winter deaths annually, primarily from hypothermia and "winter risks" such as pneumonia and influenza. Factors that predispose the elderly to hypothermia include accidental exposure to cold, CNS disorders, head trauma, stroke, endocrine disorders (particularly hypoglycemia and diabetes), drugs that interfere with heat production, malnutrition or starvation, chronic illness, forced inactivity as a result of a medical condition, low or fixed income (which discourages use of home heating), inflammatory dermatitis, and A-V shunts.

Hypothermic patients may exhibit slow speech, cold skin, confusion, and sleepiness. In early stages, vitals may reveal hypertension and an increased heart rate. As hypothermia progresses, however, blood pressure drops and the heart rate slows, sometimes to a barely detectable level. Keep in mind that the elderly patient with hypothermia often does not shiver. Check the abdomen and back to see if the skin is cool to the touch or, if your unit has a low-temperature thermometer, check the patient's core temperature.

Treatment is focused on rewarming the patient and rapid transport. Once the elderly develop hypothermia, they become progressively impaired, with their condition worsening other chronic medical problems. Remain alert for complications, most commonly cardiac arrest or ventricular fibrillation.

Hyperthermia. Age-related changes in the sweat glands and increased incidence of heart disease place the elderly at risk of heat stress. They may develop heat cramps, heat exhaustion, or heat stroke. Risk factors for severe hyperthermia include altered sensory output, inadequate liquid intake, decreased functioning of the thermoregulatory center, commonly prescribed medications that inhibit sweating (such as antihistamines and tricyclic antidepressants), low or fixed incomes (which may result in a lack of fans or air conditioning), alcoholism, concomitant medical disorders, and use of diuretics (which increase fluid loss).

Early heatstroke may present with nonspecific signs and symptoms such as nausea, lightheadedness, dizziness, headache, and high fever. Prevention strategies include adequate fluid intake, reduced activity, shelter in an air conditioned environment, and use of light clothing. If hyperthermia develops, however, rapid treatment and transport are necessary.

10. Describe the assessment and management of the elderly patient with a toxicological or substance abuse problem. pp. 907–908

Toxicological problems. Aging alters pharmacokinetics and pharmacodynamics in the elderly. Functional changes in the kidneys, liver, and GI system slow the absorption and elimination of many medications. In addition, the various compensatory mechanisms that help buffer against medication side effects are less effective in the elderly than in younger patients.

©2008 Pearson Education, Inc.
Intermediate Emergency Care: 1985, 3rd ed.

Approximately 30% of all hospital admissions are related to drug-induced illnesses. About 50% of all drug-related deaths occur in people over age 60. Accidental overdoses may occur more frequently in the aged due to confusion, vision impairment, self-selection of medications, forgetfulness, and concurrent drug use. Intentional drug overdose also occurs in attempts at self-destruction. Another complicating factor is the abuse of alcohol in the elderly.

In assessing the elderly patient, always take these steps:

- Obtain a full list of medications currently taken by the patient.
- Elicit any medications that are newly prescribed.
- Obtain a good past medical history, including prior renal or hepatic depression.
- Know your medications, their routes of elimination, and their potential side effects.
- If possible, always take all medications to the hospital along with the patient.

Substance abuse, drug abuse, alcohol abuse. In general, the factors that contribute to substance abuse among the elderly are different than those of younger people. They include age-related changes, loss of employment, loss of spouse or partner, malnutrition, loneliness, moving from a long-loved home, and multiple prescriptions.

The elderly who become physically and/or psychologically dependent upon drugs or alcohol are more likely to hide their dependence and less likely to seek help than other age groups. Common signs and symptoms of drug abuse include memory changes, drowsiness, decreased vision/hearing, orthostatic hypotension, poor dexterity, mood changes, falling, restlessness, and weight loss. Pertinent findings for alcohol abuse include mood swings, denial and hostility (when questioned about alcohol), confusion, history of falls, anorexia, insomnia, visible anxiety, and nausea.

Treatment follows many of the same steps as for any other patient with a pattern of substance abuse. DO NOT judge the patient. Manage the ABCs and evaluate the need for fluid therapy or medications to accommodate withdrawal. Transport the patient to the hospital for further evaluation and referral.

11. Describe the incidence, morbidity/mortality, risk factors, prevention strategies, pathophysiology, assessment, need for intervention and transport, and management of the elderly trauma patient. pp. 909–911

Trauma is the leading cause of death among the elderly. Older patients who sustain moderate to severe injuries are more likely to die than their younger counterparts. Post-injury disability is also more common in the elderly than in the young. Contributing factors to the high incidence and severity of trauma among the elderly include slower reflexes, arthritis, diminished eyesight and hearing predisposing them to accidents (especially falls), high risk for criminal assault (due to physical state and vulnerability), osteoporosis (muscle weakness increases the chance of fractures), reduced cardiac reserve (decreases the ability to compensate for blood loss), decreased respiratory function (increases the likelihood of acute respiratory distress syndrome (ARDS)), impaired renal function (decreased ability to adapt to fluid shifts), and decreased elasticity in the peripheral blood vessels (greater susceptibility to tearing).

General assessment of an elderly patient should include determining the MOI. Leading mechanisms include falls, motor-vehicle crashes, burns, assault or abuse, and underlying medical problems such as syncope. In assessing the elderly patient remember that the BP may be deceptive since older patients usually have higher BPs compared to younger patients. Elderly trauma patients also may not exhibit an elevated pulse, which is common in shock because they are on a beta blocker. Fractures may also be obscured or concealed because of a diminished sense of pain among the elderly. One of the best indicators of shock in the elderly is an altered mental status or changes in consciousness during assessment. Elderly trauma patients who exhibit confusion or agitation are candidates for rapid transport.

Whenever assessing the elderly patient observe the scene for signs of abuse and neglect. Abuse of the elderly is as big a problem in our society as child abuse and neglect. Geriatric abuse is defined as a syndrome in which an elderly person has received serious physical or psychological injury from family members or other caregivers. Abuse of the elderly knows no socioeconomic bounds. It often occurs when an older person is no longer able to be totally independent, and the family

©2008 Pearson Education, Inc.

has difficulty upholding their commitment to care for the patient. It can occur in nursing homes and other health facilities. Signs and symptoms of geriatric abuse and neglect are often obvious. Unexplained trauma is usually the primary presentation. The average abused patient is older than 80 and has multiple medical problems, such as cancer, congestive heart failure, heart disease, and incontinence. Senile dementia is often present. In these cases, it can be hard to determine whether the dementia is chronic or acute, especially if there is an increased likelihood of head trauma from the abuse. Follow your local procedures for reporting and documenting suspected abuse.

General management of trauma to the elderly patient is similar to that of all trauma patients. However, you must keep in mind age-related systemic changes and the presence of chronic diseases. This is especially true of the cardiovascular system, respiratory system, renal system, transport considerations, and the specific injuries discussed below.

- **Cardiovascular considerations**—Recent or past MI may contribute to the risk of dysrhythmia or congestive heart failure in the trauma patient. It may also decrease the response of the heart in adjusting its rate and stroke volume to the stress of hypovolemia. The elderly trauma patient may require higher than usual arterial pressures for perfusion of vital organs, due to increased peripheral vascular resistance and hypertension. Hypotension, hypovolemia, and hypervolemia are poorly tolerated in the elderly patient.
- **Respiratory considerations**—In managing the airway and ventilation in an elderly trauma patient, you must consider the physical changes that may affect treatment. Check for dentures that may need to be removed. Keep in mind age-related changes can decrease chest wall movement and vital capacity. Age also reduces the tolerance of all organs for anoxia. Also, COPD is a widespread problem of the elderly.
- **Renal considerations**—The decreased ability of the kidneys to maintain normal acid/base balance, and to compensate for fluid changes, can further complicate the management of the elderly trauma patient. Any preexisting renal disease can decrease the kidneys' ability to compensate. A decrease in renal function, along with a decreased cardiac reserve, places the elderly injured patient at risk for fluid overload and pulmonary edema.
- **Transport considerations**—You may have to modify positioning, immobilization, and packaging of the elderly trauma patient before transport. Be attentive to physical deformities such as arthritis, spinal abnormalities, or frozen limbs that may cause pain or require special care. Recall the frailty of an elderly person's skin and avoid creating skin tears or pressure sores.

12. Describe the assessment and management of the elderly patient with:

a. Orthopedic injuries **p. 912**

The elderly suffer the greatest mortality and greatest incidence of disability from falls. Approximately 33% of the falls in the elderly result in at least one fractured bone. The most common fall-related fracture is a fracture of the hip or pelvis. Falls also result in a variety of stress fractures in the elderly, including fractures of the proximal humerus, distal radius, proximal tibia, and thoracic and lumbar bodies. In treating orthopedic injuries, remember to ask questions aimed at detecting an underlying medical condition.

b. Burns **pp. 913–914**

People age 60 and older are more likely to suffer death from burns than any other age group except neonates and infants. Factors that help explain the high mortality rate among the elderly include age-related changes that slow reaction time, pre-existing diseases that increase the risk of medical complications, age-related skin changes (thinning) that increase the severity of burns, immunological and metabolic changes that increase the risk of infection, and reductions in physiologic function and the reduced reserves of several organ systems that make the elderly more vulnerable to systemic stress.

Management of the elderly burn patient follows the same general procedures as other patients. However, remember that the elderly are at increased risk of shock. Administration of fluids is important to prevent renal tubular damage. Assess hydration in the initial hours after the burn injury by blood pressure, pulse, and urine output.

c. Head and spinal injuries **p. 914**

As people age, the brain decreases in size and weight. The skull, however, remains constant in size, allowing the brain more room to move, thus increasing the likelihood of brain injury.

©2008 Pearson Education, Inc.
Intermediate Emergency Care: 1985, 3rd ed.

Because of this, the signs and symptoms of brain injury may develop more slowly in the elderly patient, sometimes over days or weeks. In fact, the patient may often have forgotten the offending incident.

The cervical spine is also more susceptible to injury due to osteoporosis and spondylosis—a degeneration of the vertebral body. In addition, arthritic changes can gradually compress the nerve rootlets or spinal cord. Thus, injury to the spine in the elderly makes them much more susceptible to spinal cord injury. Therefore, it is important to provide older patients with suspected spinal-cord injury, especially those involved in motor vehicle collisions, with immediate manual cervical stabilization at the time of initial assessment.

13. Given several pre-programmed simulated geriatric patients with various complaints, provide the appropriate assessment, management, and transport. pp. 888–914

During your classroom, clinical, and field training, you will assess real and simulated geriatric patients and develop a management plan for them. Use the information presented in this text chapter, the information on assessment of geriatric patients in the field presented by your instructors, and the guidance given by your clinical and field preceptors to develop good patient assessment skills. Continue to refine these skills once your training ends and you begin your career as an EMT-I.

Case Study Review

Reread the case study in Chapter 27 and then read the following discussion. This case study draws attention to the importance of recognizing the vital lives led by elderly people and the need to take their complaints seriously, rather than dismissing them as normal age-related changes.

The case study puts you in the position of an EMT-I who decides to teach a student intern about the treatment of elderly patients. At the end of the call, the intern is asked: "So Andy, do you want to talk about what went right with this call and what we could have done better while we restock the ambulance?"

So let's discuss it! The complaint of abdominal pain can be caused by many different factors, most of which cannot not be resolved in an out-of-hospital setting. Even so, after reading the text, you now know that the most frequent gastrointestinal emergency in the elderly is GI bleeding, a condition that can place the elderly at a significant risk of hemorrhage and shock. The elderly are also far more intolerant of hypotension and anoxia than younger patients. Any GI emergency should be aggressively managed.

In this case, the initial assessment ruled out an immediate life threat. The general impression was that of an elderly woman with severe abdominal pain. As noted, the pain was out of proportion to the physical exam—a symptom suggestive of mesenteric infarct. Care steps included administration of high-flow oxygen, IV fluid replacement therapy with a crystalloid solution, and, most importantly, rapid transport.

It was correct to place the patient on a cardiac monitor. An ECG of atrial fibrillation is common in elderly patients. Based on the patient's vital signs, Mrs. Bombard seemed to be tolerating the dysrhythmias. The monitor helped show that the pain was not cardiac-related, though complications could result, depending upon preexisting medical conditions.

It might have been helpful to inquire in more detail about any other GI distress experienced by the patient, such as diarrhea, vomiting, and nausea. Also, a pulse oximeter might have been useful to measure the patient's oxygen saturation en route to the hospital. However, considering the patient's presentation, she was managed appropriately.

Andy's quip about a beer and taco provided a "teachable moment" in that it corrected a mistaken attitude about the aging process—the idea that an elderly patient might not live like a younger counterpart. In fact, it would have been relevant to ask just what the patient ate—and drank—at dinner. It also highlighted the problem of alcohol abuse among the elderly. They are not only exposed to the stresses of aging, but age-related systemic changes and medical problems make it more difficult for them to metabolize alcohol or many other drugs. So it would have also been relevant to ask whether Mrs. Bombard consumed alcohol on a regular basis.

©2008 Pearson Education, Inc.

Content Self-Evaluation

MULTIPLE CHOICE

_____ 1. All of the following are responsible for the growing number of elderly people in the United States—and the projected increase in the number of elderly patients treated by EMS services—EXCEPT a(n)
A. increase in the mean survival rate of older persons.
B. increase in the birth rate.
C. absence of major wars.
D. improved health care.
E. higher standard of living.

_____ 2. The study and treatment of diseases of the aged is known as
A. geriatrics.
B. ageism.
C. gerontology.
D. eldercare.
E. gerontotherapeutics.

_____ 3. The existence of multiple diseases, as may occur with the elderly, is known as
A. functional impairment.
B. dysphagia.
C. comorbidity.
D. polypharmacy.
E. senility.

_____ 4. Common complaints in the elderly include
A. fatigue, weakness, syncope.
B. fractures, drowning, diabetes.
C. GSW, croup, nausea.
D. MVC, meningitis, poisoning.
E. fever, epiglottitis, febrile seizures.

_____ 5. When compared to younger patients, the elderly experience fewer adverse drug reactions.
A. True
B. False

_____ 6. A lack of mobility can have detrimental physical and emotional effects on the elderly.
A. True
B. False

_____ 7. Which of the following is the leading cause of accidental deaths among the elderly?
A. drownings
B. fall-related injuries
C. motor vehicle collisions
D. gunshot wounds
E. poisonings

_____ 8. The inability to retain urine or feces because of loss of sphincter control or because of cerebral or spinal lesions is called
A. diarrhea.
B. involuntary elimination.
C. diuresis.
D. incontinence.
E. uremia.

_____ 9. In elderly people with cerebrovascular disease or impaired baroreceptor reflexes, efforts to force a bowel movement can lead to a transient ischemic attack.
A. True
B. False

_____ 10. All of the following factors play a part in forming a general assessment of the elderly patient EXCEPT
A. average cost of rent.
B. medication history.
C. living situations.
D. sleep patterns.
E. level of nutrition.

©2008 Pearson Education, Inc.
Intermediate Emergency Care: 1985, 3rd ed.

______ 11. One of the most common reasons that elderly patients underestimate the severity of a primary medical problem is that they have a(n)
A. shrinkage of structures in the ear.
B. clouding and thickening of lenses in the eyes.
C. lowered sensitivity to pain.
D. deterioration of the teeth and gums.
E. altered sense of taste.

______ 12. Which of the following is a byproduct of malnutrition?
A. electrolyte abnormalities
B. dehydration
C. vitamin deficiencies
D. hypoglycemia
E. all of the above

______ 13. The elderly are more prone to environmental thermal problems due to changes in the sweat glands.
A. True
B. False

______ 14. To improve communication with an elderly patient, you should try to
A. display verbal and nonverbal signs of concern.
B. dim the room lights.
C. avoid looking directly into the patient's eyes.
D. first talk to family members, then the patient.
E. remain as quiet as possible.

______ 15. Both senility and organic brain syndrome may manifest themselves with
A. distractibility.
B. excitability.
C. hostility.
D. restlessness.
E. all of the above

______ 16. When assessing an elderly person, if he or she is confused or disoriented, you can conclude that the patient is senile.
A. True
B. False

______ 17. To help reduce an elderly patient's fears, you should
A. downplay the patient's fears.
B. ignore nonverbal messages.
C. discourage the expression of feelings.
D. confirm what the patient has said.
E. instruct the patient to calm down.

______ 18. The decrease of an effective cough reflex and the activity of the ________ make the elderly more prone to respiratory infection.
A. gag reflex
B. alveoli
C. cilia
D. bronchioles
E. vagal response

______ 19. Reasons that the elderly develop pneumonia more frequently than younger people include all of the following EXCEPT a(n)
A. decreased immune response.
B. increased pulmonary function.
C. abnormal or ineffective cough reflex.
D. decreased activity of mucociliary cells.
E. decreased colonization of the pharynx by gram-negative bacteria.

______ 20. An elderly patient in an institutional setting is up to 50 times more likely to contract pneumonia than an elderly patient receiving home care.
A. True
B. False

©2008 Pearson Education, Inc.

______ 21. The usual signs and symptoms of COPD include
A. cough and wheezing.
B. dyspnea and tachypnea.
C. exercise intolerance.
D. pleuritic chest pain.
E. all of the above

______ 22. Your elderly patient is complaining of acute onset of sharp chest pain and shortness of breath. The patient was recently released from the hospital for a leg fracture. What is the most likely suspected disorder?
A. pneumonia
B. pulmonary embolism
C. heart attack
D. COPD
E. pulmonary edema

______ 23. Although all of the following can contribute to a pulmonary embolism, the condition is most frequently caused by
A. fat.
B. bone marrow.
C. blood clots.
D. tumor cells.
E. air.

______ 24. The leading cause of death in the elderly is
A. pneumonia.
B. stroke.
C. cardiovascular disease.
D. Alzheimer's disease.
E. COPD.

______ 25. The heart sounds in an elderly patient are generally louder than those in a young patient.
A. True
B. False

______ 26. All of the following are atypical presentations of a myocardial infarction seen frequently in the elderly EXCEPT
A. syncope.
B. tearing chest pain.
C. dyspnea.
D. neck or dental pain.
E. exercise intolerance.

______ 27. Assessment findings specific to the elderly such as anorexia, nocturia, dependent edema, and hepatomegaly may be found in a patient with
A. a pulmonary embolism.
B. heart failure.
C. hypertension.
D. an aneurysm.
E. syncope.

______ 28. A series of symptoms resulting from decreased blood flow to the brain that are caused by a sudden decrease in cardiac output are known as
A. autonomic dysfunction.
B. Stokes-Adams syndrome.
C. cardiac syncope.
D. dying heart muscle.
E. Marfan's syndrome.

______ 29. Injury to or death of brain tissue resulting from interruption of cerebral blood flow and oxygenation is called a(n)
A. subarachnoid hemorrhage.
B. autonomic dysfunction.
C. TIA.
D. stroke.
E. intracerebral hemorrhage.

______ 30. Common causes of seizures in the elderly include all of the following EXCEPT
A. head trauma.
B. alcohol withdrawal.
C. spinal injury.
D. stroke.
E. hypoglycemia.

______ 31. A progressive, degenerative disease that attacks the brain and results in impaired memory, thinking, and behavior is called
A. dementia.
B. Parkinson's disease.
C. delirium.
D. Alzheimer's disease.
E. aphasia.

©2008 Pearson Education, Inc.
Intermediate Emergency Care: 1985, 3rd ed.

______ 32. A chronic, degenerative nervous disease characterized by tremors, muscular weakness and rigidity, and loss of postural reflexes is called

A. Parkinson's disease.
B. Shy-Drager syndrome.
C. Alzheimer's disease.
D. sick sinus syndrome.
E. grand mal seizure.

______ 33. All of the following are forms of upper GI bleeding EXCEPT

A. peptic ulcer disease.
B. ischemic colitis.
C. esophageal varices.
D. gastritis.
E. peptic ulcer disease.

______ 34. An example of a lower GI bleeding is:

A. a Mallory-Weiss tear.
B. diverticulosis.
C. peptic ulcer disease.
D. a bowel obstruction.
E. a mesenteric infarct.

______ 35. All of the following are signs and symptoms of hypothermia in an elderly patient EXCEPT

A. confusion.
B. slow speech.
C. shivering.
D. skin cool to the touch.
E. sleepiness.

Matching

Write the letter of the term in the space provided next to the appropriate description.

A. transient ischemic attack
B. brain ischemia
C. nocturia
D. delirium
E. senile dementia
F. mesenteric infarct
G. spondylosis

______ 36. acute alteration in mental functioning that is often reversible

______ 37. excessive urination, usually at night

______ 38. death of tissue in the peritoneal fold that encircles the small intestine

______ 39. general term used to describe an abnormal decline in mental function in the elderly

______ 40. degeneration of the vertebral body

______ 41. injury to the brain tissues caused by an inadequate supply of oxygen and nutrients

______ 42. medical condition like a stroke but reversible and commonly involving syncope

©2008 Pearson Education, Inc.

Chapter 28

EMS Response to Weapons of Mass Destruction

Review of Chapter Objectives

After reading this chapter, you should be able to do the following:

1. Identify the typical weapons of mass destruction likely to be used by terrorists. pp. 918–929

The most likely weapon of mass destruction used by the terrorist, either foreign or domestic, is the conventional explosive. As terrorists gain greater funding and sophistication, however, the risk of terrorists using nuclear, biological, and chemical weapons is increasing. Terrorists may also use agents and mechanisms not yet mentioned as they search for new ways to terrify the public and bring attention to their cause. An example of this was crashing commercial airliners, laden with fuel, into large buildings.

2. Explain the mechanisms of injury associated with conventional and nuclear weapons of mass destruction. pp. 918–921

Chemical reactions in the conventional explosion release tremendous amounts of heat energy in milliseconds. This energy instantaneously creates super-heated gases and results in extreme pressure at the detonation site. This pressure moves outward rapidly, first creating a pressure wave traveling at sonic speeds and then becomes forceful blast wind. The pressure wave (called overpressure) rapidly compresses and then decompresses all with which it comes in contact. Serious injury may result to any hollow and air-filled spaces, such as those in the middle ear, the bowel, and the lungs. The blast wind can propel the explosive container parts or other debris, such as glass or wood splinters, inducing injury in those it strikes. The blast wind may also throw victims resulting in blunt trauma as they strike objects or the ground. The pressure wave and blast wind may also cause structural collapse, resulting in crushing injury and/or entrapment. Finally, the blast heat may cause serious burn injury directly or burns from combustion of material it ignites.

The nuclear weapon releases energy as atoms are broken apart and reassembled. The energy released from a relatively small bomb is thousands of times greater than a conventional explosive of equal size. The nuclear detonation injures through the same mechanisms as the conventional explosion. The resulting injuries, however, are more extensive and serious. Additionally, the nuclear detonation releases exceptional amounts of heat energy that kills most individuals in the detonation area and causes serious burns at some distance from the blast epicenter. Lastly, the detonation emits great amounts of nuclear radiation causing direct radiation exposure and energizes dust and debris causing radioactive fallout. The fallout may travel with upper air currents and fall to earth many miles from the detonation site.

©2008 Pearson Education, Inc.

3. Identify and describe the major subclassifications of chemical and biological weapons of mass destruction.

Chemical weapons **pp. 921–926**

—**Nerve agents.** Nerve agents attack the central nervous system by causing an impulse transmission overload. This results in muscle spasms, convulsions, unconsciousness, and respiratory failure.

—**Vesicants.** Vesicants are chemical agents that damage exposed skin and cause blistering. They may also damage the eyes, respiratory tract, and lung tissue and may induce general illness as well.

—**Pulmonary agents.** Pulmonary agents attack the airway and lungs, producing inflammation and pulmonary edema. Their use frequently results in nasal and throat irritation, wheezing, cough, dyspnea, and hypoxia.

—**Biotoxins.** Biotoxins are chemicals produced by living organisms and behave more like chemical agents. Botulinum is the most toxic, 15,000 times more potent than the worst of the nerve agents (VX).

Biological weapons **pp. 927–928**

—**Pulmonary or pneumonia-like agents.** Pulmonary agents are the most likely biologic agents to be used by terrorists. These agents are transmitted via the respiratory system and induce cough, dyspnea, fever, and malaise.

—**Encephalitis-like agents.** Encephalitis-like agents affect the central nervous system and present with flu-like signs and symptoms. However, these biological agents usually carry a much higher mortality rate than the flu or similar diseases.

Other biological agents **pp. 928–929**

—**Cholera and viral hemorrhagic fever.** Cholera causes profuse diarrhea, and viral hemorrhagic fever attacks the blood's ability to coagulate.

Case Study Review

Reread the case study in Chapter 28 and then read the following discussion. This case study illustrates how the events of September 11, 2001 have affected EMS professionals and their responsibilities. It highlights the need to include the possibility of terrorist acts in all aspects of emergency care decision making.

Adam and Sean have a heightened index of suspicion for a weapon of mass destruction incident that comes following the events of September 11, 2001. When presented with several patients with similar symptoms, they suspect a chemical agent release and request activation of the county's WMD plan. They also approach the scene with care, arriving upwind of the building and directing dispatch to request evacuation (thereby evacuating the building without risk to rescuers). Sean and Adam also request the fire department (their local hazmat team) to respond as well. Finally, by using a cell phone rather than using the EMS radio, they assure their suspicion of a WMD incident is not made public.

Adam and Sean direct the potential patients to their care station using the public address system, again reducing any risk to the rescuers. They establish incident command and effectively communicate pertinent information regarding the numbers and types of patients they are encountering. This helps the emergency department prepare for arrival of numerous patients with the same complaints. Before stepping from their rig, Sean and Adam don HEPA-filter masks and gloves to further protect themselves from any biologic threat.

Adam relinquishes incident command as soon as someone from the fire department arrives. He communicates his knowledge of the scene and then joins Sean in administering to the patients. Since the number of patients outnumbers the resources available, Sean and Adam provide oxygen only to the most seriously affected patients. Thankfully, the symptoms are only minor and other ambulances arrive quickly. As more information is gathered about the scene, the initial information suggests a simple furnace or chimney malfunction. However, further investigation suggests that this was truly a WMD incident involving the intentional production of carbon monoxide. The scene then becomes a crime scene and is investigated thoroughly by the police department.

©2008 Pearson Education, Inc.
Intermediate Emergency Care: 1985, 3rd ed.

Content Self-Evaluation

Multiple Choice

_____ 1. Which of the following is the most likely weapon of choice for terrorist groups?
A. conventional explosives
B. nuclear weapons
C. biological agents
D. chemical agents
E. incendiary devices

_____ 2. Terrorists are likely to target which of the following?
A. an embassy
B. a symbol of government
C. their employer
D. corporations
E. all of the above

_____ 3. The blast pressure wave is likely to injure all of the following EXCEPT
A. the lungs.
B. the ears.
C. the bowel.
D. the heart.
E. the sinuses.

_____ 4. Incendiary agents differ from conventional explosives in that they
A. have greater explosive energy.
B. cause more burn injuries.
C. consume more oxygen.
D. are dropped from a high altitude.
E. combine both explosive and nuclear damage.

_____ 5. Which of the following is the mechanism of injury associated with most deaths from a nuclear blast?
A. radiation burns
B. radiation illness
C. cancer
D. thermal burns
E. pressure injuries

_____ 6. The best way to detect radiation in the absence of a Geiger counter is
A. by a strange taste in your mouth.
B. a warm sensation in your muscles.
C. immediate nausea.
D. a tingling sensation from the exposed surface.
E. none of the above

_____ 7. Fallout associated with the nuclear detonation is not likely to be a factor until how long after the detonation?
A. 10 minutes
B. 30 minutes
C. 1 hour
D. 4 hours
E. 2 days

_____ 8. Once a victim is exposed to nuclear radiation and debris has been properly decontaminated, he poses no danger to himself or others.
A. True
B. False

_____ 9. Which of the following is a symptom associated with radiation exposure?
A. nausea
B. fatigue
C. malaise
D. hypertension
E. all of the above except D

_____ 10. Which of the following influence the delivery of a chemical weapon?
A. wind strength
B. the agent's specific gravity
C. the agent's volatility
D. precipitation
E. all of the above

©2008 Pearson Education, Inc.

______ 11. Which of the following is NOT a common sign or symptom of a nerve agent?
A. dry mouth
B. tearing eyes
C. urination
D. defecation
E. vomiting

______ 12. Blistering agents are also known as
A. organophosphates.
B. vesicants.
C. carbamates.
D. chambering agents.
E. none of the above

______ 13. Which of the following is NOT a blistering agent?
A. lewisite
B. phosgene oxime
C. botulinum
D. sulfur mustard
E. nitrogen mustard

______ 14. One of the most toxic agents known to man is
A. sulfur mustard.
B. Ricin.
C. VX gas.
D. botulinum.
E. none of the above

______ 15. Which of the following suggests a chemical agent release?
A. a strange smell
B. numerous patients complaining of the same symptoms
C. a cloud of dust or gas
D. incapacitated or dead birds and insects
E. all of the above

______ 16. Which of the following is NOT a biologic agent capable of spreading from person to person?
A. Ebola
B. smallpox
C. plague
D. anthrax
E. cholera

______ 17. A biological release can be recognized by which of the following?
A. a distinctive cloud of gas
B. a distinctive odor
C. immediate signs and symptoms
D. very distinct signs and symptoms
E. none of the above

______ 18. The most likely biologic agents to be used by terrorists are
A. pulmonary agents.
B. flu-like agents.
C. encephalitis-like agents.
D. Ebola.
E. all of the above

______ 19. Almost all bioterrorist weapons are transmitted via the respiratory route; therefore, the HEPA respirator is very effective at reducing transmission.
A. True
B. False

______ 20. Dangers of a conventional explosion used by terrorists include all of the following EXCEPT
A. the danger of a secondary explosion.
B. inability to recognize the incident.
C. radioactive contamination.
D. structural collapse.
E. all of the above

©2008 Pearson Education, Inc.
Intermediate Emergency Care: 1985, 3rd ed.

Workbook Answer Key

Chapter 1: Roles and Responsibilities of the EMT-Intermediate

CONTENT SELF-EVALUATION

MULTIPLE CHOICE

1.	E	*p. 5*	8.	D	*p. 11*	15.	C	*p. 16*
2.	A	*p. 7*	9.	A	*p. 12*	16.	E	*p. 16*
3.	A	*p. 8*	10.	B	*p. 12*	17.	B	*p. 17*
4.	E	*p. 9*	11.	E	*p. 13*	18.	D	*p. 18*
5.	E	*p. 9*	12.	B	*p. 14*	19.	D	*pp. 18–19*
6.	B	*p. 10*	13.	C	*p. 16*	20.	A	*p. 19*
7.	E	*pp. 9–11*	14.	B	*p. 16*			

DESCRIPTION

21. (at least 3) *pp. 5–7*
    - assure vehicle inspection and routine maintenance have been completed
    - assure equipment inspection and routine maintenance have been completed
    - restock medications and IV solutions as needed
    - be aware of policies and procedures of the local EMS system
    - be aware of local geography
    - be knowledgeable of communications operation
    - be aware of support services
22. (at least 3) *p. 7*
    - personal safety
    - wear seatbelt, obey posted speed limits, and watch for hazards
    - arrive in a timely manner
    - know correct location
    - request anticipated additional resources
23. (at least 5) *p. 9*
    - self-confidence
    - credibility
    - inner strength
    - in control
    - communication skills
    - willing to make decisions
    - willing to accept responsibilities
    - knowledgeable about crew member capabilities
24. (at least 3) *p. 5*
    - clean-cut
    - remained calm
    - responded promptly
    - skillful
    - solution for everything
    - compassionate
    - top-quality care
25. (at least 3) *p. 18*
    - case reviews
    - videotapes
    - cassette lectures
    - in-hospital rotations in patient care areas
    - field drills
    - mobile classrooms that bring educational presentations to outlying squads
    - self-study exercises and computer-aided instruction
    - Internet-based programs
    - periodic "teaching days" in which a variety of topics are covered in lectures and presentations

Chapter 2: Emergency Medical Services Systems

CONTENT SELF-EVALUATION

MULTIPLE CHOICE

1.	A	*p. 27*	8.	B	*p. 34*	15.	E	*p. 42*
2.	B	*p. 30*	9.	C	*p. 36*	16.	D	*p. 43*
3.	A	*pp. 32–33*	10.	B	*p. 38*	17.	E	*pp. 44–45*
4.	E	*p. 32*	11.	A	*pp. 36–37*	18.	A	*p. 45*
5.	B	*p. 33*	12.	E	*p. 38*	19.	A	*p. 46*
6.	A	*p. 33*	13.	A	*p. 39*	20.	A	*p. 48*
7.	E	*p. 33*	14.	D	*p. 39*			

SEQUENCING

21. **A.** 1, **B.** 4, **C.** 3, **D.** 2, *p. 47*

DESCRIPTION

22. *Triage protocols (at least 1) pp. 34–35*
    - guidelines to determine patient flow through the EMS system
    - guidelines to determine what type, level, and priority of EMS response
    - guidelines to allocate system resources to meet patient needs
    - guidelines to direct the patient to the facility best suited to treat his problem

    Treatment protocols (at least 2)
    - guidelines for patient care
    - direct orders by a physician (on-line)
    - standing orders (off-line)

    Transport protocols (at least 2)
    - guidelines to determine mode of transport (air or ground)
    - level of care determined by nature of illness or injury, patient condition, transport time
    - most commonly call for transport to closest appropriate facility

©2008 Pearson Education, Inc.

Transfer protocols (at least 1)
guidelines for interhospital patient transports
ensure patient travels to an appropriate facility
ensure continuity of care

23. A. Caller interrogation—asks standard questions. *p. 38*
    B. Prioritization of symptoms—determines level of response.
    C. Selection of an appropriate response—types of personnel, number of vehicles, mode of response.
    D. Lifesaving pre-arrival instructions—first aid techniques while units are responding.

SPECIAL PROJECT

Research—Basic Life Support

Hypothesis: You should formulate a theory to be proved or disproved. (For example: Correct instruction in blood pressure determination will improve student accuracy.)

Literature Review:
magazines—*JEMS, Emergency,* etc.;
journals—*Annals of Emergency Medicine,* etc.;
textbooks—Basic level, Paramedic, etc.

Study methods: Your sample study method should be similar to this:
Had six EMTs take blood pressure readings on one another. They all used the same sphygmomanometer and stethoscope and applied the procedure in a quiet room. Each of the EMT's readings were compared with the average for each person on whom they took the readings. The EMTs repeated the experiment after the group received instruction on the correct procedures for determining blood pressure.

Conclusion: Your sample conclusion should be similar to this in wording:
During the first attempt to determine blood pressure, 70 percent of the readings were within the plus-or-minus 12 percent of the average blood pressure reading of the patient. Repeating the study after instruction increased the percentage of readings within 12 percent of average to 80 percent. A valid conclusion is that proper instruction in correct procedures improves the accuracy of blood pressure readings.

Chapter 3: Medical-Legal Considerations of Emergency Care

CONTENT SELF-EVALUATION

MULTIPLE CHOICE

1. C *p. 54*	6. B *pp. 58–60*	11. B *p. 63*
2. E *p. 55*	7. B *p. 60*	12. D *p. 64*
3. D *p. 56*	8. E *p. 61*	13. A *p. 66*
4. B *p. 57*	9. D *p. 62*	14. A *p. 66*
5. E *p. 57*	10. B *p. 63*	15. A *p. 68*

DESCRIPTION

16. *pp. 61–62* Negligence is the failure of the EMT-Intermediate to meet the standard of care when he or she had the duty to act and when his or her actions contribute to the harm suffered by the patient.
    Res ipsa loquitur is a form of negligence in which the nature of the events suggests that the EMT-Intermediate caused harm to the patient. The burden to prove innocence becomes the responsibility of the EMT-Intermediate.
17. *p. 63* The patient is unconscious.
    The patient is unable to communicate.
    The patient is mentally impaired.
    The patient is a young child.
18. *pp. 52–53* The patient is an elderly, thin male.
    He has a history of emphysema.
    He is on 3 L of oxygen per minute via nasal cannula.
    He has a bedside nebulizer.
    His respiratory rate is 6 and very shallow.
    His pulse is weak and rapid.
    The patient's daughter requested no resuscitation.
    No valid DNR was found.
    The patient's wife requested resuscitation.
    The crew discussed DNR, and rejected the daughter's request.
    Respiration was assisted via a bag-valve (BVM) unit.
    Patient's color improved with mechanical ventilation.
    Endotracheal tube placement was confirmed by bilaterally equal breath sounds and end-title CO_2 measurement.
    An IV was established.
    An albuterol treatment was administered via ET.

SPECIAL PROJECT

Answers will depend upon your state's requirements. Please confirm your answers with your instructor.

Chapter 4: Medical Terminology

CONTENT SELF-EVALUATION

MEDICAL TERM DISSECTION *pp. 76–78*

	Prefix	Combining form	Suffix
1.	myasthenia	muscle	weakness
2.	cephalgia	head	pain
3.	percuss	through	shake violently
4.	cyanosis	blue	condition
5.	hyperflexion	over	bending
6.	pathology	disease	study
7.	tachypnea	rapid	breathing
8.	rhinorrhea	nose	flow
9.	dysuria	difficult	urination
10.	hypertrophy	over	nourishment
11.	osteocyte	bone	cell
12.	hypoxemia	low oxygen	blood
13.	adrenal	toward	kidney
14.	hepatomegaly	liver	enlarged

©2008 Pearson Education, Inc.
Intermediate Emergency Care: 1985, 3rd ed.

	Prefix	Combining form	Suffix
15.	abduct	away	guide
16.	otoscope	ear	examine
17.	perinatal	around	birth
18.	antecubital	before	elbow
19.	dissect	twice	cut
20.	epicardium	above	heart
21.	postpartum	after	birth
22.	intervertebral	between	spinal bones
23.	neuroplasty	nerve	repair
24.	hemothorax	blood	thorax
25.	polyphagia	frequent	eating

ANATOMICAL LOCATIONS

MATCHING

26. G *p. 80*
27. E *p. 80*
28. F *p. 83*
29. H *p. 83*
30. D *p. 80*
31. A *p. 80*
32. C *p. 80*
33. I *p. 83*
34. B *p. 83*
35. J *p. 80*

SPECIAL PROJECT

Acquire a pocket medical dictionary and look up the pronunciation and meaning of the words listed in the chapter review.

Chapter 5: Documentation

CHAPTER SELF-EVALUATION

MULTIPLE CHOICE

1. E *p. 91*
2. B *p. 91*
3. A *p. 92*
4. B *p. 93*
5. B *pp. 95–96*
6. C *p. 101*
7. A *p. 101*
8. D *pp. 101–102*
9. C *p. 102*
10. B *pp. 102–105*
11. B *p. 104*
12. A *p. 104*
13. E *p. 104*
14. A *p. 105*
15. C *p. 105*
16. B *p. 105*
17. D *p. 105*
18. E *pp. 105–106*
19. B *pp. 106–107*
20. A *p. 106*
21. E *p. 107*
22. D *p. 107*
23. E *pp. 107–108*
24. A *p. 108*
25. E *p. 108*
26. B *p. 109*
27. A *p. 109*
28. D *p. 110*
29. E *pp. 110–113*
30. C *p. 113*

MATCHING *pp. 96–100* (Table 5–1)

31. P *p. 96*
32. Y *p. 96*
33. L *p. 96*
34. T *p. 96*
35. A *p. 96*
36. E *p. 96*
37. B *p. 97*
38. O *p. 97*
39. U *p. 97*
40. X *p. 97*
41. M *p. 97*
42. J *p. 97*
43. Q *p. 98*
44. G *p. 98*
45. R *p. 98*
46. V *p. 98*
47. I *p. 99*
48. N *p. 99*
49. F *p. 99*
50. C *p. 99*
51. W *p. 99*
52. K *p. 100*
53. S *p. 100*
54. D *p. 100*
55. H *p. 100*

SPECIAL PROJECTS
Documentation: Radio Report/Prehospital Care Report

Radio message from the scene to medical direction: Unit 21 to medical direction. We are attending a male victim of a one-car crash. He was initially unconscious but is now conscious, alert, and oriented. He has a small contusion on his forehead and a small welt on his neck. He was stung by a bee and has had a previous allergic reaction. Vitals are BP 110/76, pulse 90 and strong, respirations 30, and O_2 saturation of 94 percent. There are audible wheezes, and he is complaining of "a lump in the throat." He is on 12 L of O_2 via nonrebreather and has one IV of LR running TKO. A cervical collar has been applied and spinal immobilization is underway.

Follow-up radio message to Community Hospital: 0.3 mg epinephrine SQ and 50 mg Benadryl IM have been administered. Current vitals are BP 122/78, pulse 68 and strong, respirations 22 and regular, O_2 saturation 98%. Breath sounds are now clear. ETA is 10 minutes.

Ambulance run report form: Please review the accompanying form (on the next page) and check to be sure the form you completed includes the appropriate information. Note that you should include most, if not all, of the information listed on the accompanying sample form. If you have not done this, please review the narrative in the Workbook and determine what is missing from your version. Assure that no important details are left out of the report.

©2008 Pearson Education, Inc.

Address: **2145 E. Brookline Drive**	Location: **Wildwood & Elm** Enrt **18:32**
City: **Rochester** St: Zip:	Call Origin: **Dispatch** Scne **18:45**
Age: **28** Birth: / / Sex: [X][F]	Type: Emrg[X] Non[ ] Trnsfr[ ] LvSn **19:02**
Nature of Call: **One-car auto accident**	ArHsp **19:25**
Chief Complaint: **Head injury—allergic reaction/bee sting**	InSv **19:55**

Description of Current Problem:

Pt. was apparently stung by a bee, then struck a tree with his auto. Found unconscious, then awoke. Contusion on his forehead where it hit the windshield and a small welt on his neck. Pt. complains of a lump in his throat and mild dyspnea. Mild wheezes on auscultation. Pt. reports previous life-threatening allergic reaction, has a prescribed kit but it is at home. Assessment otherwise unremarkable.

Trauma Scr: **16** Glasgow: **15**

Medical Problems

Past		Present
[ ]	Cardiac	[ ]
[ ]	Stroke	[ ]
[ ]	Acute Abdomen	[ ]
[ ]	Diabetes	[ ]
[ ]	Psychiatric	[ ]
[ ]	Epilepsy	[ ]
[ ]	Drug/Alcohol	[ ]
[ ]	Poisoning	[ ]
[X]	Allergy/Asthma	[X]
[ ]	Syncope	[ ]
[ ]	Obstetrical	[ ]
[ ]	GYN	[ ]

Other:

On Scene Care: **O_2, C-Collar, Spinal Imm.**	First Aid: **None**
IV – TKO LR w/ 16 ga R forearm	
0.3 mg Epi SQ, 50 mg Benadryl IM	
	By Whom?

02 @ **12** L **18:52** Via **NRB**	C-Collar **18:50**	S-Immob. **18:52**	Stretcher **18:55**

Allergies/Meds: **Bee sting, no other allergies known**	Past Med Hx: **Bee sting and reaction 2 yrs ago no other history noted.**

Time	Pulse		Resp.		BP S/D	LOC	ECG
18:52	R: **90**	[X][i]	R: **30**	[s][l]	**110/76**	[X][v][p][u]	**Normal Sinus Rhythm**
Care/Comments: **IV initiated via protocol – 16 ga R forearm, audible wheezes, SaO_2 94%**							
18:59	R: **78**	[X][i]	R: **24**	[s][l]	**118/88**	[X][v][p][u]	**Normal Sinus Rhythm**
Care/Comments: **Epi & Benadryl administered, SaO_2 98%, wheezes gone**							
19:02	R: **68**	[X][i]	R: **22**	[s][l]	**122/78**	[X][v][p][u]	**Normal Sinus Rhythm**
Care/Comments: **SaO_2 98%**							
19:20	R: **86**	[X][i]	R: **24**	[s][l]	**122/80**	[X][v][p][u]	**Normal Sinus Rhythm**
Care/Comments: **Wheezes reduced, SaO_2 98%**							

Destination: **Community Hospital**	Personnel: Certification
Reason: [X]pt [ ]Closest [ ]M.D. [ ]Other	1. **Your Name** [X][E][O]
Contacted: [X]Radio [ ]Tele [ ]Direct	2. **Mike Grailing** [X][E][O]
Ar Status: [X]Better [ ]UnC [ ]Worse	3. **n/a** [P][E][O]

©2008 Pearson Education, Inc.
Intermediate Emergency Care: 1985, 3rd ed.

Crossword Puzzle

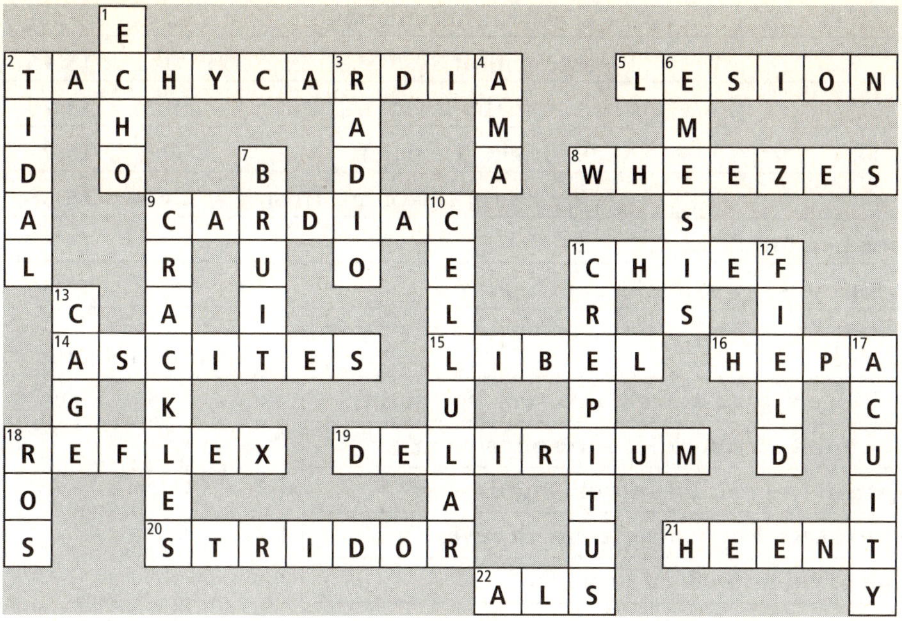

Chapter 6: EMS Communications

CONTENT SELF-EVALUATION

<u>MULTIPLE CHOICE</u>

1. E *p. 121*
2. C *pp. 124–125*
3. B *p. 125*
4. C *p. 125*
5. C *p. 127*
6. E *p. 128*
7. B *p. 129*
8. B *p. 129*
9. C *p. 131*
10. E *p. 132*
11. E *p. 133*
12. D *p. 134*
13. A *p. 134*
14. E *p. 134*
15. E *pp. 135–136*

<u>SEQUENCING</u>

16. A. 3, B. 4, C. 1, D. 2 *p. 121*

<u>DESCRIPTION</u>

17. (any 2) *p. 132*
    - establish technical standards for radio equipment
    - license and allocate radio frequencies
    - monitor radio frequencies to assure appropriate usage
    - check station licenses and station records
    - license and regulate technical personnel who repair and operate equipment
18. (any 3) *p. 132*
    - direct the appropriate vehicle to the appropriate address
    - monitor and coordinate system communications
    - obtain information necessary for the EMS response
    - instruct the caller in first aid measures
    - maintain records of the complete response
    - help assure provider safety

SPECIAL PROJECT

Your verbal reports should include most of the following elements.

Radio message from the scene to medical control:

Unit 89 to Receiving Hospital

We are at the ball field treating a 13-year-old male who collapsed while playing baseball. He is currently unresponsive to all but painful stimuli, is cool to the touch and sweating profusely. Vitals are BP 136/98, pulse 92 and strong, respirations 24 and regular, and pupils equal and slow to react. ECG is showing normal sinus rhythm. No physical signs of trauma noted and past medical history is unknown. Oxygen is applied at 4 liters via nasal cannula. Expected ETA 20 minutes.

Follow-up radio message to medical control:

One IV in left forearm running TKO with NS. Patient now responding to verbal stimuli. Vitals BP 134/96, pulse 90 and strong, respirations 24, ECG—NSR. ETA, 10 minutes.

Ambulance run report form:

Please review the next page and ensure that your form includes the appropriate information. Note that you should include most, if not all, of the information listed on the example form. If not, please review the narrative in the workbook and determine what you are missing. Ensure that no important details are left out of the report.

Date **Today's Date**	Emergency Medical Services Run Report	Run # **912**

Patient Information | **Service Information** | **Times**

Name: **Thompson, Jim**	Agency: **Unit 89**	Rcvd	**15:15**
Address: **Unknown**	Location: **Ballfield**	Enrt	**15:16**
City: St: Zip:	Call Origin: **Dispatch**	Scne	**15:22**
Age: **13** Birth: / / Sex: [X][F]	Type: Emrg[X] Non[ ] Trnsfr[ ]	LvSn	**15:38**
Nature of Call: **Unconscious person**		ArHsp	**15:57**
Chief Complaint: **Unconsciousness—possible heat exhaustion**		InSv	**16:15**

Description of Current Problem:

The patient collapsed while playing baseball on a very hot, sunny day. Pt. was found to be cool & diaphoretic, unresponsive to verbal stimuli, and responsive to painful stimuli. Pupils were normal in size but slow to react. Physical assessment reveals no apparent signs of trauma or other medical problem.

Trauma Scr: **n/a** Glasgow: **6**

Medical Problems

Past		Present
[ ]	Cardiac	[ ]
[ ]	Stroke	[ ]
[ ]	Acute Abdomen	[ ]
[ ]	Diabetes	[ ]
[ ]	Psychiatric	[ ]
[ ]	Epilepsy	[ ]
[ ]	Drug/Alcohol	[ ]
[ ]	Poisoning	[ ]
[ ]	Allergy/Asthma	[ ]
[ ]	Syncope	[ ]
[ ]	Obstetrical	[ ]
[ ]	GYN	[ ]

Other: **Unknown**

On Scene Care: **provided oxygen, removed patient from sun and heat. Attempted IV in right forearm (unsuccessful) started IV in left forearm w/ 16 ga NS – TKO**

First Aid: **pillow was placed under head**

By Whom? **bystanders**

02 @ **12** L **15:27** Via **NRB**	C-Collar **n/a** :	S-Immob. **n/a**	Stretcher **15:37**

Allergies/Meds: **Unknown**

Past Med Hx: **Unknown**

Time	Pulse	Resp.	BP S/D	LOC	ECG
15:27	R: **92** [X][i]	R: **24** [s][l]	**136/98**	[a][v][X][u]	**Normal Sinus Rhythm**
Care/Comments: **Pt. unresponsive to all but painful stimuli**					
15:37	R: **90** [X][i]	R: **24** [s][l]	**134/96**	[a][X][p][u]	**Normal Sinus Rhythm**
Care/Comments: **Pt. became responsive to verbal stimuli**					
15:45	R: **88** [X][i]	R: **24** [s][l]	**132/90**	[X][v][p][u]	**Normal Sinus Rhythm**
Care/Comments: **Pt. became fully concious, alert, and oriented**					
:	R: [r][i]	R: [s][l]	/	[a][v][p][u]	
Care/Comments:					

Destination: **Receiving Hospital**	Personnel: Certification
Reason:[ ]pt [X]Closest [ ]M.D. [ ]Other	1. **Your Name** [X][E][O]
Contacted: [X]Radio [ ]Tele [ ]Direct	2. **Steve Phillips** [P][X][O]
Ar Status: [X]Better [ ]UnC [ ]Worse	3. **n/a** [P][E][O]

©2008 Pearson Education, Inc.
Intermediate Emergency Care: 1985, 3rd ed.

Chapter 7: Human Body Systems

CONTENT SELF-EVALUATION

MULTIPLE CHOICE

1.	A	*p. 141*	36.	A	*p. 170*
2.	A	*p. 141*	37.	C	*p. 170*
3.	C	*pp. 141–142*	38.	D	*pp. 170–171*
4.	C	*p. 142*	39.	B	*p. 173*
5.	A	*p. 142*	40.	C	*p. 174*
6.	E	*p. 143*	41.	B	*p. 175*
7.	D	*p. 143*	42.	D	*pp. 174–175*
8.	E	*p. 143*	43.	A	*p. 177*
9.	E	*p. 143*	44.	C	*p. 178*
10.	D	*p. 143*	45.	D	*p. 178*
11.	A	*p. 144*	46.	A	*p. 178*
12.	E	*p. 144*	47.	B	*p. 180*
13.	B	*p. 145*	48.	A	*p. 180*
14.	A	*p. 146*	49.	B	*pp. 180–181*
15.	B	*p. 146*	50.	E	*p. 180*
16.	A	*p. 147*	51.	E	*p. 181*
17.	C	*p. 147*	52.	A	*p. 181*
18.	C	*p. 149*	53.	C	*p. 181*
19.	B	*p. 150*	54.	B	*p. 183*
20.	B	*p. 150*	55.	B	*pp. 183–184*
21.	B	*p. 150*	56.	A	*p. 183*
22.	E	*p. 152*	57.	E	*p. 184*
23.	A	*p. 154*	58.	A	*p. 187*
24.	B	*p. 155*	59.	C	*p. 187*
25.	C	*p. 147*	60.	E	*p. 187*
26.	B	*p. 157*	61.	B	*p. 188*
27.	E	*p. 160*	62.	C	*p. 191*
28.	C	*p. 160*	63.	D	*p. 191*
29.	C	*p. 161*	64.	B	*p. 191*
30.	A	*p. 222*	65.	A	*p. 193*
31.	C	*p. 164*	66.	C	*p. 194*
32.	C	*p. 166*	67.	D	*p. 194*
33.	A	*p. 169*	68.	A	*p. 194*
34.	D	*p. 157*	69.	A	*p. 194*
35.	E	*p. 228*	70.	C	*p. 194–195*

Chapter 8: General Patient Assessment and Initial Management

CONTENT SELF-EVALUATION

MULTIPLE CHOICE

1.	B	*p. 205*	18.	C	*p. 214*	35.	A	*p. 228*
2.	E	*p. 206*	19.	E	*p. 215*	36.	E	*p. 229*
3.	C	*p. 206*	20.	C	*p. 217*	37.	A	*p. 230*
4.	B	*p. 206*	21.	A	*p. 217*	38.	D	*p. 230*
5.	A	*p. 207*	22.	C	*p. 217*	39.	B	*p. 232*
6.	C	*p. 207*	23.	C	*p. 217*	40.	B	*p. 233*
7.	A	*p. 207*	24.	D	*p. 217*	41.	C	*p. 233*
8.	E	*p. 207*	25.	A	*p. 219*	42.	D	*p. 236*
9.	E	*p. 207*	26.	B	*p. 220*	43.	B	*p. 237*
10.	C	*p. 209*	27.	E	*p. 220*	44.	C	*p. 238*
11.	A	*p. 210*	28.	A	*p. 221*	45.	D	*p. 239*
12.	D	*p. 214*	29.	B	*p. 222*	46.	B	*p. 239*
13.	B	*p. 214*	30.	E	*p. 222*	47.	E	*p. 239*
14.	A	*p. 214*	31.	E	*p. 224*	48.	B [A]	*p. 239*
15.	B	*p. 214*	32.	C	*p. 228*	49.	B	*p. 240*
16.	D	*p. 214*	33.	D	*p. 229*	50.	D	*p. 241*
17.	E	*p. 214*	34.	B	*p. 229*	51.	B	*p. 242*

52.	D	*p. 242*	55.	A	*p. 246*	58.	E	*p. 253*
53.	B	*p. 243*	56.	A	*p. 248*	59.	E	*p. 255*
54.	A[D]	*p. 244*	57.	A	*p. 250*	60.	B	*p. 256*

LISTING

61. Scene Size-up
62. Initial Assessment
63. Focused History and Physical Examination *p. 205*
64. Detailed Physical Examination
65. Ongoing Assessment

SPECIAL PROJECT: p. 209

Your verbal reports should include most of the following elements.

Radio message from the scene to medical control:
Unit 89 to Receiving Hospital

We are at the ball field treating a 13-year-old male who collapsed while playing baseball. He is currently unresponsive to all but painful stimuli, is cool to the touch and sweating profusely. Vitals are BP 136/98, pulse 92 and strong, respirations 24 and regular, and pupils equal and slow to react. ECG is showing normal sinus rhythm. No physical signs of trauma noted and past medical history is unknown. Oxygen is applied at 4 liters via nasal cannula. Expected ETA 20 minutes.

Follow-up radio message to medical control:
One IV in left forearm running TKO with NS. Patient now responding to verbal stimuli. Vitals BP 134/96, pulse 90 & strong, respirations 24, ECG—NSR. ETA, 10 minutes

Ambulance run report form:
Please review the next page and ensure that your form includes the appropriate information. Note that you should include most, if not all, of the information listed on the example form. If not, please review the narrative in the workbook and determine what you are missing. Ensure that no important details are left out of the report.

Chapter 9: Advanced Airway Management, Oxygenation, and Ventilation

CONTENT SELF-EVALUATION

MULTIPLE CHOICE

1.	B	*p. 268*	20.	D	*p. 294*	39.	D	*p. 325*
2.	A	*p. 269*	21.	B	*p. 294*	40.	E	*p. 325*
3.	C	*p. 275*	22.	C	*p. 295*	41.	A	*p. 327*
4.	E	*p. 278*	23.	A	*p. 299*	42.	E	*p. 330*
5.	E	*p. 278*	24.	D	*p. 304*	43.	D	*p. 333*
6.	A	*p. 279*	25.	D	*p. 308*	44.	A	*p. 338*
7.	B	*p. 282*	26.	D	*p. 308*	45.	A	*p. 339*
8.	D	*p. 279*	27.	A	*p. 310*			
9.	D	*p. 280*	28.	D	*p. 310*			
10.	C	*p. 280*	29.	B	*p. 312*			
11.	A	*p. 281*	30.	C	*p. 312*			
12.	B	*p. 283*	31.	C	*p. 314*			
13.	B	*p. 283*	32.	A	*p. 315*			
14.	B	*p. 284*	33.	E	*p. 317*			
15.	D	*p. 284*	34.	B	*p. 318*			
16.	E	*p. 286*	35.	B	*p. 319*			
17.	A	*p. 286*	36.	B	*p. 327*			
18.	C	*p. 289*	37.	C	*p. 321*			
19.	C	*p. 291*	38.	E	*p. 322*			

©2008 Pearson Education, Inc.

LABEL THE DIAGRAM

46. *p. 268*

A. Tonsil	E. Vocal Cords
B. Tongue	F. Trachea
C. Vallecula	G. Cricoid Cartilage
D. Epiglottis	H. Esophagus

SPECIAL PROJECT

Airway Obstruction *p. 281*

1. Tongue: In the absence of muscle tone, the relaxed tongue drops back in the larynx blocking the airway.
2. Foreign body: An object, usually food, becomes lodged in the laryngopharynx and blocks the airway.
3. Trauma: Trauma may disrupt the integrity of the airway thereby allowing it to collapse or physically blocking the airway. Additionally, loose teeth or blood clots may obstruct the airway.
4. Laryngeal edema or spasm: Swelling of the laryngeal tissue may occlude the airway or spasm of the vocal cords may occur secondary to anaphylaxis, epiglottitis, or inhalation of harmful substances.
5. Aspiration: The inhalation of teeth, dentures, blood, or vomitus may occlude the airway.

SPECIAL PROJECT

Problem Solving—Airway Maintenance *p. 312*

What equipment would you prepare?		
suction	tape	10 mL syringe
laryngoscope	stethoscope	water-soluble gel
stylet	endotracheal tube	Magill forceps

How would you check your equipment?

Laryngoscope Check blade—bright white and non-flickering *p. 312*

Tube cuff Inflate with 10 mL—will it hold air? *p. 321*

One larger and one smaller tube available

What would you ask the ventilator to do prior to your attempt?

Properly ventilate the patient.

Identify the steps of the procedures you're about to attempt.

1. Fill syringe with 10–15 mL air.
2. Position the patient's head. *p. 321*
3. Grasp the handle in left hand.
4. Insert blade in right side of mouth.
5. Displace tongue to left.
6. Insert blade to epiglottis.
7. Lift laryngoscope along axis of handle.
8. Visualize the vocal folds and glottis.
9. Grasp tube and pass it between the cords.
10. Inflate the cuff and auscultate.

What actions would you take to ensure the tube is properly placed?

1. Visualize, with the laryngoscope, the tube passing through the vocal folds.
2. Check the depth of the tube against the mouth.
3. Auscultate all lung fields for bilaterally equal breath sounds.
4. Auscultate epigastrium for gurgling sounds.

What should you do if the tube is misplaced?

If the tube is placed in the esophagus, leave it in place, hyperventilate the patient and attempt to place another tube in the trachea. Reauscultate and assure the tube is properly placed. *p. 325*

Chapter 10: Fluids and Shock

CONTENT SELF-EVALUATION

MULTIPLE CHOICE

1.	A	*p. 347*	13.	C	*p. 355*	25.	B	*p. 364*
2.	A	*p. 348*	14.	C	*p. 355*	26.	E	*p. 365*
3.	B	*p. 349*	15.	E	*p. 356*	27.	A	*p. 365*
4.	C	*p. 350*	16.	D	*p. 357*	28.	E	*p. 365*
5.	B	*p. 350*	17.	D	*p. 357*	29.	B	*p. 366*
6.	A	*p. 351*	18.	B	*p. 360*	30.	E	*p. 367*
7.	B	*p. 351*	19.	B	*p. 361*	31.	C	*p. 368*
8.	C	*p. 352*	20.	C	*p. 361*	32.	E	*p. 368*
9.	B	*p. 352*	21.	B	*p. 361*	33.	B	*p. 368*
10.	B	*p. 352*	22.	D	*p. 365*	34.	B	*p. 369*
11.	D	*p. 352*	23.	C	*p. 362*	35.	A	*p. 369*
12.	A	*p. 353*	24.	D	*p. 363*			

Chapter 11: Venous Access and Medication Administration

CONTENT SELF-EVALUATION

MULTIPLE CHOICE

1.	E	*p. 378*	31.	A	*p. 396*	61.	A	*pp. 413,414*
2.	B	*p. 378*	32.	B	*p. 397*	62.	C	*p. 414*
3.	E	*p. 379*	33.	A	*p. 398*	63.	D	*p. 413*
4.	A	*p. 380*	34.	C	*p. 397*	64.	B	*p. 415*
5.	C	*p. 381*	35.	B	*p. 398*	65.	A	*p. 417*
6.	E	*p. 381*	36.	C	*p. 398*	66.	D	*p. 415*
7.	D	*p. 381*	37.	C	*p. 399*	67.	C	*p. 419*
8.	E	*p. 381*	38.	A	*p. 399*	68.	D	*p. 419*
9.	E	*p. 381*	39.	A	*p. 400*	69.	D	*p. 417*
10.	B	*p. 382*	40.	A	*p. 400*	70.	B	*p. 419*
11.	A	*p. 382*	41.	E	*p. 400*	71.	A	*p. 422*
12.	D	*p. 383*	42.	C	*p. 403*	72.	E	*p. 422*
13.	C	*p. 384*	43.	D	*p. 403*	73.	B	*p. 425*
14.	A	*p. 384*	44.	A	*p. 403*	74.	D	*p. 425*
15.	A	*p. 385*	45.	B	*p. 403*	75.	B	*p. 426*
16.	E	*p. 385*	46.	D	*p. 403*	76.	B	*p. 429*
17.	B	*p. 406*	47.	E	*p. 404*	77.	C	*p. 427*
18.	B	*p. 386*	48.	A	*p. 404*	78.	A	*p. 429*
19.	D	*p. 389*	49.	A	*p. 404*	79.	E	*p. 429*
20.	B	*p. 389*	50.	C	*p. 404*	80.	A	*p. 429*
21.	B	*p. 389*	51.	D	*p. 405*			
22.	B	*p. 389*	52.	A	*p. 405*			
23.	A	*p. 390*	53.	C	*p. 405*			
24.	C	*p. 390*	54.	B	*p. 406*			
25.	C	*p. 390*	55.	B	*p. 407*			
26.	B	*p. 393*	56.	B	*p. 407*			
27.	E	*p. 394*	57.	A	*p. 409*			
28.	D	*p. 395*	58.	A	*p. 409*			
29.	D	*p. 395*	59.	E	*p. 409*			
30.	B	*p. 396*	60.	C	*p. 413*			

©2008 Pearson Education, Inc.
Intermediate Emergency Care: 1985, 3rd ed.

Chapter 12: Pharmacology

CONTENT SELF-EVALUATION

MULTIPLE CHOICE

1.	D	*p. 434*	13.	A	*p. 439*	25.	B	*p. 443*
2.	A	*p. 434*	14.	A	*p. 440*	26.	A	*p. 443*
3.	B	*p. 434*	15.	C	*p. 440*	27.	A	*p. 443*
4.	A	*p. 434*	16.	C	*p. 440*	28.	D	*p. 444*
5.	B	*p. 434*	17.	C	*p. 440*	29.	E	*p. 446*
6.	B	*p. 435*	18.	C	*p. 440*	30.	E	*p. 446*
7.	C	*p. 437*	19.	A	*p. 441*			
8.	C	*p. 437*	20.	D	*p. 442*			
9.	A	*p. 438*	21.	E	*pp. 442–443*			
10.	C	*p. 438*	22.	A	*p. 443*			
11.	B	*p. 438*	23.	D	*p. 443*			
12.	D	*p. 438*	24.	B	*p. 443*			

SPECIAL PROJECT

Drip Math Worksheet 1 *p. 451*

1. R = 15 drops/min
V = ?
T = 25 min
D = 60 drops/ml
V = R × T = 15 drops/min × 25 min

$$V = \frac{15 \text{ gtts} \times 25 \text{ min}}{\text{min}}$$

$$V = 375 \text{ gtts/D} = \frac{375 \text{ gtts} \times \text{ml}}{60 \text{ gtts}}$$

$$= \frac{375 \text{ ml}}{60} = \mathbf{6.25} \text{ ml}$$

2. R = V/T = 250 ml/60 min
V = 250 ml
T = 60 min
D_1 = 60 drops/ml
D_2 = 10 drops/ml

A. $$R = V/T = \frac{250 \text{ ml}}{60 \text{ min}} = \frac{4.17 \text{ ml}}{\text{min}}$$

$$= \frac{4.17 \cancel{\text{ml}} \times 60 \text{ gtts}}{\text{min} \times \cancel{\text{ml}}} = \frac{\mathbf{250 \text{ gtts}}}{\mathbf{min}}$$

B. $$R = V/T = \frac{250 \text{ ml}}{60 \text{ min}} = \frac{4.17 \text{ ml}}{\text{min}}$$

$$= \frac{4.17 \text{ ml} \times 10 \text{ gtts}}{\text{min} \times \text{ml}} = \frac{\mathbf{41.7 \text{ gtts}}}{\mathbf{min}}$$

3. R = 32 drops/min
V = 50 ml
T = ?
D = 45 drops/ml
R(ml) = R(min) × D
R(ml) = 32 drops/min × 45 drops/ml

$$R(\text{ml}) = \frac{32 \text{ gtts} \times \text{ml}}{45 \text{ gtts} \times \text{min}} = \frac{32 \text{ ml}}{45 \text{ min}} = 0.71 \text{ ml/min}$$

$$T = V/R = \frac{50 \text{ ml}/0.71 \text{ ml/min}}{0.71 \text{ ml}}$$

$$= \frac{50 \text{ ml} \times \text{min}}{0.71} = 50 \text{ min} = \mathbf{0.70 \text{ min}}$$

4. R = 4 gtts/sec × 60 sec/min

$$= \frac{4 \text{ gtts} \times 60 \cancel{\text{sec}}}{\cancel{\text{sec}} \times \text{min}} = 240 \text{ gtts/min}$$

V = ?
T = 45 min
D = 10 drops/ml
V = R × T = 240 gtts/min × 45 min

$$= \frac{240 \text{ gtts} \times 45 \text{ min}}{\text{min}} = 10{,}800 \text{ gtts}$$

$$V = 10{,}800 \text{ gtts/D} = \frac{10{,}800 \text{ gtts}/10 \text{ gtts/ml}}{10 \text{ gtts}}$$

$$= \frac{10{,}800 \text{ ml} \times \text{ml}}{10} = \mathbf{1{,}080 \text{ ml}}$$

5. R = ?
V = 1.5 ml/min
T = 1 min
D_1 = 60 drops/min
D_2 = 45 drops/min
D_3 = 10 drops/min

A. $$R = V/T = \frac{1.5 \text{ ml}}{1 \text{ min}} = \frac{1.5 \text{ ml} \times D}{1 \text{ min}}$$

$$= \frac{1.5 \cancel{\text{ml}} \times 60 \text{ gtts}}{\text{min} \times \cancel{\text{ml}}} = \mathbf{90 \text{ gtts/min}}$$

B. $$R = V/T = \frac{1.5 \text{ ml}}{1 \text{ min}} = \frac{1.5 \text{ ml} \times D}{1 \text{ min}}$$

$$= \frac{1.5 \cancel{\text{ml}} \times 45 \text{ gtts}}{\text{min} \times \cancel{\text{ml}}} = \mathbf{67.5 \text{ gtts/min}}$$

C. $$R = V/T = \frac{1.5 \text{ ml}}{1 \text{ min}} = \frac{1.5 \text{ ml} \times D}{1 \text{ min}}$$

$$= \frac{1.5 \cancel{\text{ml}} \times 10 \text{ gtts}}{\text{min} \times \cancel{\text{ml}}} = \mathbf{15 \text{ gtts/min}}$$

Drug Math Worksheet 1 *p. 450*

1. Dh = 1 mg
Vh = 5 ml
Dd = 0.5 mg
Va = ?

$$Va = \frac{Vh \times Dd}{Dh} = \frac{5 \text{ ml} \times 0.5 \cancel{\text{mg}}}{1 \cancel{\text{mg}}}$$

$$= \frac{2.5 \text{ ml}}{1} = \mathbf{2.5 \text{ ml}}$$

2. Dh = 80 mg
Vh = 4 ml
Dd = 40 mg
Va = ?

$$Va = \frac{Vh \times Dd}{Dh} = \frac{4 \text{ ml} \times 40 \cancel{\text{mg}}}{80 \cancel{\text{mg}}}$$

$$= \frac{16\cancel{0} \text{ ml}}{8\cancel{0}} = \mathbf{2 \text{ ml}}$$

3. A. Dh = 1 g (1,000 mg)
Vh = 1,000 ml
Dd = 1 mg
Va = ?

$$Va = \frac{Vh \times Dd}{Dh} = \frac{1{,}000 \text{ ml} \times 1 \text{ mg}}{1 \text{ g}}$$

$$= \frac{1{,}\cancel{000} \text{ ml} \times 1 \cancel{\text{mg}}}{1{,}\cancel{000} \cancel{\text{mg}}} = \frac{1 \text{ ml}}{1} = \mathbf{1 \text{ ml}}$$

B. Dh = 1 g (1,000 mg)
Vh = 10,000 ml
Dd = 1 mg
Va = ?

©2008 Pearson Education, Inc.

$$Va = \frac{Vh \times Dd}{Dh} = \frac{10{,}000 \text{ ml} \times 1 \text{ mg}}{1 \text{ g}}$$

$$= \frac{10,\cancel{000} \text{ ml} \times 1 \cancel{\text{mg}}}{1,\cancel{000} \cancel{\text{mg}}} = \frac{10 \text{ ml}}{1} = 10 \text{ ml}$$

4. Desired dose = patient weight

$$\times 0.2 \text{ mg/kg} = \frac{6 \cancel{\text{kg}} \times 0.2 \text{ mg}}{\cancel{\text{kg}}} = 1.2 \text{ mg}$$

Dh = 6 mg
Vh = 2 ml
Dd = 1.2 mg
Va = ?

$$Va = \frac{Vh \times Dd}{Dh} = \frac{2 \text{ ml} \times 1.2 \cancel{\text{mg}}}{6 \cancel{\text{mg}}}$$

$$= \frac{2.4 \text{ ml}}{6} = 0.4 \text{ ml}$$

CHAPTER 13: Cardiac Emergencies

CONTENT SELF-EVALUATION

MULTIPLE CHOICE

1. C *p. 468*
2. C *p. 469*
3. A *p. 470*
4. E *p. 471*
5. B *p. 471*
6. E *p. 472*
7. A *p. 474*
8. E *p. 474*
9. A *p. 475*
10. D *p. 475*
11. B *p. 476*
12. B *p. 477*
13. A *p. 479*
14. B *pp. 480–481*
15. B *p. 481*
16. D *pp. 481–482*
17. B *p. 488*
18. E *p. 489*
19. E *pp. 489–490*
20. C *p. 492*
21. C *p. 494*
22. E *p. 495*
23. D *p. 497*
24. C *p. 499*
25. A *p. 502*
26. A *p. 502*
27. C *p. 503*
28. D *p. 508*
29. A *p. 509*
30. A *p. 510*
31. E *p. 511*
32. D *p. 513*
33. B *p. 514*
34. D *p. 515*
35. D *p. 516*
36. E *p. 518*
37. A *p. 518*
38. D *p. 521*
39. E *p. 522*
40. A *p. 523*

MATCHING

41. B *p. 470*
42. G *p. 470*
43. D *p. 470*
44. A *p. 470*
45. H *p. 470*
46. C *p. 470*
47. F *p. 471*
48. E *p. 471*
49. B *p. 472*
50. C *p. 472*
51. A *p. 472*

LABEL THE DIAGRAMS

Figure 1

52. D *p. 469*
53. A *p. 469*
54. B *p. 469*
55. C *p. 469*
56. F *p. 472*
57. E *p. 469*

Figure 2 ***p. 472***

58. C
59. D
60. F
61. G
62. E
63. B
64. A

Figure 3

65. C *p. 486*
66. B *p. 483*
67. E *p. 483*
68. F *p. 487*
69. A *p. 483*
70. D *p. 484*

MATCHING

71. C *p. 510*
72. D *p. 513*
73. B *p. 513*
74. F *p. 518*
75. E *p. 513*
76. A *p. 508*
77. G *p. 516*
78. H *p. 522*

SPECIAL PROJECT
ECG Interpretation pp. 482–489

Rhythm 1: *Regularity:* regular
Rate: 50 beats per minute
P Waves: uniform and upright; regular P–P interval
PRI: .12 seconds and constant
QRS: .08 seconds
Interp: Sinus Bradycardia

Rhythm 2: *Regularity:* regular underlying rhythm interrupted by an ectopic
Rate: 58 beats per minute
P Waves: uniform; regular P–P interval
PRI: .20 seconds
QRS: .10 seconds in underlying rhythm; .18 seconds in ectopic; ectopic has bizarre configuration
Interp: Sinus Bradycardia with one PVC

Rhythm 3: *Regularity:* regular underlying rhythm interrupted by ectopics
Rate: 75 beats per minute
P Waves: uniform; regular P–P interval
PRI: .18 seconds
QRS: .12 seconds in underlying complex; .12 seconds in ectopics; ectopics have bizarre configuration
Interp: Sinus Rhythm (with wide QRS) with two PVCs

Rhythm 4: *Regularity:* regular
Rate: 136 beats per minute
P Waves: uniform and upright; regular P–P interval
PRI: .16 seconds and constant
QRS: .06 seconds
Interp: Sinus Tachycardia

Rhythm 5: *Regularity:* regular
Rate: 107 beats per minute
P Waves: upright and uniform
PRI: .12 seconds
QRS: .08 seconds
Interp: Sinus Tachycardia

Rhythm 6: *Regularity:* regular
Rate: 51 beats per minute
P Waves: uniform and upright; regular P–P interval
PRI: .24 seconds and constant
QRS: .10 seconds
Interp: Sinus Bradycardia with First Degree Heart Block

Rhythm 7: *Regularity:* totally chaotic baseline
Rate: cannot be determined
P Waves: none
PRI: none
QRS: none
Interp: Ventricular Fibrillation

Rhythm 8: *Regularity:* slightly irregular
Rate: approximately 30 beats per minute
P Waves: uniform and upright; irregular P–P interval
PRI: .18 seconds and constant
QRS: .08 seconds
Interp: Sinus Bradyarrhythmia

©2008 Pearson Education, Inc.
Intermediate Emergency Care: 1985, 3rd ed.

Rhythm 9: *Regularity:* slightly irregular
Rate: 150 beats per minute
P Waves: none visible
PRI: none
QRS: .20 seconds
Interp: Ventricular Tachycardia

Chapter 14: Respiratory Emergencies

CONTENT SELF-EVALUATION

MULTIPLE CHOICE

1.	C	*p. 531*	11.	A	*p. 541*
2.	A	*p. 534*	12.	A	*p. 542*
3.	C	*pp. 535–536*	13.	D	*p. 542*
4.	B	*p. 538*	14.	A	*p. 542*
5.	E	*p. 538*	15.	A	*pp. 542–543*
6.	B	*p. 539*	16.	A	*p. 543*
7.	B	*p. 541*	17.	C	*p. 543*
8.	D	*pp. 540–541*	18.	D	*p. 543*
9.	D	*p. 541*	19.	C	*p. 544*
10.	D	*p. 541*	20.	A	*p. 544*

Chapter 15: Gastrointestinal Emergencies

CONTENT SELF-EVALUATION

MULTIPLE CHOICE

1.	B	*p. 550*	5.	E	*p. 555*	9.	D	*p. 559*
2.	D	*p. 550*	6.	E	*p. 555*	10.	B	*p. 560*
3.	C	*p. 551*	7.	B	*p. 555*			
4.	D	*p. 554*	8.	D	*p. 558*			

Chapter 16: Toxicologic and Overdose Emergencies

CONTENT SELF-EVALUATION

MULTIPLE CHOICE

1.	B	*p. 564*	5.	D	*p. 568*	9.	B	*p. 570*
2.	E	*pp. 566–567*	6.	A	*p. 568*	10.	B	*p. 575*
3.	D	*p. 569*	7.	A	*p. 570*			
4.	B	*p. 567*	8.	E	*p. 574*			

Chapter 17: Allergic Reactions and Anaphylaxis

CONTENT SELF-EVALUATION

MULTIPLE CHOICE

1.	D	*p. 579*	5.	C	*p. 580*	9.	C	*p. 582*
2.	B	*p. 579*	6.	B	*p. 580*	10.	D	*p. 582*
3.	A	*p. 578*	7.	D	*p. 581*			
4.	C	*p. 580*	8.	D	*p. 581*			

Chapter 18: Neurologic Emergencies

CONTENT SELF-EVALUATION

MULTIPLE CHOICE

1.	C	*p. 588*	5.	E	*p. 592*	9.	B	*p. 598*
2.	D	*p. 590*	6.	A	*p. 594*	10.	D	*p. 598*
3.	B	*p. 590*	7.	A	*p. 595*			
4.	B	*p. 597*	8.	B	*p. 599*			

Chapter 19: Diabetic Emergencies

CONTENT SELF-EVALUATION

MULTIPLE CHOICE

1.	C	*p. 607*	6.	C	*p. 615*	11.	A	*p. 617*
2.	B	*p. 608*	7.	A	*p. 616*	12.	A	*p. 617*
3.	E	*p. 608*	8.	C	*p. 616*	13.	A	*p. 617*
4.	C	*p. 608*	9.	D	*p. 617*	14.	B	*p. 617*
5.	D	*p. 613*	10.	E	*p. 617*	15.	E	*p. 618*

Chapter 20: Environmental Emergencies

CONTENT SELF-EVALUATION

MULTIPLE CHOICE

1.	A	*p. 623*	5.	A	*p. 530*	9.	E	*p. 638*
2.	E	*pp. 625–626*	6.	D	*p. 632*	10.	E	*p. 638*
3.	B	*p. 529*	7.	B	*p. 636*			
4.	A	*p. 529*	8.	E	*p. 634*			

Chapter 21: Behavioral Emergencies

CONTENT SELF-EVALUATION

MULTIPLE CHOICE

1.	B	*pp. 644–645*	6.	B	*p. 648*	11.	C	*p. 651*
2.	B	*p. 645*	7.	E	*p. 649*	12.	A	*p. 652*
3.	C	*p. 645*	8.	E	*p. 650*	13.	A	*p. 653*
4.	C	*p. 646*	9.	A	*p. 649*	14.	B	*p. 656*
5.	D	*p. 646*	10.	C	*p. 651*	15.	B	*p. 656*

MATCHING

16.	A	*p. 649*	18.	F	*p. 649*	20.	C	*p. 649*
17.	E	*p. 649*	19.	D	*p. 652*	21.	B	*p. 649*

Chapter 22: Gynecological Emergencies

CONTENT SELF-EVALUATION

MULTIPLE CHOICE

1.	D	*p. 664*	6.	A	*p. 666*	11.	C	*p. 666*
2.	B	*p. 664*	7.	D	*p. 666*	12.	B	*p. 667*
3.	C	*p. 664*	8.	B	*p. 668*	13.	A	*p. 668*
4.	B	*p. 664*	9.	D	*p. 667*	14.	A	*pp. 668–669*
5.	C	*p. 665*	10.	E	*p. 667*	15.	D	*p. 669*

©2008 Pearson Education, Inc.

Special Project
Problem-Solving: Abdominal Pain

1. Focused history elements: *p. 664*
   - Sample and OPQRST
   - Obstetric history: gravida, parity, abortion
   - Gynecologic history: past ectopic pregnancies, surgical procedures
   - History of trauma
   - Last menstrual period (LMP)
   - Form of birth control and regularity of use
2. Differential diagnosis possibilities:
   - PID *p. 666*
   - Ruptured ovarian cyst *p. 666*
   - Endometritis *p. 667*
   - Ectopic pregnancy *p. 667*

Chapter 23: Trauma Emergencies

CONTENT SELF-EVALUATION

MULTIPLE CHOICE

1. A *p. 675*
2. B *p. 679*
3. D *pp. 675–676*
4. C *p. 676*
5. E *p. 676*
6. B *p. 676*
7. E *p. 678*
8. D *p. 679*
9. E *pp. 681–682*
10. C *p. 682*
11. A *p. 684*
12. E *p. 688*
13. C *p. 690*
14. D *p. 696*
15. B *p. 696*
16. A *p. 696*
17. B *p. 698*
18. B *p. 700*
19. B *p. 701*
20. C *p. 700–701*
21. A *p. 710*
22. E *p. 716*
23. B *p. 718*
24. C *p. 719*
25. D *p. 722*
26. A *p. 723*
27. E *p. 723*
28. B *p. 724*
29. B *p. 724*
30. E *p. 724*
31. D *p. 727*
32. D *p. 727*
33. D *p. 727*
34. E *p. 727*
35. C *p. 728*
36. A *p. 728*
37. A *p. 730*
38. D *p. 731*
39. E *pp. 730–731*
40. D *p. 731*
41. C *p. 732*
42. E *p. 732*
43. C *p. 732*
44. A *p. 732*
45. A *p. 732*
46. B *p. 732*
47. C *p. 733*
48. A *p. 734*
49. A *p. 734*
50. C *p. 736*
51. B *p. 739*
52. C *p. 740*
53. B *p. 742*
54. C *p. 742*
55. D *p. 742*
56. E *p. 742*
57. E *p. 743*
58. E *p. 744*
59. B *p. 745*
60. B *p. 745*
61. B *p. 746*
62. B *p. 747*
63. E *p. 746–747*
64. A *p. 748*
65. E *p. 748*

SPECIAL PROJECT
Drip Math Worksheet 2

1. R = 120 drops/min; V = ?; T = 35min; D = 10 drops/mL

$$V = R \times T = 120\ \text{gtts/min} \times 35\ \text{min}$$

$$V = \frac{120\ \text{gtts} \times 35\ \text{min}}{\text{min}} = 4200\ \text{gtts}$$

$$V = \frac{4200\ \text{gtts}}{10\ \text{gtts}} = 420\ \text{gtts} \times \text{mL} \qquad \mathbf{= 420\ mL}$$

2. R = 45 drops/min; D = 60 drops/mL; D′ = 45 drops/mL

$$R(\text{mL}) = R(\text{min})/D = 45\ \text{drops/min}/60\ \text{drops/mL}$$

$$R(\text{mL}) = \frac{45\ \text{gtts} \times \text{mL}}{60\ \text{gtts} \times \text{min}} = \frac{45\ \text{mL}}{60\ \text{min}} = 0.75\ \text{mL/min}$$

$$R(\text{min}) = R(\text{mL}) \times D' = 0.75\ \text{mL/min} \times 45\ \text{drops/mL}$$

$$R(\text{min}) = \frac{0.75\ \text{mL} \times 45\ \text{gtts}}{\text{mL} \times \text{min}} = 33.75\ \text{gtts/min} \qquad \mathbf{= 0.56\ drops/sec}$$

$$R(\text{sec}) = 33.75\ \text{drops}/60\ \text{sec}$$

3. R = ?; V = 100 mL; T = 115 min; D = 60 drops/mL

$$R = V/T = 100\ \text{mL}/115\ \text{min} = 0.87\ \text{mL/min}$$

$$R(\text{min}) = R(\text{mL}) \times D = 0.87\ \text{mL/min} \times 60\ \text{drops/min}$$

$$R(\text{min}) = \frac{0.87\ \text{mL} \times 60\ \text{gtts}}{\text{min} \times \text{mL}} \qquad \mathbf{= 52\ drops/min}$$

4. R = ?; V = 45 > 100 mL; T = 60 min

$$R = V/T = 45\ \text{mL}/60\ \text{min} = 0.75\ \text{mL/min}$$

$$R' = V/T = 100\ \text{mL}/60\ \text{min} = 1.67\ \text{mL/min}$$

$$R(60) = \frac{0.75\ \text{mL/min} \times 60\ \text{gtts/mL}}{\text{min} \times \text{mL}}$$

$$= 0.75\ \text{mL} \times 60\ \text{gtts} \qquad \mathbf{= 45\ drops/min}$$

©2008 Pearson Education, Inc.
Intermediate Emergency Care: 1985, 3rd ed.

$$D = 60 - 45 - 10 \text{ drops/mL } R(\text{min}) \qquad R'(60) = \frac{1.67 \text{ mL/min} \times 60 \text{ gtts/mL}}{\text{min} \times \text{mL}} = 100.2 \text{ drops/mL}$$

$$= 1.67 \text{ mL} \times 60 \text{ gtts}$$

$$= R(\text{mL}) \times D$$

$$R(45) = \frac{0.75 \text{ mL/min} \times 45 \text{ gtts/mL}}{\text{min} \times \text{mL}} = 0.75 \text{ mL} \times 45 \text{ gtts} = 33.75 \text{ drops/min}$$

$$R'(45) = \frac{1.67 \text{ mL/min} \times 45 \text{ gtts/mL}}{\text{min} \times \text{mL}} = 1.67 \text{ mL} \times 45 \text{ gtts} = 75 \text{ drops/mL}$$

$$R(10) = \frac{0.75 \text{ mL/min} \times 10 \text{ gtts/mL}}{\text{min} \times \text{mL}} = 0.75 \text{ mL} \times 10 \text{ gtts} = 7.5 \text{ drops/min}$$

$$R'(10) = \frac{1.67 \text{ mL/min} \times 10 \text{ gtts/mL}}{\text{min} \times \text{mL}} = 1.67 \text{ mL} \times 10 \text{ gtts} = 16.7 \text{ drops/mL}$$

5. $R = ?$ $\qquad R = V/T = 150 \text{ mL}/65 \text{ min} = \frac{150 \text{ mL}}{65 \text{ min}}$ $= \mathbf{2.3\ mL/min}$
   $V = 150 \text{ mL}$
   $T = 65 \text{ min}$

Chapter 24: Obstetrical Emergencies

CONTENT SELF-EVALUATION

MULTIPLE CHOICE

1. D *p. 766*
2. D *p. 766*
3. D *p. 768*
4. E *p. 770*
5. C *pp. 773–776*
6. B *pp. 774–776*
7. A *p. 774*
8. A *p. 774*
9. C *p. 774*
10. B *p. 777*
11. E *p. 777*
12. A *p. 779*
13. C *p. 771*
14. B *p. 779*
15. C *p. 781*
16. B *p. 786*
17. C *p. 789*
18. B *p. 786*
19. B *p. 790*

MATCHING

21. D *p. 766*
22. E *p. 766*
23. A *p. 776*
24. C *p. 766*
25. B *p. 766*
26. G *p. 779*
27. H *p. 769*
28. I *p. 766*
29. F *p. 779*

Chapter 25: Neonatal Resuscitation

CONTENT SELF-EVALUATION

MULTIPLE CHOICE

1. B *p. 796*
2. B *p. 800*
3. C *p. 797*
4. D *p. 798*
5. E *p. 800*
6. A *p. 798*
7. A *p. 798*
8. B *p. 799*
9. D *p. 804*
10. B *p. 808*

SPECIAL PROJECT

APGAR SCORE

Part I: Total score = 4 See Table 24–1

Part II: From top to bottom, items should read—oxygen, bag-mask ventilation, chest compressions, intubation, medications *p. 798*

Part III: Total score = 9 See Table 24–1

Chapter 26: Pediatric Emergencies

CONTENT SELF-EVALUATION

MULTIPLE CHOICE

1. C *p. 813*
2. C *p. 813*
3. B *p. 816*
4. C p. 820
5. E *p. 820*
6. A *p. 820*
7. B *p. 820*
8. B *p. 820*
9. B *p. 822*
10. B *p. 823*
11. E *p. 826*
12. E *p. 827*
13. A *p. 828*
14. D *p. 829*
15. D *p. 829*
16. E *p. 833*
17. C *p. 832*
18. A *p. 837*
19. C *p. 839*
20. D *p. 840*
21. A *p. 842*
22. C *p. 842*
23. B *p. 847*
24. C *p. 850*
25. E *pp. 851–852*
26. C *p. 849*
27. A *p. 853*
28. D *p. 855*
29. B *p. 854*
30. A *p. 856*
31. B *p. 862*
32. C *p. 866*
33. C *pp. 869–870*
34. C *p. 870*
35. B *p. 870*
36. A *p. 871*
37. D *p. 873*
38. E *p. 874*
39. D *p. 877*
40. C *p. 880*

SPECIAL PROJECT

BURNS

1. 45% *p. 873*
2. 40½% *p. 873*
3. Sample answer: The modified rule of nines for the pediatric patient gives less body surface area to the legs and more to the head of a toddler. *p. 873*
4. "rule of palm" *p. 873*

©2008 Pearson Education, Inc.

Chapter 27: Geriatrics Emergencies

CONTENT SELF-EVALUATION

MULTIPLE CHOICE

1. B	*p. 888*	19. B	*p. 897*
2. A	*p. 888*	20. A	*p. 897*
3. C	*p. 889*	21. E	*p. 898*
4. A	*p. 889*	22. B	*p. 898*
5. B	*p. 889*	23. C	*p. 898*
6. A	*pp. 889–890*	24. C	*p. 899*
7. B	*p. 890*	25. B	*p. 899*
8. D	*p. 891*	26. B	*p. 900*
9. A	*p. 891*	27. B	*p. 900*
10. A	*p. 892*	28. C	*p. 901*
11. C	*p. 892*	29. D	*p. 902*
12. E	*p. 892*	30. B	*p. 902*
13. A	*p. 892*	31. D	*p. 903*
14. A	*p. 893*	32. A	*p. 903*
15. E	*p. 894*	33. B	*pp. 904–905*
16. B	*pp. 894–895*	34. B	*p. 905*
17. D	*p. 895*	35. C	*p. 906*
18. C	*p. 897*		

MATCHING

36. D *p. 903*
37. C *p. 900*
38. F *p. 905*
39. E *p. 903*
40. G *p. 913*
41. B *p. 902*
42. A *p. 901*

Chapter 28: EMS Response to Weapons of Mass Destruction

CONTENT SELF-EVALUATION

MULTIPLE CHOICE

1. A	*p. 918*	11. A	*p. 922*
2. E	*p. 922*	12. B	*p. 923*
3. D	*p. 918*	13. C	*p. 923*
4. B	*p. 919*	14. D	*p. 924*
5. D	*p. 921*	15. E	*p. 925*
6. E	*p. 921*	16. D	*p. 927*
7. C	*p. 919*	17. E	*p. 927*
8. A	*p. 921*	18. A	*p. 928*
9. E	*p. 921*	19. A	*p. 929*
10. E	*p. 922*	20. B	*p. 930*

©2008 Pearson Education, Inc.
Intermediate Emergency Care: 1985, 3rd ed.

EMERGENCY DRUG CARDS

The following pages contain prepared 3″ × 5″ index cards. Each card represents one of the drugs commonly used by the EMT-Intermediate. They identify the name and class of the drug, a brief description, its indications, contraindications, precautions, common dosages, and routes of administration.

Detach and cut out the cards and review each one in detail. Be sure that your instructor identifies which drugs are used in your system and which need to be modified to indicate your system's specific indications, contraindications, precautions, doses, and methods of administration. You may also wish to prepare cards for the drugs used in your system that are not included in this card set.

Once your cards are prepared, begin to familiarize yourself with all the information contained on the card when presented with the drug name. You will notice that the drug name appears on the back of each card. Working on just a few cards each week and then reviewing them as your course progresses will help you commit to memory the essential information you must know about each drug.

ACETYLSALICYLIC ACID (ASA) Aspirin

Class: **Analgesic, Platelet Inhibitor, Anti-inflammatory**
Actions: Blocks platelet aggregation.
Indications: Chest pain suggestive of an MI. Signs and symptoms of ischemic stroke.
Contraindications: Hypersensitivity to drug.
Precautions: GI bleeding and upset stomach.
Side Effccts: Heartburn, nausea and vomiting.
Dosage/Route: 160 to 325 mg PO (chewable).

©2008 Pearson Education, Inc.

ADENOSINE (Adenocard)

Class: **Antidysrhythmic**
Actions: Slows atrioventricular conduction, can interrupt re-entrant atrioventricular pathways and slows the SA node rate.
Indications: Narrow, complex paroxysmal supraventricular tachycardia.
Contraindications: Hypersensitivity, 2nd- and 3rd-degree heart block, sick sinus node.
Precautions: It may cause transient dysrhythmias. Hypotension. Asthma.
Side Effects: Facial flushing headache, chest pain, shortness of breath, dizziness, nausea. Asystolic period following administration.
Dosage/Route: 6 mg rapidly (over 1 to 2 sec) IV. If ineffective, 12 mg in 1 to 2 min, may be repeated. Ped.: 0.1 mg/kg (over 1 to 2 sec) IV, then 0.2 mg/kg in 1 to 2 min to max 12 mg.

©2008 Pearson Education, Inc.

ALBUTEROL (Proventil, Ventolin)

Class: **Sympathomimetic Bronchodilator**
Actions: Selective $beta_2$ agonist causing relaxation of bronchial smooth muscle, decreasing airway resistance and increasing vital capacity.
Indications: Bronchospasm in asthma and COPD.
Contraindications: Hypersensitivity to the drug.
Precautions: The patient may experience tachycardia, anxiety, nausea, cough, wheezing, and/or dizziness. Vital signs and breath sounds must be monitored; use caution with elderly, cardiac, or hypertensive patients.
Side Effects: Tremors, anxiety, dizziness, headache, insomnia, palpitations, tachycardia, hypertension.
Dosage/Route: Two inhalations (90 mcg) via metered-dose inhaler (2 sprays) or 2.5 mg in 2.5 to 3 ml NS via nebulizer, repeat as needed. Ped.: 0.15 mg/kg in 2.5 to 3 ml NS via nebulizer, repeat as needed.

©2008 Pearson Education, Inc.

ACETYLSALICYLIC ACID (ASA) Aspirin

ADENOSINE (Adenocard)

ALBUTEROL (Proventil, Ventolin)

AMIODARONE (Cordarone)

Class: **Antidysrhythmic**

Actions: Prolongs the duration of the action potential and refractory period. Acts on all cardiac tissue and blocks sympathetic stimulation.

Indications: Life-threatening ventricular and supraventricular dysrhythmias such as ventricular tachycardia and fibrillation.

Contraindications: Severe SA dysfunction. 2nd and 3rd degree heart block and hypotensive bradycardia.

Precautions: Heart failure

Side Effects: Nausea, hypotension anorexia, malaise, fatigue, tremors, pulmonary toxicity, ventricular ectopy.

Dosage/Route: Arrest from VF or VT: 300 mg. Persistent VF or VT: 150 mg IV over 10 min. Maximum 2.2 grams/24 hours. Ped.: 5 mg/kg IV/IO, to maximum 15 mg/kg.

©2008 Pearson Education, Inc.

ATROPINE SULFATE

Class: **Parasympatholytic**

Actions: Blocks acetylcholine receptors. Increases heart rate. Decreases gastric secretions.

Indications: Hemodynamically significant bradycardia, bradyasystolic arrest, and organophosphate poisoning.

Contraindications: None in the emergency setting.

Precautions: Use with caution in myocardial ischemia.

Side Effects: Palpitations, tachycardia, headache, dizziness, anxiety, dry mouth, papillary dilation, blurred vision, urinary retention (older men).

Dosage/Route: Symptomatic bradycardia: 0.5–1 mg IV. Repeat 3 to 5 min to 0.04 mg/kg. Ped.: 0.02 mg/kg IV. Minimum 0.1 mg. Asystole: 1 mg IV. May repeat 3 to 5 min up to 0.04 mg/kg.

Organophosphate poisoning: 2 to 5 mg IV every10 to 15 min.

©2008 Pearson Education, Inc.

DEXTROSE 50% IN WATER ($D_{50}W$)

Class: **Carbohydrate**

Actions: Dextrose is a simple sugar that the body can rapidly metabolize to create energy.

Indications: Hypoglycemia.

Contraindications: None in hypoglycemia.

Precautions: Tissue damage at injection site. Can cause severe neurologic symptoms in thiamine deficiency.

Side Effects: Warmth and pain at injection site.

Dosage/Route: 25 gm $D_{50}W$ (50 ml) IV. Ped.: 2 ml/kg of a 25% solution IV

©2008 Pearson Education, Inc.

AMIODARONE (Cordarone)

ATROPINE SULFATE

DEXTROSE 50% IN WATER ($D_{50}W$)

DIAZEPAM (Valium)

Class: **Benzodiazepine, Antianxiety, Anticonvulsant, Sedative/Hypnotic**
Actions: Exact sedative mechanism unknown. Suppresses the spread of seizure activity.
Indications: Status epilepticus, premedication prior to painful procedures, and acute anxiety.
Contraindications: Hypersensitivity to the drug, shock and coma.
Precautions: Elderly or very ill patients, or COPD.
Side Effects: Drowsiness, fatigue, confusion, dizziness, hypotension, tachycardia, blurred vision, nausea, respiratory depression.
Dosage/Route: Seizures: 5 to 10 mg IV/IM. Ped.: 0.5 to 2 mg IV/IM.
Acute anxiety: 2 to 5 mg IM. Ped.: 0.5 to 2 mg IM.
Premedication: 5 to 15 mg IV. Ped.: 0.2 to 0.5 mg/kg IV.

©2008 Pearson Education, Inc.

DIPHENHYDRAMINE (Benadryl)

Class: **Antihistamine (H_1 receptor antagonist)**
Actions: Blocks histamine receptors with significant anticholinergic activities.
Indications: Anaphylaxis, allergic reactions, and extrapyramidal reactions.
Contraindications: Hypersensitivity to the drug or similar drugs.
Precautions: Use with caution in asthma, seizure disorders, hypertension, and in older adults and young children.
Side Effects: Drowsiness, dizziness, disturbed coordination, palpitations, tachycardia, dry mouth, urinary retention, and wheezing.
Dosage/Route: 25 to 50 mg IV/IM. Ped: 2 to 6 yrs 6.25 mg IV/IM, 6 to 12 yrs, 12.5 to 25 mg.

©2008 Pearson Education, Inc.

EPINEPHRINE (Adrenalin) 1:1,000

Class: **Sympathomimetic**
Actions: Acts on both alpha and beta adrenergic receptors and imitates the actions of the sympathetic nervous system.
Indications: Allergic reactions.
Contraindications: Hypersensitivity to the drug.
Precautions: Repeated injections may cause tissue necrosis. Avoid IV administrations.
Side Effects: Nervousness, restlessness, anxiety, tremors, palpitations, hypertension, dysrhythmias, MI, nausea, vomiting.
Dosage/Route: Allergic reactions: 0.3 to 0.5 mg of 1:1,000 SC Ped.: 0.01 mg/kg of 1:1,000 SC.

©2008 Pearson Education, Inc.

DIAZEPAM (Valium)

DIPHENHYDRAMINE (Benadryl)

EPINEPHRINE (Adrenalin) 1:1,000

EPINEPHRINE (Adrenalin) 1 to 10,000

Class: **Sympathomimetic**

Actions: Acts on both alpha and beta adrenergic receptors and imitates the actions of the sympathetic nervous system.

Indications: To restore rhythm in cardiac arrest and severe allergic reactions.

Contraindications: Hypersensitivity to the drug.

Precautions: Repeated injections can cause tissue necrosis, monitor vital signs and ECG.

Side Effects: Nervousness, restlessness, anxiety, tremors, palpitations, hypertension, dysrhythmias, MI, nausea, vomiting.

Dosage/Route: Arrest: 1 mg IV/IO every 3 to 5 min (ET: 2.0 to 2.5 mg 1:1,000 in 10 mL NS). Ped.: 0.01 mg/kg 1:10,000 IV/IO every 3 to 5 min. ET doses 0.1 mg/kg 1:1,000. Allergic reactions: 0.3 to 0.5 mg of 1:1,000 SC/5 to 15 min as needed or 0.5 to 1 mg of 1:10,000 IV if SC dose ineffective or severe reaction. Ped.: 0.01 mg/kg of 1:1,000 SC/10 to 15 min or 0.01 mg/kg of 1:10,000 IV if SC dose ineffective or severe.

©2008 Pearson Education, Inc.

FUROSEMIDE (Lasix)

Class: **Loop Diuretic**

Actions: Inhibits reabsorption of sodium and chloride in the Loop of Henle. Venodilator thus decreasing cardiac preload.

Indications: Congestive heart failure and pulmonary edema.

Contraindications: Hypersensitivity to furosemide or the sulfonamides.

Precautions: Infants, elderly, and cardiogenic shock associated with acute MI.

Side Effects: Postural hypotension, dizziness, fluid and electrolyte imbalances, nausea, pruritis.

Dosage/Route: 40 to 120 mg slow IV. Ped.: 1 mg/kg slow IV.

©2008 Pearson Education, Inc.

GLUCAGON

Class: **Hormone, Antihypoglycemic**

Actions: Causes a breakdown and release of stored glycogen and inhibits the synthesis of glycogen from glucose. Increases heart rate, AV conduction, and cardiac contractility similar to catecholamines, but through a different mechanism.

Indications: Hypoglycemia without IV access and to reverse beta-blocker overdose.

Contraindications: Hypersensitivity to glucagon.

Precautions: Effective only if there are sufficient stores of glycogen in the liver.

Side Effects: Dizziness, hypotension, nausea, and vomiting.

Dosage/Route: Hypoglycemia: 1 mg IM/SQ repeat/15 to 20 min. Ped.: Neo/infant: 0.025–0.03 mg/kg IM/SQ/IV (max 1 mg.). Child: 0.03–0.1 mg/kg IM/SQ/IV (max. 1 mg). Beta-blocker overdose: 50 to 150 mg/kg IV over 1 min. Ped.: 50 to 150 mg/kg IV over 1 min.

©2008 Pearson Education, Inc.

EPINEPHRINE (Adrenalin) 1 to 10,000

FUROSEMIDE (Lasix)

GLUCAGON

IPRATROPIUM (Atrovent)

Class: **Anticholinergic**

Actions: Anticholinergic agent, chemically related to atropine, which acts on the bronchial smooth muscles causing bronchodilation. It also dries airway secretions.

Indications: Bronchospasm associated with asthma, COPD, and acute attacks of bronchospasm.

Contraindications: Hypersensitivity to the drug or atropine or its derivatives.

Precautions: Should not be used as primary treatment of bronchospasm. It should be used in conjunction with beta agonists or similar bronchodilators.

Side Effects: Blurred vision, bitter taste, dry mouth, nausea, constipation, hoarseness, urinary retention.

Dosage/Route: 0.5 mg in 2.5 to 3 mL NS via nebulizer or 2 sprays from a metered dose inhaler. Ped.: 125 to 250 mcg in 2.5 to 3 mL NS via nebulizer, or 1 to 2 sprays a metered-dose inhaler.

©2008 Pearson Education, Inc.

ISOETHARINE (Bronkosol)

Class: **Sympathomimetic Bronchodilator**

Actions: Selective beta$_2$ adrenergic agonist that relaxes the bronchial smooth muscles, decreasing airway resistance and increases vital capacity.

Indications: Bronchospasm in asthma and COPD.

Contraindications: Hypersensitivity to the drug.

Precautions: Use with caution in patients with myocardial ischemia (note to measure peak flow before and after treatment).

Side Effects: Tremors, anxiety, dizziness, headache, insomnia, palpitations, tachycardia, hypertension.

Dosage/Route: 1 to 2 sprays via metered dose inhaler, 0.5 mL in 2 to 3 ml saline via nebulizer. Ped.: 0.01 mL/kg of 1% solution (max 0.5 mL) diluted in 2 to 3 ml NS by nebulizer.

©2008 Pearson Education, Inc.

LEVALBUTEROL (Xopenex)

Class: **Sympathomimetic Bronchodilator**

Actions: Selective beta$_2$ adrenergic agonist that causes relaxation of bronchial smooth muscles, thus decreasing airway resistance and increasing vital capacity.

Indications: Bronchospasm associated with reversible obstructive airway disease (asthma, chronic bronchitis, emphysema).

Contraindications: Patients with known hypersensitivity to the drug.

Precautions: Use with caution in patients with cardiac ischemia. Try and measure peak flow before and after treatment.

Side Effects: Tremors, anxiety, dizziness, headache, insomnia, palpitations, tachycardia, hypertension.

Dosage/Route: Nebulizer: 0.63 mg in 3.0 mL normal saline every 6–8 hrs. Ped.: $<$12 yrs 0.31 mg in 3.0 mL normal saline 3 times per day.

©2008 Pearson Education, Inc.

IPRATROPIUM (Atrovent)

ISOETHARINE (Bronkosol)

LEVALBUTEROL (Xopenex)

LIDOCAINE (Xylocaine)

Class: **Antiarrhythmic**

Actions: Suppresses automaticity in the His/Purkinje system, elevates the threshold for ventricular fibrillation and lowers the threshold for defibrillation and cardioversion.

Indications: Ventricular tachycardia (with and without a pulse) and ventricular fibrillation.

Contraindications: Hypersensitivity to the drug, supraventricular dysrhythmias, 2nd- and 3rd-degree heart blocks, and bradycardias.

Precautions: Hepatic or renal disease, CHF, marked hypoxia, respiratory depression, and shock.

Side Effects: Drowsiness, dizziness, restlessness, confusion, bradycardia, conduction disorders, blurred vision, nausea, vomiting.

Dosage/Route: VT/VF Cardiac arrest: 1 to 1.5 mg/kg IV repeated every 3 to 5 min up to 3 mg/kg, follow conversion with a drip of 2 to 4 mg/min. Ped.: 1 mg/kg IV, repeat/3 to 5 min up to 3 mg/kg, follow conversion with a drip of 20 to 50 mcg/kg/min.
VT w/pulse: 1 to 1.5 mg/kg slow IV. May repeat at one-half dose every 5–10 min until conversion up to 3 mg/kg. Follow conversion with an infusion of 2 to 4 mg/min.
Ped.: 1 mg/kg, followed by a drip at 20 to 50 mg/kg/min.

©2008 Pearson Education, Inc.

METAPROTERENOL (Alupent)

Class: **Sympathomimetic Bronchodilator**

Actions: Selective $beta_2$ adrenergic agonist that causes relaxation of bronchial smooth muscles, thus decreasing airway resistance and increasing vital capacity.

Indications: Bronchospasm associated with reversible obstructive airway disease (asthma, chronic bronchitis, emphysema).

Contraindications: Patients with known hypersensitivity to the drug.

Precautions: Use with caution in patients with cardiac ischemia. Try and measure peak flow before and after treatment.

Side Effects: Tremors, anxiety, dizziness, headache, insomnia, palpitations, tachycardia, hypertension.

Dosage/Route: 0.65 mg via metered dose inhaler (2 sprays); 0.2 to 0.3 mL in 2.5 to 3 ml NS via nebulizer. Ped.: 0.1 to 0.2 mL/kg (5% solution) in 2.5 to 3 mL NS via nebulizer.

©2008 Pearson Education, Inc.

MORPHINE SULFATE (Morphine)

Class: **Narcotic Analgesic**

Actions: Acts on opiate receptors in the brain causing analgesia and sedation.

Indications: Moderate to severe pain and in MI and to reduce venous return in the acute MI and pulmonary edema.

Contraindications: Hypersensitivity to opiates, undiagnosed head injury, hypotension, or volume depletion.

Precautions: Do not use in asthma, COPD, or severe respiratory failure.

Side Effects: Respiratory depression, disorientation, hypotension, bradycardia

Dosage/Route: Pain: 2.5 to 15 mg IV; 5 to 20 mg IM/SQ. Ped.: 0.05 to 0.1 mg/kg IV; 0.1 to 0.2 mg/kg IM/SQ.
Reduce preload: 1 to 2 mg/6 to 10 min to response.

©2008 Pearson Education, Inc.

LIDOCAINE (Xylocaine)

METAPROTERENOL (Alupent)

MORPHINE SULFATE (Morphine)

NALOXONE (Narcan)

Class: **Narcotic Antagonist**

Actions: Blocks opiate receptors thus negating the effects of opiates.

Indications: Narcotic overdose.

Contraindications: Hypersensitivity to the drug, non-narcotic-induced respiratory depression.

Precautions: Titrate to increase respirations as too large a dose may induce withdrawal.

Side Effects: (narcotic withdrawal) tremors, agitation, runny nose, diarrhea.

Dosage/Route: 0.4 to 2 mg IV/IM (2 to 2.5 times the dose ET), repeated/2 to 3 min as needed up to 10 mg. Ped.: 0.01 mg IV/IM (2 to 2.5 times the dose ET) repeated/2 to 3 min as needed up to 10 mg.

©2008 Pearson Education, Inc.

NITROGLYCERIN (Nitrostat)

Class: **Nitrate**

Actions: Potent vasodilator with anti-anginal, anti-ischemic and antihypertensive effects.

Indications: To increase coronary perfusion and decrease chest pain in angina and MI and to reduce preload in acute pulmonary edema.

Contraindications: Hypersensitivity, hypotension, and shock.

Precautions: Use with caution in patients with possible head injury, increased ICP shock and in patients taking Viagra, Cialis, Levitra.

Side Effects: Headache, dizziness, postural hypotension, tachycardia, nausea, vomiting.

Dosage/Route: 1 tablet (0.4 mg) SL. May be repeated/3 to 5 min up to 3 tablets, or 1/2 to 1 inch of topical ointment on the chest wall, or 0.4 mg (one spray) SL every 3 to 5 min, up to 3 sprays.

©2008 Pearson Education, Inc.

TERBUTALINE (Brethine, Bricanyl)

Class: **Sympathetic Bronchodilator**

Actions: Selective $beta_2$ adrenergic agonist that causes relaxation of bronchial smooth muscles, thus decreasing airway resistance and increasing vital capacity.

Indications: Bronchospasm associated with reversible obstructive airway disease (asthma, chronic bronchitis, emphysema). To suppress preterm labor.

Contraindications: Patients with known hypersensitivity to the drug.

Precautions: Use with caution in patients with cardiac ischemia. Try and measure peak flow before and after treatment.

Side Effects: Tremors, anxiety, dizziness, headache, insomnia, palpitations, tachycardia, hypertension.

Dosage/Route: Two inhalations with a metered-dose inhaler, repeated once in 1 min or 0.25 mg SQ repeated in 15 to 30 min. up to 0.5 mg in 4 hours. Ped: 0.005 to 0.01 mg/kg (max. 0.4 mg) every 15 to 20 min. up to 2 doses.

©2008 Pearson Education, Inc.

NALOXONE (Narcan)

NITROGLYCERIN (Nitrostat)

TERBUTALINE (Brethine, Bricanyl)

VASOPRESSIN (Pitressin)

Class: **Hormone, Vasopressor**
Actions: Inhibits water secretion by the kidneys and a potent vasodilator in higher doses.
Indications: To increase peripheral vascular resistance in arrest (CPR).
Contraindications: None in the emergency setting.
Precautions: Few in the emergency setting.
Side Effects: Infrequent with low doses.
Dosage/Route: Arrest: 40 IU IV (once).

©2008 Pearson Education, Inc.

VASOPRESSIN (Pitressin)